CANCER:

how and why it may be wiped out

FIRST EDITION
Library of Congress Catalog Card No.: 77-70955
International Standard Book No.: 0-912760-37-0

Published by the Roberts Cancer Research Publications, Inc.
in cooperation with Valkyrie Press, Inc.
St. Petersburg, Fla.

Dedicated to
Dr. Khem M. Shahani
without whose creative
research and cooperation
this book would not
have been possible.
And
with appreciation
expressed to
Marjorie Schuck
for
exceptional workmanship.

TABLE OF CONTENTS

TABLE OF CONTENTS

FOREWORD

The Challenge of this Book

This book offers a challenge to debate.

The basis of the proposed debate is this:

Optimistic forecasts are offered that 90% of cancer may be wiped out within ten years, by presently acceptable methods through improved techniques. Such is the gist of a statement by Dr. Luther Brady, chairman of the department of radiation therapy and nuclear medicine at the Hahnemann Medical College in Philadelphia in the November 2, 1976 issue of the *National Enquirer.* (The nature of the material makes this magazine a medical journal in the foregoing instance.)

This book challenges such forecast.

According to this book, at least two major defects in human evolutionary development make impossible the prevention and arrest of cancer with acceptable predictability by present methods, with whatever improvement. And even with the elimination of such defects, supplementary diet must be adequate.

It is not the purpose of this book, however, to prove, per se, that the foregoing is right or wrong. It is the purpose of this book to recommend that the cancer problem not be restricted to supposition, turned into official regulation, thereby making determination in human terms, all but impossible.

History offers many examples of tragedy coming out of regulation by supposition. The "official" view of Aryan superiority by Adolph Hitler, Chief of State, represents the most flagrant. Others are less obvious, but perhaps as little in the public interest.

At one time, pasteurization was outlawed by the State of New York. The FDA attempted to legalize the introduction of vitamin C into "imitation" milk while precluding its use in milk from a cow. Homogenization of milk was once outlawed.

"To err is human," and the badge of authority does not change this.

If cancer is to die at all, it will die in the marketplace, according to this book. But presently, it cannot, because of "official" assumptions, despite promises instead of public protection. The record shows that cancer is becoming a worse threat, insofar as prevention is concerned, especially.

I do not involve the scientists I have cited in any way in the debate I suggest. My premise is that those who suffer from cancer need protection by Constitutional Amendment.

This issue I will debate with any individual or group providing the money to pay for whatever means of communication are chosen. I would appreciate the help of any able to supply supportive evidence, especially in terms of personal experience.

Write me, or order book, or both:

J. GORDON ROBERTS
P.O. Box 1662
Clearwater, FL 33517

INTRODUCTION

THE TEST OF A CANCER CURE

It is unlikely that anyone with the benefit of breast-feeding in infancy, who followed dietary law as prescribed in the Bible, strictly throughout life, might ever get cancer, possibly save through some inordinate pollution.

The test of a cancer cure should be the same as a test for cure of obesity: prevention.

Obesity may be eliminated by literally cutting off fat, by shortening the digestive tract, by appetite-depressants; by feeding vitamin pills, water, and no food for months.

Such methods may eliminate obesity and be considered necessary under some conditions. But no one would accept them as an answer to obesity.

The proof of an answer to obesity lies in its capacity to prevent obesity, with no other answer to be considered acceptable.

The ultimate answer to cancer may hardly require any less. However, valuable research may be in solving specific problems, its total value would seem to necessitate the yard-stick indicated as a measure.

This book shall examine many approaches to cancer with the foregoing gauge in mind, in the hope that it may induce more complete orientation of research, and perhaps help those who actually have cancer or fear that they may have it, or fear getting it. It offers a perspective which should be considered by all concerned.

A PRESCRIPTION DESCRIPTION OF THIS BOOK

This book offers the cancer patient something to do besides feel hopeless. It shows that there are alternatives, as a needed source of hope, for one thing. It shows the different approaches from different parts of the world, indicating that somebody is doing something to help him.

And it might offer help in helping himself.

The book offers nineteen examples of cancer inhibition to a degree suggesting permanent cure . . . by unusual methods, including the use of bacteria by Bulgarians.

This book suggests no continuing cure without attention to irritants which may be carcinogenic, within our environment and our way of life. It suggests no vaccination against irritants.

This book raises the question of need to establish enzymatic adequacy, especially as an essential part of cooperation with nature, to prevent cancer, or arrest it.

Figures indicate that virtually everyone may conceivably have cancer before the end of the century, without effective counter effort, as cancer appears to metastasize throughout society, as within the individual.

This book offers information, not judgments. However, each of us must make a judgment, as the following illustrates:

A friend of mine has had two operations for the same kind of cancer. He is hoping for a "cure" with no change in his way of life. This book offers no "cure" in the sense of what this man desires, nor even suggests one.

Unrelated as this may seem, the controversy over how to deal with cancer amounts to a question of ethics within the universe, a theological question, if you please.

Do you eliminate cancer by destroying something or by cooperation with benevolent forces? How do people divide themselves on this issue?

People who either have cancer, themselves, or are involved with loved ones who do, met in a regular meeting in Tampa, Florida, on January 16, 1976.

Robert W. Stickle of Cleveland, Ohio, a man presumably cured of cancer, addressed the group. As I interpret his *Malignant Melanoma Case History*, he had one instance of minor surgery and three majors, including muscle and skin graft.

With a background in architecture, he described himself as a "half-assed architect" following surgery.

On April 15, 1973, further surgery was recommended but refused. His case was recited in both Tampa and Clearwater, Florida.

The details of this case shall be covered later, but not in this prescription description, to avoid losing the thread of purpose here.

Hope to help such as attended the Tampa meeting inspires this book. Those in attendance objected to requiring the public to accept checkups which could not, of course, prevent cancer, with surgery, chemotherapy, and radiation the only answers to damage already done.

This group declared itself to represent a rising tide of indignation within this country over such answers as the only ones available, with less than adequate interest in alternatives, on the part of those who should take major responsibility for public health.

The congregation concerned with cancer expressed no antagonism, however, toward anyone, merely the desire to take all possible steps to remain alive, or help someone else remain alive.

The discussion brought out the disillusioned belief that a pill might no more be found to cure cancer, than to cure sin; that in both instances, a way of life must be found.

Mr. Stickle declared that some people did not really want to live.

"Such might often be true," he said, "when the husband

telephones for the wife or the wife calls for the husband, seeking help."

This book is not written for those who wish to die, but for those who wish to live.

The assumption underlies this book that whatever may be needed to prevent or inhibit cancer must certainly be considered basic to any arrest of cancer; adequate enzymes, for example. Such adequacy may not be taken for granted, for some reasons which may surprise you.

Enzymes are proteins acting as catalysts in nearly all aspects of physical survival. Just how they operate is not fully clear even to the scientists most learned in this field. Even so, much more information shall be furnished further on.

To the knowledge of this writer, no meaningful minimal requirements for enzymes have ever been established. Should such be established, as has been done at least tentatively with minerals and vitamins, it is possible that there would be no more cancer, or even heart attacks, for reasons to come.

Possible enzymatic conflicts, and the significance ascribed to them, shall be discussed later.

Enzymatic adequacy requires that all necessary nutrients, including trace minerals and vitamins, be present in the diet, but that the system be not overloaded with calories, especially in relation to other nutrients; nor with any one kind of food.

Also needed are adequate roughage and proper intestinal flora: wholesome bacteria. Whether bacteria may act through enzymes completely or in part, or independently, or just how, has not been made clear to me through any literature I have read. They may be necessary, for example, in the production of Vitamin B^{12}. However, the need for proper bacteria is there.

Exercise may represent far more importance than recognized, for reasons to be adduced. Proper chewing of food may be critically important, conceivably as important as proper nutrition, itself. The evidence shall be reviewed as we proceed.

Such review is not easy, even for reading, but especially for writing, for these reasons:

Scientific research is necessarily isolated in its area of examination and limited to the specific and precise. It is hard to relate to a life style, or even a broad view, however relevant, basically.

Interpretation of material for readers is often done to solicit funds, an end requisite for research, but hardly conducive to objectivity.

Interpretations to sell something often create alarm, without calming it.

Much material written to sell books has text so jealously guarded as to be almost useless as a basis for comparisons or studying relationships. Authors and inventors do need protection; so I merely state the problem, rather than try to solve it here.

"Authoritative" work on cancer barely touches upon nutrition, by and large, if at all.

Material from Bulgaria, nevertheless, I can quote in its entirety, material indicating "cures" under certain conditions. In no manner could this material be paraphrased in a meaningful way. To get the most from the report, one must read the entire manuscript, as quoted, even though written to meet scientific requirements, primarily, and styled accordingly.

To obtain permission for such quotation of copyright material in this country, the one making the request would certainly be required to offer assurances that the material express the ideology of the publisher. The Russian-Bulgarian material describes a specific, doctor-patient relationship such as established the results for the report. Even so, such relationship is not emphasized in this book.

Therefore, I suggest no conflict with the foregoing or its

authorship, when I propose that the elimination of cancer must depend upon a better relationship with the benevolent forces of nature than may be established solely by any one-to-one relationship.

Once cancer occurs, some knowledgeable person must certainly be consulted, preferably a physician. In fact, the approach described here does not preclude any method which has proved itself effective; surgery, chemotherapy, radiation, or, for that matter, fasting, balanced diet, natural foods, or any unorthodox method for which success may be claimed in any instance for any rational reason.

The point I make here is that such catholic approach might hardly obtain permission to reproduce the Bulgarian material, were it published in the United States, and copyrighted.

Even though the material contained in this book is copyrighted to prevent its possible use in advertising, I suggest that scientific material, used for comparisons in a problem whereby the human race is threatened with extinction, should not be fenced in, like a private game preserve.

In relation to openness, Dr. Herbert M. Shelton, author of the *Hygienic System* is like a breath of spring. Apparently, his material is open to anyone and worth the while of anyone interested in cancer to study.

On the other hand, this book shall not follow the ludicrous premise that the medical profession has done nothing right in all the years of its existence.

Questions relating to cancer remain unanswered, nevertheless, and shall be raised herein, with reasons given for their adduction.

For example, what about the destruction of enzymes through heating most of the food we eat, whether or not such heating be necessary for our protection?

What about intestinal flora and its effect upon essential enzymes? May we take internal ecology for granted?

Just how much pollution of our environment may we endure, irrespective of what we do, internally, to protect ourselves?

Although the one beset with cancer may have alternatives — conceivably, even workable "cures" — the best protection, obviously, is prevention; protection now before cancer strikes, if possible.

CANCER:

how and why it may be wiped out

By The Man Who Helped Wipe Out Rickets

J. GORDON ROBERTS

Valkyrie Press, Inc.

CHAPTER 1

A POSSIBLE RELATIONSHIP BETWEEN LACTOBACILLI AND VITAMIN C

"Scurvy and the Cancer Problem" by Irwin Stone in the *American Laboratory*, September, 1976, illustrates a possible relationship between cancer and a profound evolutionary shortage of human vitamin C, as compared with mammals which produce their own vitamin C.

"Lactose and Lactase" by Norman Kretchmer, *Scientific American,* October, 1972, demonstrates that the majority of peoples throughout the world are short of the enzyme, lactase, necessary to digest sweet, cow's milk satisfactorily.

Those areas of the world with a long history of dairy farming appear to show either more lactase in the human digestive tract, or better adjustment to shortage, or, conceivably, both.

In either case, vitamin C or lactase, a nutritional shortage may occur, based upon evolutionary development.

According to Dr. Charles Chapple, quoted in my book in connection with birth defects, estrogen may inhibit scurvy as well as vitamin C, and rickets as well as vitamin D. Yet estrogen is neither, by most authorities at least.

Should the enzyme, lactase, work synergistically, or in some catalytic way, with vitamin C, how might it work? The souring of milk produces B vitamins. By reciting a few alternative explanations, I do not pretend to exhaust the list, or make a case for any suggestion.

Lactase might simply produce vitamin C. Or the bacteria required to produce glucose and galactose might simply produce vitamin C, as well as lactase.

Symbiotic bacteria might enable the body to produce its own vitamin C for a limited time.

Symbiotic bacteria may act in some mysterious fashion

as does estrogen.

Symbiotic bacteria may enhance the production of estrogen or some other hormone with similar effect.

Symbiotic bacteria may encourage production of enzymes working as hormones.

Dr. Khem M. Shahani of the Food Science Department at the University of Nebraska is working on this problem. Unfortunately, the scientific answer may not be easy to find. But somehow lactase and vitamin C appear to work toward the same goals. Or perhaps that statement goes too far.

In any case, some symbiotic bacteria appear to inhibit cancer. According to Stone, the same appears to be true of vitamin C.

It is at least possible that market milk from cows, protected as completely as feasible by symbiotic lactobacilli, and fortified with at least 10,000 units of vitamin C per quart (as a preventive measure) might wipe out cancer as fully as vitamin D wiped out rickets, with the condition that the environment, itself, be not polluted inordinately.

As with rickets and vitamin D milk, such hypothesis might be proved or disproved only in the marketplace, through freedom of information and freedom of action on the part of the public, liberties which should now be subject to examination and review.

CHAPTER 2

WHY AND HOW SOME BACTERIA MAY INHIBIT CANCER

Out of nurturing in my bathtub may come at least one way to inhibit cancer to some degree.

Before shoving this material aside as ludicrous, look at some solid evidence and the theory outlining where to look.

The approach to the problem of cancer represents the unusual to an unusual degree. One aspect of the approach represented the spiritual, the desire to prove that the Universe is ruled by a Benevolent Force. (Many people are mentally sick because of believing the opposite.)

Dr. W. H. Thompson of the University of Nebraska at Omaha, encouraged me. He is a psychologist. Inasmuch as I tend to freeze on tests, such encouragement doubly inspired me.

Based upon such inspiration, I developed a new system of logic and mathematics to approach the problem of cancer, founded upon training by the Institute of General Semantics.

I will not try in this treatise, to describe my mathematics. I will point out that, following my system, I looked first to see where cancer was not, rather than where it was.

The significance of this kind of search is clearly illustrated by Dr. Charles C. Chapple, formerly of Omaha and a co-worker with Dr. Richard Ogborn of the Veterans Administration.

In 1972, an article, *Developmental Defects,* by Dr. Chapple, was published by the National Foundation - March of Dimes. In an Addendum, referring to my approach, Dr. Chapple points out that cancer at birth appears to be rare indeed.

Thus is described the starting point in the search for at least one way to inhibit cancer, conceivably.

Much in advance of Dr. Chapple's interest, and that of Dr. Ogborn, Dr. E. L. MacQuiddy entered the picture in the early sixties.

At eighty years of age, Dr. MacQuiddy lost his sight, but not his insight. Using the kind of logic described previously, I told Dr. MacQuiddy where he might expect to find certain bacteria. He checked the medical books tò find the bacteria described which I could not name. This turned him into an enthusiastic supporter.

He sought the support of Dr. Khem Shahani of the Food Science Department of the University of Nebraska, without whose research this book would not have been possible.

Dr. MacQuiddy looked into the kind of bacteria which might possibly help protect the newly-born infant from unwarranted cell proliferation, as I had done. He found that bifidus bacteria, acidophilus, and Doderlein's bacteria, are much alike.

Doderlein's bacteria I had described with its locale, to Dr. MacQuiddy.

Bifidus bacteria is normally found in human milk. According to some scientists, it may turn into acidophilus upon exposure to air.

Acidophilus is a lactobacillus. It sours milk.

What may bacteria, which sours milk, do for human health?

According to Norman Kretchmer, in "Lactose and Lactase," *Scientific American,* October, 1972, on the basis of human population, world-wide, most people are intolerant to lactose, which is milk sugar, the carbohydrate found in milk. But souring breaks the lactose down into glucose and galactose, which most people can tolerate.

So bacteria which sours milk may have a symbiotic or mutually beneficial relationship with human beings. Some bacteria may sour milk, may survive within the human digestive tract, especially bifidus and acidophilus. Moreover, lactase, the enzyme within the human system which breaks down lactose, is found in connection with such culture organisms.

Relative to cancer, the question comes down to just how far a symbiotic or mutually beneficial relationship may go. A "true" answer to cancer must probably involve understanding of cells down to their electronic interchange, an area of interest to such scientists as Dr. Denham Harman of Omaha.

A shortcut would be most welcome, according to just about everybody, if not everybody.

Some of Dr. Shahani's work has previously been reported in the *Omaha World Herald.* Some efforts were checked at Sloan-Kettering Institute.

On June 3, 1966, Dr. Shahani sent a report to me at Roberts Dairy that *L. Acidophilus* may inhibit the growth of at least some bacteria. Anti-cancer effect was considered inconclusive at that time.

Antitumor Activity of Yogurt Fractions, a thesis prepared under the supervision of Dr. Shahani by Robert Elvin Farmer, came out in October, 1974. *Lactobacillus bulgaricus* and *Streptococcus thermophilus,* yogurt culture, were the bacteria used.

Authorities indicate such bacteria will not survive in the human digestive tract. However, mice were used. Moreover, the possible significance of transforming lactose into glucose and galactose might hardly be affected.

Within the report is the following statement:

"As shown in Table 3, the feeding of yogurt inhibited the total tumor cell count by 27.3 to 29.7%, and the DNA content by 25.1 to 28.8%."

As to innoculation: "The results presented in Table 7 revealed that only the solids fraction inhibited the tumor growth by 30 to 42%, and the super-activity fraction showed no inhibitory activity."

In 1961, Dr. I. G. Bogdanov and P. Pophistor of Bulgaria and Russia, presented to the International Cancer Congress in Moscow, a paper, "Experimental and Clinical Studies on the Anti-Cancer Action of Anti-bioticum Bulgaricum" as already indicated, another paper by I. G. Bogdanov and P. G. Daler and associates in October, 1975.

Dr. Shahani declares that he wrote Dr. Bogdanov several times in 1972 and 1973, finally receiving papers from Bogdanov in March of 1975, along with a request for Shahani's work.

Regarding specific kinds of cancer treated in human subjects (five kinds), the Bulgarian report reads:

"Incompletely purified concentrations of filtrates from cultural liquids containing *A. bulgaricus,* when applied locally within the tissue of the tumor, exert an evidently inhibitory and disintegrative action on the cancer tissue."

The Bulgarian's work with human subjects has been offered. It shows no conflict with work in the United States, known to me.

The 1974 Nebraska report by Farmer, deals, of course, with mice. It includes a table, "Effect of Inoculating Different Fractions of Yogurt Culture Upon Tumor Cell Proliferation as Determined by DNA Content." The table lists inhibition as ranging between 30 and 44%.

Separately, however, the two bacterial types in yogurt produce inhibition listed at 34.5 and 34.8% for *L. Bulgaricus* and 21.5 and 20.4% for *S. thermophilus,* a combined total exceeding 50%, for whatever significance this might have. It might have much significance if multiple curdling may prove to have any kind of multiple effect.

And this leads back to my bathroom in Florida. I learned that the commercial culturing of buttermilk uses up only 20% of the lactose, or milk sugar. In my experiments following my exile from Omaha in 1972, I discovered, among other things, that ordinary buttermilk may be cultured a second time with *L. bifidus* or *L. acidophilus,* at body temperature.

I used my finger for a thermometer. Anybody can do this. Just watch for the buttermilk to curdle a second time.

Ordinary buttermilk, by the way, is cultured at a temperature of 70 degrees Fahrenheit, usually, at least.

I have applied for a patent on the commercial use of the idea just expounded. Outside the obvious motive of obtaining money to continue research, why else?

When Vitamin D milk was introduced into the United States, 80% of American infants suffered from rickets, even though many people, and probably a majority, knew that cod liver oil would prevent or cure rickets.

Cod liver oil does not taste good to most people. Neither does acidophilus buttermilk, cultured singly. Should bacteria have any benefit, it might well primarily be preventive. But this prospect may never be tried without a product of good flavor, just as Vitamin D milk substituted for cod liver oil.

At least, it should break down lactose, milk sugar.

In the *1976 Yearbook of Science and the Future,* published by *Encyclopedia Britannica,* Stephen L. Wolfe describes "The Living Cell." He speaks of bacterial repressors, which again raises the question as to just how far symbiosis, cooperation with friendly bacteria, might go.

Whatever the outcome, beginning with the gratis training in nutrition given me by Dr. Victor E. Levine of Creighton University in the early thirties, this episode in Omaha and Nebraska demonstrates a willingness to cooperate beyond the call of duty and with no hope of reward, which is one of the most remarkable aspects of this entire tale. Hopefully, letters such as the following may be followed by many, many others.

CHAPTER 3

PATIENT REPORTS ON BACTERIA

March 9, 1975

To Whom It May Concern:

In April 1970, I consulted Dr. Porter Crawford of Largo, Florida, a specialist in skin diseases and skin cancer, because of an apparent bleeding mole on my left shoulder. He immediately urged me to have a surgeon look at the mole for further diagnosis and possible surgical removal. Dr. Carl H. Calman of Clearwater, Florida, upon seeing the growth, placed me in Morton Plant Hospital, where he removed the mole and, when it was found to be malignant, removed much of the adjacent area in an attempt to contain the disease. The actual diagnosis of my problem was a malignant nevus melanoma.

At my first consultation with Dr. Calman, I was told that my chances for survival were about 50-50 or slightly better, due to the speed and extent of the surgery. He further stated that if there had been no recurrence within five years, I could feel more comfortable about the survival probability. Immediately after the meeting with Dr. Calman, I reported the diagnosis to Mrs. J. Gordon Roberts, who relayed the information to Mr. Roberts.

To improve my general health, Mr. Roberts began supplying acidophilus milk to me at that time and has continued to the present. My original consumption was four ounces each day, increasing to about eight ounces through the years. I have had the opportunity to drink the acidophilus approximately 50-60 percent of the days during the five years since my operation. In addition to the acidophilus milk, I attempted to improve the nutritional quality of my diet by selecting foods more wisely, taking natural vitamins, minerals, amino acids, etc., and reducing my consumption of beef. My only other preventive measure was to reduce my exposure to the sun on the advice of Dr. Soloman Garb of the American Medical Center at Denver. I consulted Dr. Garb at the suggestion of Mr. Roberts.

During the five years since the nevus melanoma was diagnosed, I have had three complete physicals and one insurance examination. Dr. B. J. Hood of Clearwater, Florida, who performed the three complete physicals, found my health to remain excellent, and, in fact, led him to say, "Whatever you're doing you should certainly keep it up." It should be noted that exercising was not one of the things I was doing because of the nature of my work. Dr. Hood checked fifteen constituents of my blood and found that all remained within the desirable range with a tendency toward improvement except for a slight increase in the cholestoral level.

Personal characteristics which may be of interest are:

Age now:	44
Weight:	155 lbs.
Height:	6 ft. 1 in.
Health:	Excellent
Smoke:	No (Never)
Alcoholic Intake:	Very moderate

Sincerely,

* * *

January 6, 1972

Dear Sir:

This is in reply to your letter of December 29, 1971. I wish to express my very deepest appreciation and thanks to Mr. Gordon Roberts and to Roberts Dairy Company for providing my wife, Caroline, with the Company's special acidophilus cultured milk.

In August, 1971, a diagnosis was rendered by Mrs. ------'s doctors, while she was a patient in Charleston General Hospital. It was based upon exploratory surgery in the abdominal cavity. This diagnosis was that Mrs. ------ had an extensive malignant tumor lying behind the right kidney and extending in the abdominal cavity to an area to the left of the spinal column. The operating doctors reported that the tumor could not be removed by surgery. Tissue specimens were removed for biopsy and the incision was sutured. Pathological examination identified the tumor as a reticulum cell sarcoma.

Within approximately two weeks of the date of diagnosis, Mrs.------ was admitted as a patient in the National Cancer Institute of the National Institutes of Health at Bethesda, Maryland. Tests and examinations there confirmed the identity of the tumor, established that the bone marrow was not involved, and resulted in the discovery of a secondary growth, or "daughter tumor," at the base of the neck on the left side. This growth, upon discovery, was described as being about the size of a ping pong ball.

NCI determined to proceed on a course of treatment by chemotherapy. The drugs to be used were Cytoxan, Vincristine, Procarbizine, and Prednosone. The administration of the drugs was to be on the basis of a 14-day cycle, with the Cytoxan to be given by intravenous injection (along with Vincristine), on days 1 and 8 of each cycle, at the rate of 650 milligrams per square meter of body area; Vincristine on the same days at the rate of 1.4 milligrams per square meter; Procarbizine, 100 milligrams per day orally; Prednosone, 40 milligrams per day for 14 days during cycles 1 and 4. Between each 14-day cycle, a period of 14 days would elapse during which no drugs were administered.

Immediately after the diagnosis of Mrs.------'s condition made at Charleston General Hospital, I talked with Mr.

Gordon Roberts on the phone. At that time, he told me that he would send me some of your acidophilus milk to be included in Mrs.------'s diet. Beginning some time in August, she began to include in her diet from eight to twelve ounces of acidophilus milk per day. This continued for a period of about three weeks, to approximately September 6, when she was admitted to NCI at Bethesda as a patient. From September 6 to September 16 she remained as a patient in NCI. During that period she had no acidophilus milk. On September 16, she was advised by the doctors at Bethesda that the tumor node in her neck had reduced in size from approximately that of a ping pong ball to less than the size of a pea; that in the doctors' opinion, a relative reduction in the tumor in the abdominal cavity had also occurred, and that she would be placed on an outpatient basis, to return to NCI on two successive Mondays of each month (following a 14-day period during which no drugs were taken or injected). Since that date, Mrs.------ has returned to Bethesda, as prescribed, for intravenous injection of Cytoxan and Vincristine. Also since that date, she has followed the routine of including the acidophilus milk in her diet. She has taken at least eight ounces of acidophilus milk each day during the period, except those days when she is at NCI.

In December of 1971, the attending physician at NCI told Mrs.------ that he could find no swelling lump or other indication available through external examination of either the abdominal tumor or the tumor which had been discovered in her neck. Upon her original admission in NCI, the abdominal tumor was quite apparent as a hard lump or mass which could be felt through the back muscles or through the front muscles of the abdomen. On her last visit to NCI on Monday, January 3, the attending physician told Mrs.------ that her chemotherapy course of treatment would cease on January 10, 1972, and that thereafter, a determination would be made, probably in March, as to whether or not a further course of treatment should be followed.

I think that I should add that Mrs.------'s physician in Charleston, in August and immediately following the operation which resulted in the discovery of the tumor, told her that she should take 3,000 milligrams of Vitamin C per day, plus 1,000 milligrams of Vitamin E. She has been taking these vitamins on a practically regular basis ever since that date, except during the period of time that she was a patient in NCI (as an inpatient).

Your interest in this matter is very greatly appreciated, and the assistance in the way of acidophilus milk you have given to Mrs.------ is most deeply appreciated.

Sincerely,

* * *

Downers Grove, Illinois 60515
July 19th, 1975

Dear Sir:

I am taking this occasion to write this letter to you so that you may benefit from some information which became known to me a few weeks ago, when returning to the Veterans Administration Hospital in Hines, Illinois, for a followup appointment. It was at this facility, four years ago, that I received treatment for bronchogenic carcinoma.

The doctors assigned to the treatment of my problem after first performing a thoracostomy, decided that my tumor was too advanced, and that further surgery was not advisable. After a week or so, following this exploratory operation, a series of twenty-six radiation treatments were initiated. About half these treatments were as an outpatient, since I lived less than an hour away from the treatment center. I believe that unit used to treat my chest tumor was called a "Betatron."

By the time I received my first exposure to the Betatron, I was in such a condition that I could not lie down in a horizontal position, as it would be impossible for me to breathe. It was necessary for me to sit in an upright position, while the attendants rotated the machine to a ninety-degree attitude. This arrangement lasted through the first six treatments. After the sixth or seventh treatment, enough progress had been made in shrinking the tumor that I could now lie horizontally for the three or four minutes of radiation exposure. Somewhere during these next few treatments, I was also able to turn over onto my stomach side, so that the tumor could be radiated from the backside.

It was shortly after my last exposure to the Betatron on the 26th of October, 1971, that I began to receive shipments of acidophilus milk from Mr. J. Gordon Roberts' Dairy in Omaha, Nebraska. It was through a very close and dear friend of mine, who lives in Florida, that my plight was brought to the attention of Mr. Roberts. To my recollection, these shipments lasted over a period of three to four months.

Since the last Betatron treatment in October, 1971, I have had no further radiation or drug therapy. I have returned to the hospital on frequent followup appointments. Thoracic x-rays and blood chemistry work are completed during these visits. Examination for lymph and liver enlargement are performed by palpitation. Also, my weight is checked at every visit.

To this date, apparently the tumor has been shrunk and at least temporarily, arrested, for which I am most grateful. I do suffer from a circulation difficulty, which I understand I will have for the rest of my life. It occurs whenever I bend over, overstrain myself, or rise too fast. I have been told it is part of the symptoms known as the "Superior Vena Cava Syndrome." I have no disturbing pain in my body, other than I'm sure a good many men approaching their fifties experience. I entered the hospital in September, 1971, weighing two hundred and fifteen pounds. After surgery and radiation, my weight dropped to one hundred and seventy pounds. My weight today is a testament to my lack of will power. It is two hundred, twenty-five, and holding.

Now I'm sure the patient is the last one to know, and probably that is for the best. But it is just recently that I have learned the true name of my illness and that the prognosis four years ago was very poor indeed. I learned a month ago that the radiologist, who first saw me in September, 1971, had given me less than six months to live. This same doctor examined me at my last followup visit, and informed me that, as of this date, I am the only patient treated for bronchogenic carcinoma, in their department, who is still living, and that he believes it is through an act of God.

Needless to say, the heavy smoking habit I was a slave to, was discontinued almost four years ago. Not one cigarette has been lighted since two days before the thoracostomy. I mention this point only to state that the most likely cause for my cancer has been removed, and that this information may be helpful in your overall evaluation.

It is for you to assemble the above information in such a way that perhaps, with other cases and knowledge you possess, a pattern will emerge. I can only pray that this pattern can be discovered in time to help my dear friend, Mr. Howard W. Duke, who is suffering from astrocytoma, and whose prognosis is poor.

Respectfully yours,

* * *

July 19, 1975

Dear Gordon:

Enclosed is a letter which I am mailing to Dr. Shahani today in the hope that the information, which I just recently discovered, may be helpful to his research program.

I have had no information about Howard's current condition, but I'm praying that satisfying progress is being made.

The foregoing letters are not sufficient to offer any kind of adequate scientific proof, for many, many reasons. They are offered only to indicate a possibility.

* * *

On a cruise with my wife, I had an awesome experience with healing. In 1967, the *Constitution* went all the way to Odessa, Russia, its last cruise since that time. The event occurred on Sunday morning, as announced by church music arising from the ship's auditorium.

As my wife and I were patrolling the deck on this Sunday, my wife screamed: "I can't see."

"What is wrong?" I asked, unstrung.

"Half the world is black," she said. "The bottom part is so black I can see nothing."

With little if any hesitation, I took her down to the ship's auditorium where church services were about to start. I seated her. I put my hand across her eyes, in prayer.

"God, in the name of Jesus, pray make her see."*

Without a moment's hesitation, she said: "I see! I see!"

I was flabbergasted, not by what happened, being a born-again Christian, but by what happened with me involved. I feel that I am not as good a Christian as I should be, completely unworthy.

In connection with those with arrested cancer, related to me or my efforts in any way, I have tried, where I felt I might, to appeal to the same Force as with my wife. I do not suggest that my appealing was perfect.

Even so, I do not know what division, if any, may be made, completely separating the physical and the spiritual.

These testimonials are not offered as scientifically acceptable evidence, but as straws of hope. For other material I have offered as much validation as I can.

I do appreciate those unselfish people who have permitted me to use their material.

*As I remember this incident.

CHAPTER 4

HOW A MAN NAMED CHEATHAM CHEATED DEATH

"Health and The Shangri-La
by R. J. Cheatham

"I recovered from cancer and I should like to tell you how it happened: –

"April 14, 1948 – a day I will always remember . . . I had gone to a hospital for an examination of what I had considered to be a minor problem. It was a lump on my right chest which had developed into an open running sore. After an extensive examination, x-rays, and a biopsy, the physicians came forth with a diagnosis of malignant melanoma or cancer on the right chest area. The physicians recommended an immediate operation.

"The Operation

"It never occurred to me that I should question the physician's diagnosis, so we proceeded to make arrangements for admission to the hospital the following day. The operation was performed at the Hines Veterans Administration Hospital in Hines, Illinois, a suburb of Chicago. I was in the operating room for over five hours and the surgeons removed the entire surface of the right side of my chest, leaving the bones covered with only a little skin and a scar seventeen inches long. The next three months I spent in the hospital recuperating from the operation and trying to regain my health by following the orthodox procedures. Every few hours I received a shot of penicillin and on alternate hours a pill or some other type of medication. Interspersed with the medications were the typical hospital meals. Finally, on July 30,

1948, I was released from the hospital with instructions to eat a 'well-balanced diet' and a warning from the Chief Surgeon that I should not expose my body to the sunshine under any circumstances.

"Search for Truth

"It was while recuperating in the hospital that I found time to think about my cancer condition and its causes. I began to question the physicians, surgeons, nurses, and the other patients. After considerable questioning, I found that mine had been a very serious condition, the chances of recovering from the operation about fifty-fifty and further, that the maximum life expectancy after such an operation was only about five years.

"I then tried to find out what the cause was and what I could do to prevent any further problems. The answers I received from the physicians and surgeons did not seem to satisfy me, and I found myself embarked upon a search to find an answer that would satisfy my now curious mind and possibly save my life.

"During the next two years I ran the gamut of practically all of the so-called 'healing professions.' I took their prescribed medicines, pills, shots, drugs, and accepted their treatments of massage, adjustments, vibrations, x-rays, colonics, and a host of other 'cures.' In spite of being continually 'cured' by all this medical science, my condition did not actually seem to improve. To the contrary, on returning to the hospital for routine examinations the surgeons found more lumps and began to operate again to remove sections for biopsy or examining purposes. Hearing of the third death among my cancer-ridden hospital roommates did not improve my mental outlook. To make matters worse, one insurance company cancelled my life insurance and other companies flatly refused to provide me with any insurance at any price.

Reflecting on the past, and the obvious inability of the orthodox methods to help my condition, I lost confidence in all the physicians and their efforts to 'cure' me.

"About this time (1950) I began to frequent the health food stores where I purchased their various products as well as magazines and books. Any book I could find on the subject of health improvement was studied thoroughly from cover to cover. Every health lecturer who came to town found me in attendance to listen, to buy his products and books, to take his courses, and to ask questions. As time went by, I became familiar with most of the people speaking on health improvement and I knew what their point of view was. Fortunately, from each of these I was able to glean a little truth and I put into practice the ideas that made sense to me.

"Natural Hygiene

"One evening I noticed an advertisement in the newspaper about a lecturer who was going to speak on the subject of how to improve health through Natural Hygiene. This was something new to me, so I made it a point to be at the meeting if for no other purpose than to determine what he had to sell and what was his point of view. I had been through the mill and by this time was a true skeptic. But the principles of Natural Hygiene, or the laws of Nature, with their simplicity, logic, and common sense impressed me. By the time the lecture was over, I felt sure that here was the answer to health and disease, to living or dying.

"Having found what promised to be the answer, I purchased book after book and attended many lectures on the subject. Later I was privileged to attend one of the Annual International Conventions of the American Natural Hygiene Society. After attending the many classes and lectures given by the leading professional and lay hygienists on the many facets of Natural Hygiene, after listening and participating in the question-and-answer periods and after talking with many people who had followed this way of life, any doubts or reservations I might have had were completely eliminated.

"To put it briefly, the study of Natural Hygiene taught me that cancer, or any other disease, is not a chance thing, that disease isn't something that you accidentally catch, but is the result of definite causes. Disease is not harmful but rather the vital action of the body trying to correct itself and is actually beneficial. One should not interfere with disease by the use of palliative and suppressive drugs, medications, and treatments, but one should assist this eliminative effort of the body by complete rest and fasting if possible.

"Natural Hygiene teaches that if we want to have good health, it is necessary to eliminate the causes of poor health. It teaches that the human body must have adequate sunshine, fresh clean air, pure uncontaminated water, regular exercise, sufficient rest and sleep, bodily cleanliness, and mental and emotional poise. Further, that we must provide the body with fresh, unprocessed natural foods at the proper time, in the proper quantities, and in the proper combinations.

"After the Convention, I resolved to do everything I could to help communicate the knowledge of this better way of life to the rest of the world. Becoming active as an officer of the local Detroit Chapter of the American Natural Hygiene Society probably helped me more than anything else to develop sufficient self-control and self-discipline to put into practice the hygienic principles necessary to restore my own health. Each year I have managed to get to the Annual Convention wherever it was held. It was my pleasure to be appointed Convention Manager for the 1959 International Convention which was held in Detroit, Michigan. Then, during 1959-60, I was privileged to serve as National President and General Manager of the American Natural Hygiene Society.

"The Results of Better Living

"Having told you about my experience in Natural Hygiene, let me tell you a little about the results of living this better way of life. After giving my body a chance to rehabilitate itself through fasting, working out a daily exercise program, arranging my time so that I could get plenty of rest and sleep, planning for regular sun and air baths, and correcting my diet by eliminating dead substances such as meat, fish, fowl, white bread, white sugar, salt, coffee, soda pops, chewing gum, spices, condiments, etc., and substituting plenty of live foods, such as fresh succulent salads, fresh vegetables, fresh fruits and fresh nuts; I found that I was able to eliminate the eye glasses which I had worn for about ten years. When I took the test for renewing my driver's license, the examiner passed me without question. An insurance company examination found me qualified for a larger policy. My physical examinations have revealed no further lumps or problems. Mrs. Cheatham and I have had four additional children since the operation. These children have been brought up from birth in this better way of life. They are all lovely children . . . all pictures of health . . . and without the 'benefit' of any medications, shots or treatments of any kind. Incidentally, our last three children were born at home with myself in attendance for the delivery.

"Perhaps most important, over twenty-five years have passed since my cancer operation. Those who were with me, in the same hospital, with similar conditions and orthodox care, have long since passed away. Not only am I alive, in spite of the operation, but I now feel better than I can ever remember feeling, and I look forward to many more healthy, wonderful years.

"A Plan Developed

"In order to pursue my new interest in Natural Hygiene,

I decided to sell the successful business which I had owned and operated in Detroit, Michigan, for almost ten years, and move to Florida so that I would have a more desirable climate for myself and family. Soon after making this decision, I received the honor of being elected the first lay National President of the American Natural Hygiene Society. I then took it upon myself to make a lecture tour of the United States to visit all the local Chapters of the American Natural Hygiene Society and also the vegetarian-hygienic resorts and institutions which were in existence at that time. It was during this tour that I first began thinking of trying to locate, organize and develop a place where these wonderful laws of Nature could be taught, lived and practiced. I began a new search, for a location at which to establish an hygienic institute. In order to prepare myself for this new work I intensified my study of Natural Hygiene, obtaining and studying every single work of Dr. Herbert M. Shelton and all the other leaders of the Hygienic movement. In addition, I took extensive courses, obtaining diplomas in Naturopathy, Homeopathic Medicine, Osteopathy Life Science, and Metaphysics.

"My search for a suitable location lasted for over two years, taking me all over the United States, through Canada, the Bahama Islands, Jamaica and Mexico, until I found a place in Orange City, Florida, which was formerly a monastery. This we called The Paragon Health Resort, and we operated it for about four years. Still, not being completely satisfied, we continued the search and finally found exactly what we were looking for in Bonita Springs, Florida, The Shangri-La Natural Hygiene Institute, Bonita Springs, Florida 33923-CF."

CHAPTER 5

HOW MILK MAY HELP PROTECT OR FAIL TO PROTECT AGAINST CANCER

Taken from General Semantics Bulletin 38-39-40
1976

The theory that sweet milk may "cause" cancer is based upon the possibility that cancer may result when the enzymatic system is overwhelmed at some point, or in some way. (The theory that milk may help is based upon enzymatic adequacy.)

Of course I have not read all the reports on cancer research, but none I have read, whether based upon cigarette smoking or hydrocarbons in the air, may preclude the possibility of the foregoing suggested cause.

Most of the people in the world lack the lactase to cope with sweet milk, even by the standard of clinical observation, much less sub-clinical result, according to "Lactose and Lactase," by Norman Kretchmer, *Scientific American,* October, 1972.

Carbohydrates, proteins, and fats are digested according to different time schedules, in different parts of the digestive tract. Food combinations in themselves may cause enzymatic conflicts. Emotional upsets may delay digestion in such fashion as to imitate shortage of lactase.

At body temperature, pasteurized milk does not curdle normally; it turns into a putrefactive mess. With digestive delays resulting from enzymatic conflict, or emotional disturbance, the same toxic material could result from pasteurized milk within the digestive tract.

Even though *Lactobacillus Bulgaricus* and *Streptococcus Thermophilus* presumably do not survive within the human digestive tract, "the feeding of yogurt inhibited the total" (mice) "tumor cell count by 27.3 to 29.7%, and the DNA content by 25.1 to 28.8%," according to "Antitumor Activity of Yogurt Fractions" by Robert Elvis Farmer, a thesis presented to the Graduate College of the University of Nebraska in partial fulfillment of requirements for the degree of Master of Science, Department of Food Science and Technology, under the supervision of Dr. Khem M. Shahani, Lincoln, Nebraska, October, 1974.

"Erhlich ascities tumor (Line E-182, generation F-72) was elected for use in this study."

"Male Swiss mice weighing about 25 gm were selected for use in this investigation."

The foregoing indicates a possible relationship of symbiotic cellular nature with bacteria which produce lactase. Such bacteria, especially acidophilus and bifidus, also are helpful in the maintenance of a healthy intestinal flora, which might be interrupted in some ways under some conditions, by pasteurized milk.

The possible need of market milk for bacterial protection should be given much more attention and study than offered until now.

CHAPTER 6

OVERLOOKED ASPECTS OF ENVIRONMENT WHICH MAY RELATE TO CANCER

Pasteurization in Relation to Environment

In fairness, let us look to possibilities other than the pasteurization of milk, for causing cancer.

Whatever deleterious to health has occurred since the turn of the century, either within environment outside ourselves, or our way of life, mathematically, there would almost seem to be a corollary between diseases of the heart and cancer, according to figures prepared by the American College of Underwriters. Take, for example, the figures for 1900-04 and 1960-64:

Cancer deaths per 100,000 more than doubled.

Diseases of the heart more than doubled. Cancer increased by 2.222; diseases of the heart by 2.495. But –

A footnote shows some change in the manner of reporting occurred in 1950. If we allow for changes indicated by the footnote, cancer has increased by 2.199 or 219.9%, and diseases of the heart by 2.289 or 228.9%, a difference percentagewise of nine out of more than 200% change over a span of sixty years.

Let us compare 1950-54 with 1960-64. In 1960-64, cancer is up by not quite five percent, and diseases of the heart by slightly more than four percent. Cancer appears to be gaining on diseases of the heart, so late figures would also seem to indicate. Nevertheless, the possibility of broad areas of common cause should not be overlooked.

Possible enzymatic shortage through snacks rather than fruits and vegetables and the heating of foods, generally, including milk, may not represent the only adverse change, as we shall see. However, enzymes are destroyed at 122 degrees Fahrenheit, according to Carlson Wade in *Helping Your*

Health with Enzymes. Pasteurization requires a temperature of at least 145 degrees or more, depending upon the time of heating.

Some bacteria, such as acidophilus, may have an antibiotic effect, destroying the likes of salmonella. Cattle are tested for tuberculosis and brucellosis. The question should be raised as to whether or not the pasteurization of milk, at this point in time, should represent a legal requirement.

Especially is this true inasmuch as colostrum (the product of the cow for the first seven days of lactation), may possibly combine with cultured milk to offer some measure of protection against cancer.

On the other hand, should such measures be undertaken with maximum effectiveness, by no means would all the steps have been taken for complete enzymatic nourishment, much less total health.

For example, let us consider exercise.

A stagnant pool of water and a stagnant blood supply may have more in common than one would imagine.

In one sense, a person is alive to the extent that he burns up oxygen. Exercise forces the body to use more oxygen than it would otherwise.

In terms of generalization, a man at rest circulates about a gallon of blood a minute . . . the entire blood supply circulates throughout the tissues about once a minute. Hard exercise may speed circulation by eight or nine times . . . fifty-five feet a minute as compared to 450, through large arteries.

Inasmuch as an individual may weigh one hundred pounds or three hundred, figures of this kind may hardly apply exactly to the reader. Nevertheless, the principle involved would apply generally.

Presumably, as with a stream of water, a fast current eliminates waste faster than a sluggish creek.

Muscles which are not used tend to atrophy, become unsuitable for use. Should the same principle apply to the circulatory system, the more it is used, the better.

Usually exercise is related to health only when some individual who is completely out of shape will become inspired to do unaccustomed exercise, and die of a heart attack. Under such conditions, from one point of view, exercise is blamed for what should in fairness, be blamed upon lack of exercise.

Anyone involved in an automobile accident, after not driving for twenty years, may hardly blame his difficulty upon too much driving.

For the one fit to do it, hard exercise will induce sleep better than anything short of hard drugs. Arduous exercise limits the use of drugs in most people who do it, which, in itself, would justify the activity. Any product consumed which is not metabolized, with the possible exceptions of table salt and roughage, may threaten well-being to some degree, however necessary by reason of some physical contingency.

Quite often, medication may be a calculated risk, however inescapable, which should be taken only when justified, certainly not as a habit. Thus, prescriptions are required.

Without the habit of exercise, the habit of some kind of medication is likely to take its place. And medication is likely to induce even more unnatural rest, when "rest" may represent the last thing the individual may actually need.

For example, some researchers have found that those who do hard physical work are far less likely to accumulate cholesterol, even on a high cholesterol diet. And this does not mean that a high cholesterol diet should be followed. As a matter of fact, cholesterol and diet are taken up further on.

Nor do I suggest that the entire problem of cholesterol may be handled by exercise. I do suggest that the increases in cancer and diseases of the heart are close enough that a healthy heart should not be disregarded as possibly being related to protection against cancer.

According to enthusiasts, exercise increases the glandular activity. Logically, it would almost have to do this for the body to handle the increased flow of blood. Some say that exercise may increase the size of the coronary arteries. Exercise increases the size of other muscles.

A study of primitive people indicates that childbirth is much easier for the primitive woman accustomed to hard work.

Exercise appears to slow down the pulse rate. A Soviet scientist is quoted as saying that exercise may improve eyesight.

Exercise illustrates an area of possible health improvement, conceivably related to cancer, which may be critically important, yet never proved in the laboratory as related to cancer.

Even if mice could be induced to take some kind of involuntary exercise . . . as in a laboratory . . . such exercise might hardly be compared with voluntary human exercise. Some areas of cancer study, if conducted at all, must necessarily be conducted by accurate surveys covering large numbers of people. The laboratory is simply not suitable for all kinds of testing.

Yet the only testing considered valid in connection with cancer, based upon reports, is laboratory testing. And it is at least possible that a complete answer to cancer may never be found in a laboratory, however vital and indispensable such research may be, especially as a guide.

Because of uncertainty as to who may or may not get cancer, and because of uncertainty as to what form of nutritional shortage might be involved in one suffering from cancer, conclusive proof in relation to food would almost necessitate studies of large groups of people. In the foregoing sense, new approaches to nutritional requirement might conceivably be helpful.

In any case, it would appear stupid for anyone wishing

to inhibit cancer as a protective measure or for any reason, to continue unnecessarily any practice which may be related, even remotely, to bringing on a condition which might be conducive to cancer.

An outline follows later.

CHAPTER 7

CANCER OF THE COLON SUGGESTS AN APPROACH TO PREVENTION

Dennis P. Burkitt wrote "Epidemiology of the Cancer of the Colon and Rectum," printed by The American Cancer Society in *Cancer,* Vol. 28, No. 1, July, 1971.

The author points out that cancer of the bowel and lung cancer are of recent development, both rare in developing countries.

The author borrows from Doll, R.: The geographical distribution of cancer, *British Journal of Cancer* 23: 1-8, 1969, when he informs us that the incidence of cancer in Kampala (Uganda) is 3.5 as compared with Connecticut, 51.8 for men 35-64 years of age.

Borrowing from other sources, he illustrates that large bowel cancer and colon diverticula are three times as common in industrialized Sweden as in "more rural" Finland.

He suggests that there is a well recognized association between bowel cancer and ulcerative colitis and that association between bowel cancer and hemorrhoids has been accepted.

He declares: "There is clear correlation between intestinal transit time and stool bulk, and the fiber content of food."

He offers: "It can be concluded that diet affects intestinal transit time, and the bulk, consistency and bacterial flora of the feces."

He postulates that altered bacterial flora may lead to degradation of bile salts with resultant formation of carcinogens.

As an hypothesis: "It seems likely that bacterial changes will be accepted as probable causative factors in bowel cancer, though the reasons for the bacterial changes may be disputed."

He declares that cancer may be suppressed in germ-free rats, and offers experimental evidence from the United States and Japan to support this contention.

He concludes: "In view of the evidence, it seems justifiable to issue a warning against the removal of so much of the unabsorbable fiber from our food, and the associated over-ingestion of refined carbohydrates."

In the opinion of this writer, such warning would certainly appear justified. On the other hand, such material does not include other differences which may be involved in differing results, such as differences in vitamin and mineral consumption with concomitant effect upon enzymatic action.

Such material does not cover the order in which food is consumed, nor the presence or absence of food conflicts, such as suggested in the listing of minerals and vitamins.

It does not explain why newly born infants throughout the world are almost entirely free of any cancer, with no roughage whatever in their diet.

Of course adults may not be compared totally with newly born infants. But conceivably these other factors may not be disregarded either, rationally. And infants are offered a kind of bacterial protection in mother's milk which might hardly be usual in the adult diet, even though it might suggest supplementation, to help offset environmental contingencies.

Let us, by the way, take a look at what some of these environmental contingencies are. For the last thing I wish to do with this book is to convince anyone that some kind of overall Salk vaccine, except for cancer rather than polio, is likely to emerge as a total answer because of multiple causes, if for no other reason.

One of the principal causes of cancer may consist of a search primarily for a cure for cancer, rather than an answer. A workable answer must probably require cooperation worldwide. Otherwise, the world might well decimate itself of human beings, without bombs or even bows and arrows.

At present "developing" countries are developing cancer, as statistics indicate.

A study of how chemical carcinogens may induce cancer may indicate, at least, one facet of the complexity of cancer. I suggest the following book for anyone seriously interested in cancer, for whatever reason. It is for sale by the Superintendent of Documents, U.S. Government Printing Office, Washington, D.C., 20402, for $1.50.

More on the foregoing in the Appendix.

CHAPTER 8

ALCOHOLISM, CANCER, AND DIET

Dealing with the relationship between food and emotional problems is *Pschodietetics, Food as the Key to Emotional Health,* by E. Cheraskin, M.D., D.M.D., and W. M. Ringsdorf, Jr., D.M.D., M.S., with Arlene Brecher, published by Stein and Day, New York, 1974.

The book points out that alcoholism may be turned on and off in rats by diets high in nutritional value as compared with diets high in carbohydrates, but low in vitamins and minerals.

It points out that the diets of many teenagers will cause alcoholism in rats.

Tests indicate that alcoholism may be related to hypoglycemia, low blood sugar, induced by high levels of refined sugar, which bounce the blood sugar level up and down, caffeine, and nicotine, according to the material in the book, and other sources.

According to this book, diets high in vitamins and other needed nutritional factors may at least reduce greatly the torment of the alcoholic struggling to leave liquor alone, possibly struggling against a nutritional shortage, according to the material presented here.

The book warns against more than 10% of the diet as empty calories.

The dietary requirements to protect against alcoholism may be similar to those which may protect against cancer, if not the same. However, personally, I would not subscribe completely to all the recommendations in this book, as related to cancer. I could be wrong in some areas, as could the authors, inasmuch as omniscience is unlikely to be found anywhere.

Even so, the material on alcoholism contained in the

foregoing book was presumably extrapolated from scientific research.

If true in principle regarding alcoholism, perhaps the same principle applies to cancer.

In fact, theoretically, a diet and way of life adequate to protect against cancer should minimize, at the least, alcoholic compulsion. No one trying to cure himself of cancer through changing his way of life would dream of loading his system with nicotine and caffeine in copious quantities. Excesses in these areas may make sick a normal person, without either cancer or alcoholic compulsion.

Although I would never suggest other than complete abstinence, I would also suggest that normalizing the diet may help anyone.

If diet be involved in human emotion, human relations may be influenced at least as much by diet as by political ideology, with implications as to crime, and war and peace.

Resolving the question of dietary effect upon cancer might have some effects not subject to anticipation. For a diet protective against cancer might be protective in other areas as well, should such a diet be feasible.

Perhaps more effort should be made to find out.

The book also offers another point of extreme importance to health, mental and physical. Change can be painful. Even dieting can be painful, from the standpoint of change alone. Part of the success of weight-watchers depends, in effect, upon group therapy.

The discovery of cancer is a shocking change for anyone. If for no other reason, change offers a reason for the existence of the International Association of Cancer Victims and Friends. In Clearwater, Florida, 33516, the local chapter may be reached through Peter Reuter, 1950 Sandra Drive. Each group should identify itself.

"Sanity of the Soviets:
The Communist Approach to Mental Illness
by William F. O'Neill, Ph.D. and George D. Demos, Ph.D.

"Sanity is invariably a cultural concept. For the primitive Mundugumors of New Guinea, paranoia is a group norm. For the docile Arapesh who live nearby, a genial and succoring 'other-direction' is the sought-after cultural ideal. In a similar sense, the normal Yurok Indian cries to his gods 'like a baby'; he hallucinates in his meditation 'like a psychotic'; he acts 'like a phobic' when confronted with contamination; and he tries to act avoidant, suspicious, and stingy 'like a compulsive neurotic.' Ultimately, then, and as anthropologist Dorothy Lee so acutely observes:

" 'The world view of a particular society includes that society's conception of man's own relation to the universe, human and non-human, organic and inorganic, secular and divine, to use our own dualisms. It expresses man's view of his own role in the maintenance of life, and of the forces of nature.' "

The above appeared in the publication *ETC: a review of general semantics,* Volume 33, Number 1, March 1976.

The following article appear in the *Bulletin of Atomic Scientists,* April, 1976, page 6:

"In the 15th century the religious reformer Jan Hus formulated the ethical groundwork of scientific thought, and was tried for heresy, condemned and burned at the stake at Constance for his search for and defense of truth.

"In the 17th century, John Amos Comenius, the founder of modern pedagogy, was forced to emigrate from Czechoslovakia and spend the rest of his life abroad because of his beliefs."

The approach to cancer, itself, must involve a critical examination of the nationality of whatever approach is to be considered.

CHAPTER 9

THE LAW OF THE MINIMUM

Further on, the material in this book shall really reach far out, into consideration of time, itself, as a wave. Inasmuch as no sort of clock is to be offered as a cure for cancer, such speculation should produce ridicule at worst, and contemplation, at best.

Effort shall be made to circumscribe the cancer phenomenon with mathematical description, hypothetically describing what may occcur.

But now let us consider "The Law of the Minimum" by Dr. Herbert M. Shelton, *Hygienic System,* Volume II, Fifth Edition, 1969, published by Dr. Shelton's Health School, San Antonio, Texas, page 98:

"The metabolic process by which an apple, a tomato or a portion of cabbage is made into hair, or muscle or nerve, or some of the cells of the eyes, or into a hormone of some of the ductless glands is beyond our present comprehension, although a few steps in this process are supposed to be known. What we do know is that if the foods we eat are to be made into tissues and secretions, they must contain adequate amounts and due proportions of all the elements needed in the production of these things.

"Just as we cannot make concrete with cement alone or with sand alone, but must, if our concrete is to be good, have due proportions of both, so, if we are to have good structures in our bodies, we must have adequate amounts and proper proportions of all the food elements that go into the construction of these structures.

"To make the best use of any food elements, such, for example, as the proteins, certain other food substances and possibly a variety of them must be available in the diet in definite proportions. No food element is of itself of more importance in the body than another. It is only by the combination of all the necessary ones that the whole may be obtained.

"Liebig laid down a 'law of the minimum' in these words: 'The development of living beings is regulated by the supply of whichever element is least bountifully provided.'

"The law of the minimum implies that the nutritive value of any food-mixture, however abundant most of the food elements therein may be, is limited by the minimum quantity of any essential element it may contain; unless, as it happens in certain food constituents, the lacking factor may be synthesized from some of the more abundant food elements, fat from sugar, for example.

"Calcium cannot be utilized in producing enamel in the absence of phosphorus. If phosphorus is present in inadequate amounts, the enamel will be of poor quality. If iron is lacking, there will also be poor enamel. If any one of the vitamins is lacking poor enamel is the result.

"The united 'action' of minerals, proteins, vitamins, etc., in the production of tissues and fluids in the body is called 'synergistic action.' Since they do not act, but are used, it may be more correct to say that the body makes correlated use of them. At any rate, a knowledge of the 'synergistic action' of the food elements and vitamins is of vast importance and helps to make clear to us the Law of the Minimum.

"Tooth enamel is made up largely of calcium and phosphorus with small quantities of iron. But the fusion of these substances into enamel requires the presence of vitamins A, C and D. At least half a dozen elements and factors are essential to the production of this tissue. In the absence of either of these factors the enamel of the teeth cannot be made. It is folly to feed much calcium in an effort to produce good teeth and to ignore the other essential elements of the teeth.

"Many different tissues are being built and repaired in the body at all times. These tissues are constantly engaged in a wide variety of activities. This means that there is a continuous use of vitamins, minerals, amino acids, sugars and fatty acids in the body. Consuming an abundance of a single vitamin or of a single mineral is not sufficient to meet the needs of the many 'synergistic actions' that are in constant process in the body. All of the vitamins and all of the minerals are required. If all the nutritive elements are present in adequate quantities and in due proportions, all the synerrgisms of all the minerals, vitamins, amino acids, sugars, etc., are at work piling up their benefits.

"It is well to keep in mind that these 'synergistic actions' are far more complex and broader than our description of them would indicate. The many functions of the body are also synergistic. The function of one part of the body is dependent upon the functions of all other parts. Feeding vitamin B in certain forms of nervous trouble with the aim of remedying the nervous impairment, and ignoring the correlated functions of the body that support nerve function, is doomed to failure. All of the 'synergistic chemical actions' in all parts of the body must be adequately provided for before the actions of any part can be ideal. This is the thing that makes specific diets so unsatisfactory.

"The work of potassium in promoting the formation of proteins, fats and glycogen, is not essentially unlike the work ascribed to vitamins. Zinc is thought to be connected with the action of the vitamins, which it seems to be able to replace to some extent, at least in the animal organism. Lithium is also thought to influence metabolism in a way not unlike that of the vitamins. The same is true of copper, nickel and of arsenic. It should be borne in mind that little is known about the offices of zinc, lithium, copper, nickel and arsenic in the body and that experimenters, carrying out their experiments, have wholly neglected these elements.

"In plant life and growth the Law of the Minimum has long been known. If perfect growth is to be procured in plants, these must find a certain minimum of each of several elements in the soil in which they are grown. If only half the needed amount of potassium, for example, is present, then, regardless of how abundant all the other soil elements may be, their normal utilization is reduced one-half. The rate of growth of the plant and its ultimate development are correspondingly depressed.

"Prof. Osterhout showed that seeds placed in distilled water grow better than when placed in water containing but one salt, and that each salt exerts a specific toxic effect according to its chemical nature. He found that one salt 'counteracts' the effects of another.

"An excess of nitrogen in the soil retards the formation of grain, roots and tubers and gives rise to sickly plants. Nitrogen excess in the soil of rose beds leads to the production of soft, sappy tissues, a luxuriant growth of leaves, and roses with little or no perfume.

"Plant processes, from germination to ripening of their seed, are a drama of physiological minerals and gases. Without a sufficiency of lime or potash in the soil, acids, sugars and starches cannot be formed; without iron no chlorophyll and no albumen can be formed. Without silica no fibre or plant skeleton, etc. Each mineral plays a definite role in the growth of healthy plants.

"The actual amount of potassium requisite for plant growth is very small compared with the needed amount of carbon or nitrogen. But if this relatively small quantity is not available the utilization of other constituents in tissue growth or repair is always deficient.

"If one essential food element, which normally should compose one per cent of the food eaten, is present in only half this amount, then, the body will only be able to utilize the other elements, in tissue building, in the same reduced quantity.

"The organic whole – the unit – is official to animal nutrition. Not the sum total of the minerals consumed, but their relative proportions, determines the nutritive value of any given dietary.

"A certain minimum amount of organic salts is essential to optimal growth. A further increase in these, even a great increase, does not further influence growth. Not only the total quantity of these salts, but also the quantities of the individual minerals and their mutual quantitive relationships are of decisive importance in regulating the assimilation of proteins.

"If we are to have normal development the mineral elements in our diet must also be present in minimum quantities, but they must also represent proper ratios one to another. The mineral salts are most sensitive to any deficiency of any of them in the diet. Many common foodstuffs are deficient in iron and calcium, and these deficiencies reduce the ability of the body to assimilate the other elements. On the other hand, in experimental diets, any increase of one element raises the mineral requirements of all the others.

"If health and development are to follow, certain relationships must prevail between the various salts. Berg, McCarrison, McCollum and others have amply demonstrated this. Rose found that a certain relationship must prevail between calcium and magnesium if the maximum development of the body is to be attained. Between lime and potassium, lime and sodium, potassium and magnesium and between the metals on the one hand and sulphur and phosphurus on the other, an optimum ratio exists.

"The proper exploitation of both proteins and carbohydrates is determined by mineral metabolism, since they can be more readily oxidized in an alkaline medium than when an excess of bases over acid-forming foodstuffs ingested promotes the utilization of proteins. Zunts, of Berlin, showed that diabetics can more easily oxidise sugar if the body has an abundance of bases at its disposal. Abderhalden performed investigations which showed that a diet rich in bases is essential for the proper functioning of the hormones of the ductless glands.

"Without iron there can be no oxygen supply for the cells. Without copper there can be no assimilation of iron. Without sodium there is no elimination of carbon-dioxide from the tissues of the body. Every physico-chemical process of the body is correlated with others and any failure in one spells a corresponding failure in the correlated processes.

"May Mellanby says that the evidence shows that the calcium in the diet does not in itself directly control the calcification of the teeth, but that it is subservient to other dietetic factors. One of these is Vitamin A. She thinks that she has demonstrated the existence of factors in some foods, particularly in cereals, and more especially in oats, that inhibit calcification. Phosphorus is as essential to the formation of good bones and teeth as is lime.

"The present furore over vitamins has caused many exspurts to concentrate their whole attention upon these substances and almost forget the other elements of nutrition. We pick up a book or a magazine article or a report dealing with nutritional problems and we learn that a rich diet in Vitamin A does thus and so, or a diet poor in Vitamin B results in such and such effects. The minerals in the diets are particularly overlooked. Interest in vitamins is causing us to forget the importance of other food elements.

"The present over-emphasis on vitamins is as absurd as if we were similarly to over-emphasize sodium, or magnesium. To ignore the organic salts, as is so often done in our mad rush for vitamins, is as foolish as would be the ignoring of the vitamins.

"It has been demonstrated that regardless of the amount of Vitamin A supplied in the diet, if some other constituent of the diet is wholly lacking, Vitamin A can have no effect. Berg shows that a cereal diet complete in A is without effect unless sodium and calcium are added to the diet in sufficient quantities to produce an excess of bases. McCollum and his co-workers have shown that when there is an abundance of Vitamin A in the diet, the mother cannot secrete sufficient milk for her progeny, unless her food contains an adequate amount of organic salts in proper proportions.

"The absence of any one of the essential vitamins prevents the rest of them from functioning at all. If any one of them is present in but one-half or in but one-fourth the required amount, then the others, though abundantly present, will function only up to one-half or one-fourth of their full effectiveness.

"Lack of vitamins disturbs calcium metabolism. A lack of calcium or an excess of calcium in the diet renders Vitamin A of no effect. Vitamins are valuable only in the presence of each other. Calcium seems to be usable only in the presence of Vitamin A.

"McCarrison says that 'in the absence of vitamins or in their inadequate supply, neither proteins, fats nor carbohydrates nor salts are properly utilized; some are largely wasted, while others yield products harmful to the organism. In such circumstances life may be sustained for a longer or shorter period, during which the body utilizes its stores of vitamins and sacrifices its less important tissues to this end. But there is a limit beyond which such stores cannot be drawn upon, and once this is reached the cells of higher function — secretory, endocrine and nerve cells — begin to lack vigor, and to depreciate in functional capacity, although the tissues may continue to hold considerable stores of vitamins. The disintegration process is delayed or hastened, lessened in severity in one direction or increased in severity in another, according to the character of their lack of balance.'

"There are many kinds of proteins and where one is securing his protein from one source only he is likely to suffer from protein inadequacy even though he is consuming an excessive amount of protein. The biological value of the various proteins varies considerably.

"Proteins are broken down into their constituent amino-acids in the process of digestion and these amino-acids are employed in constructing new and different proteins in the body, but amino-acids may be utilized by the body only to the extent that the diet supplies other protein constituents which enable the body to synthesize them into proteins proper to man. If more amino-acids are introduced into the blood than the presence of other elements will enable the body to utilize, the amino-acid content of the blood rises and there is an increased excretion of amino-acids in the urine.

"It is at once apparent from this, that growth can proceed at an ideal rate only as rapidly as all of the essentials of growth become available to the growing organism.

"It is found, in harmony with this law, that in the case of proteins, the value of a protein or mixture of proteins for structural purposes in the body, is limited if one of the indispensable amino-acids is deficient or wholly lacking. If and when this deficiency is remedied, a deficient supply of some other indispensable amino-acid constitutes a further limitation.

"Attempts are often made to determine the value of an article of food by using as an index to its fitness, the amount of some element contained in it; let us say phosphorus. This effort is based on a misconception of the office of these elements in nutrition. To over-emphasize the importance of any of the salts — iron, calcium, potassium — or of any of the vitamins or complettins, or of protein or carbohydrate is to overlook the essential fact that these things function in nutrition only in union with the other elements.

"This law of the minimum applies even to water. It has been shown repeatedly that if water is limited to a certain extent in the diet of infants, and all the other growth essentials are adequate, growth will not take place. Children placed on dehydrated diets can be taught within a very short time to take and be content with a small amount of water. The body establishes a water balance on a very low level but does not grow.

"Many scientists have concentrated on single issues, seeking in these the secrets of life. But this concentration on one detail caused them to overlook the importance of the tout ensemble. Schaumann, for example, attempted to show that beriberi (polyneuritis) is due to the loss of a phosphorus compound in the milling of whole grains. Chamberlain checked up on his assumption and found it to be wrong. Several elements are lost in the milling of grains and the troubles resulting from consuming denatured grains grow out of the total deficiency.

"The effort to supply us with isolated vitamins and minerals is essentially a medical rather than a tropholgic procedure and harks back to the antiquated notions that there are 'specific diseases,' having specific causes and requiring specific remedies.

"Every tissue builder is dependent upon all the others. The decisive factor in development is not so much the absolute quantity of the various food elements in the diet, but their relative proportions. The organism's need for one element of food may be supplied only when all other elements are supplied in relative proportions. The diet must contain a sufficiency of all essential food elements, but there must be no great excess of any of these.

"The amount of any given element available for utilization by the body depends, not alone upon the proportions of other elements present in the diet, but also upon other factors. The organic salts enter into important reciprocal relationships, especially in the work of secretion, but also in the process of synthesizing new organic compounds, so that we are concerned with both a qualitative and a quantitive minimum. If an element is being fed in quantities that are adequate per se, but some other and antagonistic substance is also being given, the quantity of the first is thereby rendered inadequate. An adequate amount of calcium for example, would be rendered inadequate by the medical administration of acids, or by acid fermentation in the digestive tract. The calcium would be exhausted in neutralizing the acids and little or none would be left for the body. An abundance of calcium coupled with a lack of sodium means trouble, for the sodium is essential to keep the calcium in solution.

"The availability of a food element depends, not alone upon the amount and form of this element present in the food, but also upon the quantities of other elements present. The quantity of available calcium for example, does not depend wholly upon the absolute quantity of calcium in the diet, but upon the quantity of mineral bases generally present in one's food. A shortage of these bases involves a drain on the calcium for purposes of acid-neutralization, and consumes an amount of calcium which would otherwise be available for assimilation.

"After the alkaline salts have been consumed in neutralizing the acids in the foods themselves, the residue of these are available for storage in the body as a reinforcement of its alkaline reserve. The availability of the alkaline elements is proportioned to their excess over the food acids. This is the reason that our diet should at all times be preponderantly aklaline. McCarrison showed that an excess of fat or of unsaturated oleic acid in the food may cause a relative deficiency of iodine and enlargement of the thyroid.

"MacCollum, of Johns Hopkins, states in his 'Pathology' that there seems to be some relation between the deposition of calcium and the available supply of iron. Iron is not assimilated in the absence of copper.

"An excellent example of this matter, on the positive side, is the increased protein-calcium-phosphorus retention produced by the use of orange juice. The regular use of orange juice results in an increased retention of these elements out of all proportion to the amounts of these actually present in the juice itself.

"It has been found that a diet with an acid-ash residue results in a greater excretion of minerals than one with an alkaline ash. Oranges give an alkaline ash. Indeed, the addition of oranges to a decidedly acid-ash diet of much cereal, meat, and few vegetables, gives such a marked alkaline result that it shifts the reaction of the urine from a decidedly acid reaction to a decidedly alkaline one. This means increased mineral retention and also increased nitrogen assimilation.

"Drs. Miller and Newell, of Iowa State College, added an ounce and a half of orange juice daily for three months to the otherwise unchanged diet of fourteen underweight children and tabulated the results. The weight of these children increased 146 per cent of the expected gain, in contrast with only 46 per cent observed during the preceding three months.

"Dr. Cheney, of California, fed a group of undernourished children an orange a day. To another group he gave no oranges. During two different periods of two months each, the children who received the oranges gained an average of 141 and 118 per cent above the expected increases. The other group, without oranges, gained only 18 and 18 per cent above the expected gain. During the non-orange juice periods, including the preliminary days, the children gained an average of .08 pounds a day; with the oranges they gained an average of .3 pounds a day — approximately four times as much as without the fruit.

"Failure of growth may rightly be considered a deficiency disease although, on certain types of diets, both animals and man maintain good health and proportionate development, failing only to attain their normal sizes. Except for size they seem to be normal animals. This is explained by the law of the minimum given at the beginning of this chapter. Such diets contain all the needed food elements and growth is determined by the elements least bountifully supplied.

"Unfortunate experiences such as famine, war, poverty, and the ignorance that causes many people to feed upon denatured diets, prove that the laws of nutrition and growth are the same in man as in the lower animals and plants. The wise will understand.

"To secure the highest possible development from food, it must be adequate in every respect. All of the food nutrients must be present in sufficient quantities and in due proportions and in digestible and assimilable, that is available, form. This adaptation in the food is relatively more important while the child is growing most rapidly, and less important as the birth period, is receded from. Suitable variety and proper blending of foods, therefore, cannot be ignored, if we desire the highest vigor and greatest development in our children. Happily, except in isolated places and among the most poverty-stricken classes, the diet of the child may be easily controlled. Knowledge of correct feeding is needed by mothers.

"McCarrison noted that under about the same conditions of filth and squalor, the Sihks and Pathans were much larger than the Madrassis and other peoples of India. He found the Sihks and Pathans eating leafy vegetables, curds and cheese, and these are lacking in the general Indian diet.

"He fed a group of rats on the Sihk and Pathan diet and another group on the general Indian diet. The first group grew to great size; the second group remained small. He fed other groups on the customary Japanese diet, Philipino diet, Javanese diet, and the characteristic diet of the ill-nourished English working man. The results of these diets he checked with the results of the Sihk-Pathan diet. The results were the same. All groups, except those fed on the English diet, were small in size; while the latter group attained nearly the size of the group fed on the Sihk diet but had rough coats and a combative disposition.

"Experiments with Japanese school children, covering several years, show that similar additions to the regular diet of Japanese children cause them to grow to be several inches taller and several pounds heavier than the average Japanese child.

"A few years ago the *New York Times* carried the picture of three boys of the same age (eight years); one an average American boy, of average size for his age; the other two, European boys, whose growth had been stunted by inadequate food. Neither of the European boys reached to the horizontally outstretched arms of the American boy. The European boys were victims of the war that had deprived them of food. In accordance with the Law of the Minimum, the growth of these two boys was relative to the element least abundant in their diet.

"McCollum has repeatedly demonstrated that if a litter of rats is divided into two groups of four each, and one group is fed distilled water and whole wheat only, and the other group exactly the same quantities of distilled water and whole wheat, plus the addition of turnip or beet leaves, each rat in the first group will only attain the size of a large mouse; whereas, those in the second group will attain nearly double the size of those in the first group. Except as to size both groups of rats are 'normal' in all respects.

"We cannot better sum up what has gone before than in the following words of McCarrison: 'It is unwise to consider any of the essential ingredients of food, whether proteins, carbohydrates, fats, salts, water, or vitamins, as independent of the assistance derivable from their associates in the maintenance of digestive and nutritional harmony. No doubt some of these have special relations to others, as for instance that of iodine to fats, that of Vitamin B to carbohydrates, that of Vitamin A to lipoids, calcium and phosphorus holding substances, and that of Vitamin C to inorganic salts. But whatever be their special relations to one another they are all links in the chain of essential substances requisite for the harmonious regulation of life's processes; if one link be broken, the harmony ceases or becomes discord.'''

CHAPTER 10

A DIET RICH IN MINERALS AND VITAMINS

1. Total Source — Minerals

A. Except for organic vegetables, variation wide.

(1) Total mineral matter — percentage dry weight

a. Snap beans	10.45 - 4.04
b. Cabbage	10.38 - 6.12
c. Lettuce	24.48 - 7.01
d. Tomatoes	14.20 - 6.07
e. Spinach	28.56 - 12.38

B. Organic meats are rich in minerals and vitamins — especially pork liver.

C. Cereals are largely stripped of minerals and vitamins.

D. Nuts contain some minerals.

E. Milk products rich in calcium and phosphorous.

F. As a whole, modern diet must be fortified by most people not organic gardeners or bio-chemists.

G. Calcium, magnesium and seleniun, especially, allegedly, may be anti-cancerous.

2. Minerals required by a plant do not necessarily suffice for animal.

A. Plants may not require iodine.

B. Spotty fertilizers, chemically, may produce gorgeous vegetables short in essential nutrients.

C. Kwashiorkor, a disease resulting from protein shortage, may be epidemic in tropics in which plant life thrives.

3. The body can endure a shortage in vitamins longer than mineral shortage.

4. Florida soil is deficient in iron and calcium.

5. Milk products best source of calcium, but nuts, molasses, beans, peas, and cabbage, as well as soy beans, may be rich in calcium if soil is rich.

6. Phosphorous has more functions in body than any

other.

A. Body requires 1½ to 2 times as much phosphorus as calcium.

B. Milk from cow is out of balance for humans– too much calcium compared to phosphorus.

C. Rich protein foods are good sources – meat, poultry, fish and nuts, most legumes, whole grain foods and egg yolk.

D. Plant life requires phosphorus.

7. Potassium shortage may result from too much salt.

A. Peaches, currants, spinach, carrots, soy beans, lentils, bananas, apples, limes, goose and mutton, avocados, brewer's yeast, potatoes, and pecans are rich in potassium.

B. Soil requires it.

C. Manure supplies it.

8. Magnesium necessary to proper use of cholesterol.

A. Florida soil is short of magnesium.

B. Chlorophyll containing vegetables, such as cabbage, cauliflower, beets, kohlrabi, soy beans, nuts and seeds usually good sources (corn is excellent).

9. Cabbage, spinach, turnips, beets, and lettuce are anti-iodine foods – work against iodine, may cause goiter.

A. Iodine found in all seafood.

B. Found in seaweed, kelp, etc.

C. Thio-oxgzolidone works against iodine, but destroyed by cooking.

10. Manganese vital to enzyme system, to glucose utilization.

A. Vital to Vitamin B, Thiamine – high calcium and phosphorus increase need.

B. Five milligrams needed daily for reasons unknown.

C. Related to mother love of new-born child.

D. Cereal, bran, nuts, blueberries, beans, bananas, and lettuce are good sources.

11. Zinc is part of the structure of several enzymes –

blood cells could not function without it — improves exercise tolerance.

A. Maple syrup, wheat germ, mushrooms, oatmeal, carrots, yeast, liver, and especially in herring.

B. Inorganic zinc toxic.

C. Acid drinks must never be consumed from galvanized containers.

D. Alcohol flushes zinc out of liver.

12. Cobalt found in $B_{(12)}$

A. Deficiency causes anemia and may also cause depression.

B. Bacteria required to utilize — related B_{12}.

C. Sour milk rich in B_{12}.

D. Liver is the richest source of B_{12}, also kidney, muscle, meats, milk, eggs, cheese, and fish.

E. A vegetarian diet may mask shortage so that irreparable nerve damage can occur — unless precautions carefully taken.

F. Yeast, wheat germ, and soy beans offer traces of B_{12}.

G. Vitamin B_{12} and cobalt work with folic acid.

13. Chromium appears in blood — 20 parts per *billion.*

A. Chromium works with insulin in glucose utilization.

B. Chromium necessary to control cholesterol level.

C. Brewer's yeast best source.

D. Unsaturated fats a good source.

E. Meats contain more chromium than fruits and vegetables.

14. Copper works with iron to prevent anemia, also works with Vitamin C.

A. Calves' liver contains more copper than beef liver — eight times.

B. Almonds, avocados, kidney and navy beans, wheat bran, brazil nuts, bitter chocolate rich in copper.

C. Dried currants, dried lima beans, molasses, mushrooms, dried peas, pecans and walnuts, also rich in copper.

D. Cow's milk is low in both copper and iron.

15. Iodine prevents or delays hardening of the arteries, allegedly, among other things.

A. Perspiration uses up iodine.

B. Hot weather reduces use – by body.

C. Kelp, bone-meal and iodized salt sources of iodine.

D. Fish, liver the best source.

E. Other sources:

1. Abalone – 1053 parts per billion
2. Asparagus – 180-1080
3. Beans, dried – 260-1870
4. Blue fish – 260-1870
5. Catfish – 992
6. Charde, Swiss – 1370-5350
7. Codfish – 1000-5350
8. Cod liver oil – 290-1140
9. Crabmeat – 148-3150
10. Eel – 800
11. Flounder – 290-1180
12. Haddock – 290-9070
13. Halibut – 250-830
14. *Herring* – 214-1000
15. *Lobster* – 822-11000
16. Mackerel – 400-1410
17. Oysters – 1160-6000
18. Perch – 420-1420
19. Salmon – 210-2010
20. Shrimp – 875-1100
21. Spinach – 32-1079
22. Turnip tops – 340-2296

16. Selenium – tuna, herring, brewer's yeast, wheat germ, bran, broccoli, onions, cabbage and tomatoes may be good sources.

UPI, *St. Petersburg Times,* June 6, 1976:

"Dr. Gerhard N. Schrauzer of the University of California, San Diego, has experimented in providing selenium, a trace element, in a diet of mice. He said the experiment has prevented breast cancer in a strain of mice which normally exhibit almost 100 percent incidence of the disease."

17. Sulphur – nitrogen and sulphur in protein about 16 to 1.

A. Produces acid reaction.

B. Should be balanced with fruits and vegetables with alkaline reaction.

C. Sulphur contained in hormones, insulin, produced by pancreas, and the "anti-pituitory" hormone.

D. Sulphur also in vitamins, thiamine and biotin.

E. Sulfa drugs contain sulphur.

F. Foods rich in amino acids contain sulphur, such as milk, eggs, wheat, corn, beans, onions, nuts, fowl; also good sources of iodine.

G. Arthritic patients show less sulphur in finger nails.

H. Sulphur baths won't hurt and appear to help in arthritis.

18. Vanadium helps inhibit cholesterol formation, apparently, according to some writers.

A. Meat contains no vanadium in measureable amounts.

B. Fish, especially herring and sardines, are good sources.

C. Some vegetables contain some, especially kelp.

VITAMINS

1. Vitamins are of two kinds:

A. Fat – soluble – found especially in liver and eggs, destroyed by mineral oil, rancid fat.

B. Water soluble – found in fruits and vegetables.

2. Vitamin A, fat – soluble, helps fight infection. (Other

fat soluble vitamins to follow.)

A. Should take 5 to 10,000 units daily.

B. Found in carrots and other vegetables, butter fat, fish liver oil, eggs and fruit, organic meats.

1. Vegetables contain "pro-vitamins."

2. "Actual" Vitamin A is the safeguard.

3. Body stores Vitamin A.

C. Vitamin A destroyed by use of mineral oil, nitrates and nitrite in preserved meats, preservatives generally.

3. Vitamins – water soluble.

A. Inositol – isotopic glucose may be converted to inositol in animals.

1. Combats high cholesterol.

2. Contained in dried lima beans, beef brains, beef heart, liver, cantaloupe, grapefruit, peaches, peanuts, oranges, peas, raisins, wheat germ, cabbage, brewer's yeast.

B. Choline – Amino acid methionine in B_{12} removes need for it.

1. Richly contained in colostrum, extra rich starting lactation.

2. Helpful to heart and circulatory system.

C. Biotin.

1. Amount in body very small.

2. Destroyed by raw eggwhite.

3. Found in natural food supplements – brewer's yeast, wheat germ, all the organ meats.

D. Thiamine takes part in oxidation, serving as active part of co-enzyme necessary for oxidation pyruvic acid, one of the products of carbohydrate oxidation.

1. Hard physical work increases need.

2. Affects nervous tissue especially by reason of dependency carbohydrate oxidation – appears to affect ability to learn.

3. Thiamine is not appreciably stored.

4. Sweets, alcohol, tobacco reduce thiamine.

5. High heat, alkalis, especially in cooking, destroy thiamine.

6. Destruction of a "natural balance" of B vitamins prevent exact replication, and imbalance may exaggerate reduction by amount of surplus of another B vitamin.

7. Preservatives as in bread destroy thiamine.

8. Although many foods contain thiamine, brewer's yeast and soybeans are among richest sources.

9. Depletion of bakers' flour destroys most accessible source.

E. Riboflavin is an active part of several enzymes – aids metabolism.

1. Destroyed by cooking with baking soda.

2. Destroyed by light.

3. Three mg's should be minimum intake.

4. Brewer's yeast, whey, organ meats, eggwhite and milk products best sources.

F. Shortage of niacin or nicotinic acid produces pellagra, once common.

1. Three D's of pellagra – "depression, dermatitis and diarrhea."

2. Niacin helps form enzymes to assimilate sugars and starches.

3. Niacin and thiamine usually occur in the same foods.

4. Twenty-five mg's should represent minimum for safety.

5. Organ meats, peanut butter, wheat, bran and brewer's yeast richest sources – amino acid, tryptophan may substitute, from milk and eggs.

G. Pyridoxine, Vitamin B_6, found in lower levels in cancer tissue which uses amino acids differently than normal tissue – breaks down amino acids.

1. In nature, always found with other B vitamins – metabolizes fats and carbohydrates.

2. Quick cooking may not destroy if vitamin not thrown out with water.

3. Roasting or stewing meat can destroy B_6.

4. Foods richest in organ meats, bananas, dried lima beans, cabbage, molasses, dried peas, peanuts, sweet potatoes, wheat germ, brewer's yeast.

5. *Again* brewer's yeast is richest source.

6. Pyridoxine, pyridoxal and pyridoxamine three forms of B_6.

H. Pantothenic Acid – panthos means universal in Greek.

1. Operates in conjunction with other B vitamins, appears to nourish intestinal bacterial which produces other B vitamins – lactic acid bacteria growth factor.

2. Dissolves in water and may be thrown out with cooking water.

3. Lost through cooking with baking soda.

4. Organ meats, brewer's yeast, egg yolk, peanuts, best sources.

5. Five to 10 mg's required daily.

6. Dessicated liver a good supplement.

7. Growth promoting factor for yeast.

I. Pava Amino – Benzoil Acid (Pava means against).

1. Nicknamed "Paba."

2. Works against sulfa drugs – sulfa drugs work against Paba.

3. When Paba unable to function, body lacks folic acid which results in a lack of Pantothenic Acid.

4. Fits into definition of B vitamin.

A. A natural constituent of yeast, liver, and/or whole grain cereals.

B. Water soluble.

C. Cannot be stored for long in the body.

D. Growth substance for bacteria, yeast, fungi or moles.

E. Physiologically active in small amounts.

F. It causes a deficiency disease when lacking in diet.

5. Plentiful in liver, brewer's yeast, milk, eggs, rice bran, whole wheat, wheat germ, molasses, and some in beef and pork muscle meats.

J. Folic acid easily destroyed by heat or exposure to light. (An excess may be dangerous to one with cancer.)

1. Quantity of folic acids, greens probably dependent on chlorophyll.

2. Protects against some kinds of anemia and against sulfa.

3. Brings about growth and reproduction of blood cells in bone marrow.

4. Required for synthesis and breakdown of nucleic acid and other compounds.

5. Polyglutamates of folic acid interchangeable in animal metabolism but not always in bacterial metabolism.

6. In some animals vitamin synthesized by bacteria in digestive tract and absorbed into body of host.

7. Leukopenias — white cell shortage — may result from lack of folic acid.

8. Dried lima beans, cantaloupe, chicken, liver, Irish potatoes, salmon, brewer's yeast, rich sources.

4. Vitamin C — water soluble, volatile, unstable — lost by heat, agitation, time.

A. Vitamin C helpful in carrying hydrogen to cells.

B. Necessary to collagen development.

C. Required for proper storage of calcium and phosphorus.

D. Necessary for assimilation of iron and copper.

E. Minimizes bruising — aids wound healing.

F. Helps keep circulatory system in good repair.

G. May prevent hemorrhaging before and after surgical operations.

H. Contact with copper destroys Vitamin C.

I. Rich sources — brussel sprouts, dandelion greens, grapefruit, guavas, honeydew, kale, mustard greens, oranges, peppers, green and pimento, rosehips, turnip tops.

J. Require 100 to 1,000 units daily — depending upon authority — or much more.

5. Vitamin P. flavanoids — water soluble.

A. In natural foods found with Vitamin C.

B. Found in white skin and segment part of orange.

C. Ten times as much flavanoid in whole orange as in juice.

D. Lemons, grapes, plums, black currants, grapefruit, apricots, cherries, and blackberries also contain it.

E. Will sometimes straighten out infections and general health problems not cured by "C" alone.

F. Require at least 1,000 mg's daily.

6. Vitamin D. may come from food as fish liver oil or from the sun — fat soluble.

A. Food source should be natural, if possible, with accompanying Vitamin A, as in cod liver oil, to help assure sound bones and teeth.

B. Helps assimilate calcium which should be balanced by magnesium and phosphorus.

C. Four hundred units daily enough from food source.

7. Alpha tocopherol (Vitamin E) [from Greek], means bearing fertility — fat soluble.

A. Male chicks and guinea pigs suffer degeneration of testicles when deprived of Vitamin E.

B. Vitamin E prevents the oxidation of Vitamins A and C in the digestive tract — however, supplemental organic iron will negate "E" and vice versa, if consumed at same time.

C. Vitamin E appears to help heal burns.

D. Lack of Vitamin E produces muscular dystrophy in dogs.

E. Vitamin E required in cell respiration, use of oxygen.

F. Vitamin E appears at least "to hold back" aging.

G. Dr. Evan Shute uses Vitamin E to help prevent or cure heart attacks through keeping clear the circulatory system.

H. Hydrogenated fats contain no Vitamin E, by and large.

I. Nuts and grains contain Vitamin E.

J. One may allegedly take 2,000 units daily with potential benefit, no harm.

8. Vitamin I — linoleic acid.

A. Safe use of linoleic acid without developing peroxides depends upon Vitamin E.

B. See outline on cholesterol.

9. Vitamin K is synthesized within the intestinal tract provided such tract contains the right intestinal flora.

A. Antibiotics may destroy such flora.

B. If disease may interfere with production of bile, Vitamin K. may not be utilized.

C. If intestinal walls are damaged or diseased, Vitamin K may not be absorbed — same with liver.

D. Vitamin K fat soluble — subject to destructive agents, for such vitamins.

E. Vitamin K essential to coagulation, along with minerals.

F. Vitamin K rich foods — spinach, kale, alfalfa, cabbage, cauliflower, green peas, carrot tops, black strap molasses, liver, egg yolk, soybean oil, and fish liver oil.

The following list was furnished by the Committee for Freedom of Choice in Cancer Therapy, Inc., 146 Main Street, Suite 408, Los Altos, California 94022, (415) 948-9475.

Foods Containing Amygdalin

(Vitamin B-17 or Nitrilosides)

Beans
Broad Bean (Vicia Faba)
Burma beans
Chick peas
Lentils (sprouted)
Lima
Mung beans (sprouted)
Rangoon
Scarlet runner

Berries
Almost all wild berries
Blackberry
Chokeberry
Christmas berry
Cranberry
Elderberry
Raspberry
Strawberry

Grasses
Acacia
Alfalfa (sprouted)
Acuatic grass
Johnson grass
Milk weed
Sudan grass
Tunus grass
Velvet grass
Wheat grass
White clover

Grains
Oat groats
Barley
Brown rice
Buckwheat groats
Chia
Flax
Millet
Rye
Vetch
Wheat berries

***Kernels or Seeds of Fruits**

Apple
Cherry
Peach
Plum
Apricot
Nectarine
Pear
Prune

Nuts

Bitter almonds
Macadamia Nuts

**Contain highest concentration of B-17 to be found in nature.*

Seeds
Chia seed
Flax seed
Sesame seed

Miscellaneous
Bamboo shoots
Fuschia plants
Sorghum plants
Wild hydrangea
Yew tree (needles; fresh leaves)

(Caution concerning folic acid suggested in
"Update Diet Nutrition and Cancer"
by David P. Rose, M.D., Ph.D.,
Professor of Human Oncology, Wisconsin Clinical
Cancer Center, University of Wisconsin),
from *Professional Nutrition,* Vol. 8, No. 4, Oct.-Dec., 1976,
pp. 1-5

CHAPTER 11

THE NUTRITIONAL BACKGROUND OF A PROPER LEVEL OF CHOLESTEROL

1. Cholesterol is produced by the body – for pituitary adrenal and sex hormones as well as bile salts.

A. Cholesterol level has not been demonstrated to be solely a matter of diet – can be produced from light sugar, or even protein.

B. Probably cholesterol level depends upon a number of "balances" within the body – only liver produces cholesterol for blood.

2. Lecithin is considered an aid to proper cholesterol level.

A. Lecithin related to the liver, represents 73% of total liver fat.

B. Lecithin serves as a structural material for body cells especially those of the nervous system; 30% of dry weight of brain.

C. Lecithin aids in transportation of fats, helps body remove fats and cholesterol from blood as well as utilize them.

D. High fat meal triggers increase in lecithin in healthy persons; not so with one suffering from athercoslerosis.

E. Lecithin increases production of bile acids from cholesterol, thereby reducing amount in blood.

F. Lecithin requires essential new materials for manufacture.

3. Support needed for lecithin – linoleic, linolenic, and arachidonic acid needed.

A. Lecithin is found in all unrefined foods containing oil – eggs, liver, nuts, wheat and soy oil are good sources proved by experiments (with athercoslerosis).

B. Arachidonic acid necessary before lecithin may be

produced — such acid presumably found in fats not saturated.

C. Any oils, including fish oils, which contain *no* essential fatty acids help reduce blood cholesterol by decreasing its absorption.

D. The more solid fats are eaten, the greater becomes the need for linoleic acid.

1. Arachidonic and linolenic acids may be synthesized if enough linoleic acid present provided essential vitamins and minerals are present.

2. Peanut, safflower and soy oils are among richest sources of arachidonic, linoleic and linolenic acids — (equal parts of all three recommended).

E. B vitamins, choline and inositol needed — but will not drop cholesterol alone.

1. Choline may be produced from amino acid, methionine.

2. Produced only from surplus of methionine.

3. Choline and inositol richly supplied in brewer's yeast, as well as methionine — supplied also in liver, yeast, lecithin and wheat germ.

4. Milk contains all essential amino acids; so do eggs.

4. Other support needed.

A. Lecithin may not be synthesized without enzymes containing B_6 or pyridoxine — (B complex vitamins are a good source).

B. Such enzymes active only if magnesium present.

C. Magnesium found in dolomite, wheat germ, cocoa, desiccated liver, eggs, green vegetables, soy beans, and almonds.

D. The need for magnesium tremendously increased when cholesterol level is high.

5. Vitamin E necessary — as well as Vitamin B_{12} in acidophilus buttermilk.

A. Vitamin E dissolves scars on arterial walls, allegedly.

B. Reduces need for oxygen.

C. Reduces pain caused by fatty deposits.

6. Refined sugar may be quickly turned into saturated fat within body.

7. The more deficient the diet, the greater the craving for sweets and alcohol – which may turn to cholesterol.

8. Pectin from citrus rinds combats cholesterol.

9. All vitamins, including C necessary, sunshine helps utilize cholesterol.

10. Iodine in combination with Vitamin E inhibits cholesterol.

11. Stress may exaggerate cholesterol, but not with dietary precaution.

12. Experimental heart disease in animals, allegedly has been produced with diets completely devoid of cholesterol, so avoiding cholesterol appears to be not the total answer, utilization appears basic.

While we are at it, let's review vitamins and minerals and their necessity to survival, even beyond good health. It is conceivable that under some circumstances, any one of the nutritional factors described might, under specific conditions, represent an inhibitory factor against cancer.

CHAPTER 12

IS WHEN YOU EAT, WHAT YOU EAT IMPORTANT?

FOOD SELECTION

by J. Gordon Roberts

In this treatise, foods are divided into proteins, starches, fats, acid fruits, sub-acid fruits, non-starchy and green vegetables, melons, and milk products.

Milk products and eggs really do not belong with the other categorized foods, because both are conglomerates.

Although milk is a liquid, it requires more saliva than even dry food. In small children it is coagulated by rennen. In adults, presumably by pepsin, a protein enzyme, even though milk contains milk sugar and fat, among other things.

Saliva adjusts to the food consumed. For starches, saliva is alkaline. For protein, acid. One neutralizes the other.

Enzymes requiring an alkaline medium are destroyed by acid. Each enzyme requires the medium suited to it, chemically.

Saliva adjusts to the food supplied, if the food be simple enough in composition to make such adjustment possible. Without such adjustment, the load on the digestive system later on in the process must be made more onerous.

Feed a dog flesh and there is a secretion of thick, viscous saliva. Feed him dried and pulverized flesh and a copious, watery solution will pour out. The mucous secretion serves to lubricate the bolus of food, and thus facilitate swallowing.

Saliva, however, also starts the digestive process, especially in the case of starches.

Although food appears to be actually assimilated in the small intestine (toward the end of the line), and the liver, for use or storage, digestion starts much sooner.

Alkaline food, starches, for example, may start to digest in the fundus, or upper portion of the stomach. Protein is digested in the distal, or more distant, portion of the stomach. Sugar may go directly to the small intestine, like a bright brat who skips grades.

Sugar may be digested in a matter of minutes. Fats may take hours, and protein, a long time.

A mixture of sugar and fat is a race between the hare and the tortoise, in which the tortoise always wins. The hare is held back by the tortoise.

In the digestive process, however, fermentation and putrefaction are involved in this kind of "race." The "hare" becomes a stuffed rabbit in this sort of race, and about as difficult to digest.

My metaphors are deliberately mixed to simulate mixing of food. So . . .

1. Eat acids and starches at separate meals. ("Acids" refer to oranges, grapefruit, sour grapes, and the like.)

2. Eat protein foods and carbohydrates at separate meals. (Proteins are nuts, flesh foods, dry beans and peas, peanuts, cheese olives, and avocados. Potatoes and the like are carbohydrates.)

3. Eat but one concentrated protein at a meal. (Avoid steak and cheese, for example.)

4. Eat proteins and acids at separate meals. (Although proteins require acid, the acid should be generated from within, not ingested from without.)

5. Eat fats and proteins at separate meals.

6. Eat sugars and proteins at separate meals.

7. Eat starches and sugars at separate meals. (Starches require about two hours to digest, as I remember, sugars, ten minutes.)

8. Cheese and acid, for example, is tolerable. (Cheese holds back digestion to the point that acid foods have time to digest.)

9. Eat melon alone, or, at least, with other fruits, but, preferably, alone.

10. Take milk alone, preferably curdled milk, to get away from the need to coagulate the milk within the body and provide proper bacteria for breaking down milk sugar.

(Milk products may form a coating over other food which may interfere with digestion.)

CHAPTER 13

FASTING

Outside of a "natural" diet, fasting appears to represent the only "medicine" known to the animal world, other than man.

Inasmuch as human beings have more cancer than any other creature on earth, it would seem wise to consider fasting seriously. Fasting, by the way, consists of complete abstinence from food, with only water permitted.

According to its proponents, fasting may result in autolysis, the breaking down of substance within the body. Such proponents claim that it may not only break down fat, but also other substance not needed by the body, and possibly poisonous or destructive to it.

Remarkable "cures" have been claimed in its behalf. Fasting may be differentiated from starvation in that fasting allegedly covers only the elimination of unwanted material without any dangerous depletion of necessary tissue. By such definition, starvation starts only after the unwanted tissue or substance has been eliminated, when starts the breakdown of vital organs.

Proponents of fasting claim to know just when to stop the fast to preclude the possibility of danger to the patient, as a result of fasting. More later on this.

Scientific American, October, 1971, "The Physiology of Starvation" cites a woman of fifty-four who fasted 249 days, losing seventy-four pounds. It also cites the case of a twenty-year-old girl who fasted 210 days by comparison, and died. Among other tissues, part of the fibrous tissue of the heart muscle had been consumed.

Physiologically, what actually happens in fasting?

Outside of fasting, the principal fuel for vital functions is glucose, a form of sugar refined by the body from starches and other foods. For the brain, glucose is essential as oxygen. When the body is resting, the brain consumes about two-thirds of the circulating glucose, almost one and one-half times the percentage of oxygen.

Daily, the brain requires between 100 and 145 grams of glucose. The liver stores less than 100 grams, and not all of this is available. The liver stores some glucose for emergencies, for sudden stress.

The liver can supply the brain for only a few hours, out of storage. Even between meals and overnight, the liver draws on the tissues of the body, to synthesize necessary glucose, tissues such as the skeletal muscles.

Amino acids (from protein) are precursors for the synthesis of glucose. Free fatty acids, derived from triglycerides in fatty tissues may supply energy to tissues other than the nervous system, but not to the brain.

If the foregoing sources were used solely for very long, to supply energy to the nervous system, fasting would certainly be fatal within a very short time. But the body's methods of meeting the situation change.

Body fat becomes the source of energy. Fat represents nine calories per gram of body weight; protein, two, and carbohydrate, one. Eventually, in obese people, fat provides virtually all the energy needed.

Meanwhile, as weight is lost, cells shrink, by as much as 45%, according to one authority.

"Ketones" supply an energy substitute from the fatty tissues. It consists of acetoacetic acid, with derivatives acetone and beta-hydroxybutyric acid.

Ordinarily, fatty acid metabolism does not create ketones. The breakdown of body protein does not completely disappear with prolonged fasting, however. The body requires some such fat glucose, even with prolonged fasting, but such requirement may be drastically limited by ketone. Even so, obviously, the fast may not continue indefinitely.

The body, nevertheless, does make some radical adjustments. For example, the cortex of the kidney normally plays a minor role in the synthesis of glucose. By the sixth week of fasting, the kidney cortex may synthesize more glucose from amino acids than the liver does.

A change in acid-base balance in the blood occurs, which may relate to ketone production.

Sometimes crash diets may produce considerable loss of weight through loss of body liquid. But, with the possible exception of children, diseases of famine do not seem to affect those who fast, totally.

The significance of this is far beyond the capacity of this writer to suggest interpretation, even with the help of scientific material available.

We now turn to Dr. Herbert M. Shelton's *Hygienic System,* Vol. III, Fourth Edition, 1963, published by Dr. Shelton's Health School, San Antonio, Texas, Chapter V, page 98, "Autolysis," and "Physiological Rest," first paragraph, page 155.

CHAPTER 14

AUTOLYSIS – THE DIGESTION OF ONE'S OWN CELLS

"In order that we may comprehend much that takes place within the fasting organism, it is necessary that we have an understanding of the process of autolysis, which, although very common in nature, has been all but overlooked by physiologists generally. We have previously mentioned the fact that the vital or functioning tissues of the fasting organism are nourished off the food reserves stored in the body. These reserves are stored as rather complex substances, such as sugar (glycogen), fat, protein, etc., and are no more fitted for entrance into the bloodstream and use by the cells than are the fats, proteins, and carbohydrates of another animal or another food. Before they can be taken up by the circulation and assimilation by the cells, they must first be digested.

"Let us begin with a familiar example of the digestion and absorption of a part of a living organism by the organism itself. In the process of becoming a frog the tadpole grows four legs. After these are fully formed, it no longer has use for the tail that served so well in the tadpole stage, so it proceeds to get rid of it, not by shedding it as is popularly supposed, but by absorbing it. The tail is made up of muscle, fat, nerves, skin, etc. To absorb these structures, they are digested in the same way that fat and muscle are digested in the digestive tract. By the action of the appropriate enzymes the proteins and fats are broken down into their constituent amino and fatty acids. Only thus are they fit to re-enter the circulation. Only as fatty acids and amino acids can they be re-used with which to nourish other structures of the body of the frog.

"During the period when the tail of the ex-tadpole is being absorbed, the young frog does not eat. Indeed, it ceases to eat when the forelegs come into view. Fasting may be essential to the absorption of the tail, at least it hastens the process, for it compels the utilization of the tail as food with which to nourish the vital tissues of the fasting frog.

"We may liken this process to that of the eating of its skin by the toad. Toads molt several times yearly. They swallow their molted skin after they emerge from it. To make use of the molted skin, the toad must first digest it. Its proteins and fats must be reduced to simple acceptable compounds, such as amino acids and fatty acids. This is done in this instance in the stomach and intestine of the toad. But in the case of the fasting frog digesting its tail, the work is done within the tail itself.

"The thymus gland, which controls the growth of the young, is absorbed after its work is completed. Noting the manner in which the body rids itself of non-functioning or no-longer-needed structures, as in the case of this gland, it would be extraordinary were it to really turn out that there are structures in the body that are truly functionless and have been so for ages. At this point, however, our interest in this gland and its absorption is for a different lesson. It is referred to here to point out that it is broken down and absorbed by the process of autolysis. There can be no doubt that the materials of which it is composed are re-used by the organism.

"The word autolysis (a-tol-i-sis) is derived from the Greek and means, literally, self-loosing. It is used in physiology to designate the process of digestion or disintegration of tissue by ferments (enzymes) generated in the cells themselves. It is a process of self-digestion – intra-cellular digestion.

"A number of autolytic (a-to-lit-ik) enzymes are known and are included under the general terms, oxidase and peroxidases. Physiologists know that proteolytic (protein digesting) enzymes are formed within many, if not in all living tissues. Apparently every tissue turns out its own enzyme, which, probably, under all ordinary circumstances of life, is employed in the regular processes of metabolism. Under other conditions the enzymes may be employed to digest the substances of the cells themselves. In their *Textbook of Physiology* (1946 edition), Zoethout and Tuttle mention that under certain experimental conditions the unrestrained activities of the enzymes normally present in the liver (proteases, lipases, carbohydrases) digest the proteins, carbohydrates, and fats of the liver. In normal life this digestion of the liver does not occur. These various intra-cellular enzymes play a conspicuous part in the metabolism of food substances; that is, in the normal or regular function of nutrition or metabolism.

"A few familiar examples of autolysis will prepare the reader to understand its use in 'disease.' The phenomena of fasting supply many examples of the control of the body exercises over its autolytic processes. For example, tissues are lost in the inverse order of their usefulness — fat and morbid growths first, and then the other tissues. These tissues (fatty tissue, bone marrow, etc.) and food substances (glycogen) are not fit to enter the blood stream before they are acted upon by enzymes. Indeed, human fat, or human muscle, is no more fitted to enter the circulation without first being digested, than is fat or muscle from the cow or sheep. Glycogen (animal starch), stored in the liver, must be converted into a simple sugar before it can be released into the blood stream. This conversion is accomplished by enzymic action.

"The manner in which an abscess 'points' on the surface of the body and drains its septic contents on the outside is well known to every one of my readers. What is not generally known, is that this 'pointing' on the surface is possible only because the flesh between the abscess and the surface is digested by enzymes; that is, it is autolyzed and removed.

"The absorption of the bone-ring support established about the ends of a fracture is made possible by the autolytic disintegration of the bone-ring. The re-arrangement of materials in pieces of planaria and the dissolution of the pharynx in the piece containing this, to form a new one to fit the new size, as described elsewhere, is made possible by autolysis.

"Sylvester Graham had some conception of the process of autolysis and of its use in disease. He thought that it is a general law of organic life that, when, any means or from any cause, the catabolic processes exceed those of anabolism, the body always lays hold of and removes those substances which are of least use to the organism. For this reason, he said, all the morbid accumulations, such as wens (cysts), tumors, abscesses, etc., are rapidly diminished and often wholly removed under severe and protracted abstinence and fasting.

"The view of many physiologists of Graham's era was that the lymphatics throughout the body, like the lacteals in the intestines, possess, to a high degree, the power to take up from the tissues, food substances, which they convert into a chyle-like substance, but of a more refined and sublimated quality, and that this pre-digested material is returned to the general circulation to be used in all parts of the body as nutriment. Although Graham thought that the 'assimilating power' of the lymphatics (or, as they often called them, the absorbents), was real, he was of the opinion that the physiologists had magnified it. Nonetheless, he said that 'when supplies of food in the alimentary canal are exceedingly small or entirely cut off for a considerable time, the lymphatics unquestionably become much more active than usual, and prey upon the adipose and other substances of the body, forming a lymph which has many of the characteristics of chyle and blood, and which may, to some extent, in such an emergency, serve the purpose of nutrition.' He said that this does not occur in the ordinary and undisturbed operations of the organism when the digestive tract supplies adequate food materials. He, along with many other physiologists of the period, thought of lymph, under these circumstances, as being 'mainly if not entirely an excrementitious substance.'

"He did not think that there are any facts to justify the assumption that the fat thus converted into lymph is used as nutriment during a fast. He regarded fat as being more or less in the nature of uneliminated surpluses (largely of an undesirable character) that the body was forced to store because it was unable to excrete. For this reason, it is unfit for food. His view was that in a perfectly healthy state of the body, a perfect equilibrium between the processes of assimilation and dis-assimilation is maintained so that no fat accumulates.

"AUTOLYSIS IN PLANTS

"The plant kingdom teems with examples of autolysis, but a few familiar examples will suffice for our present purpose. All bulbs, of which the onion will serve as an example, maintain within themselves a new plant surrounded by sufficient food to tide it over during a period of rest, during which period it does not take up food from the soil and air. Indeed, it may be taken out of the ground and stored for long periods. The onion may begin to grow in the bin or bag in which it is stored. It sends up stems and soon almost the whole of the bulb of the onion is transformed into green blades. The bulb gradually becomes soft, and finally, there is left a mere shell, as the growing plant digests and utilizes the substance of the onion. Beets, turnips and many other tubers will grow in the same manner. By autolytic digestion of the substances in the tuber, material is provided for growth and even while out of the ground, these plants will put forth stems and leaves and grow.

"Who has not seen the housewife put a sweet potato in a jar of water and hang it up and watch it grow? It sends out stems which grow to great lengths and puts out many green leaves. Such a potato plant will continue to grow so long as there remains any of the food that was stored as sweet potato. The so-called Irish potato will also put forth stems and leaves and these will grow, drawing upon the substances stored in the potato as their sole source of food. If there is light, the leaves and stems will be white. If there is a crack several feet away through which a little light enters, these stems will grow in the direction of the source of light and will grow several feet long, if the light is that far away. By autolysis the stored food substances in the tubers are broken up and made useable by the young plant.

"The early growth of all plants from seed involves digestion of food stored in the seed. Seed, like the eggs of animals, are chiefly storehouses of food. The actual living part of the seed is almost microscopic in size.

"A rose cutting or a fig cutting placed in the soil and watered, will put forth roots and leaves and grow. Both the leaves and the roots are grown from materials within the cutting. Cut a begonia leaf into small pieces and properly tend these and each piece will grow into a new begonia plant. The substances of the fragment of the leaf are used out of which to build a new plant. These are instances of the autolysis, redistribution and reorganization of materials contained within the part.

"AUTOLYSIS IN ANIMALS

"At the very commencement of life, autolysis is an essential process. The embryonic development of animals in eggs involves digestion of the food stored in the eggs. Eggs, however large or small, contain a living germ that is microscopic in size which is the only living part of the egg. The remainder of the egg consists of stored food material out of which the evolving animal constructs its organs and parts. This food substance is no more suited to the use of the evolving embryo than it is suited to the use of the adult animal. Before it can be used in making tissue, it must be digested. This digestion is achieved by enzymes produced by the embryo.

"The fasting salamander, the tail of which has been cut off, grows a new tail. It draws upon its general food stores for materials out of which to construct the new tail. These materials must first be broken down (digested) by the process of autolysis and then transferred to the growing tail. Here we watch a process that is somewhat the reverse of that seen in the frog that is absorbing its tail. Here materials are taken from the body and used in producing a tail; there materials are taken from the tail and used with which to nourish the body.

"The enormous growth of the gonads of fasting salmon is accomplished by transferring materials from the body of the salmon to the testicles. Autolysis is necessarily the first step in this transfer of materials. The body is not only able to build tissue, it can also destroy tissue. It can not only digest and utilize the tissues of other organisms, it can digest and use its own tissue.

"AUTOLYSIS DURING PUPAL SLEEP

"The period of pupal sleep in the life of insects is a period of great and complex organizational changes, resulting in a new and radically different insect. The larvae of insects devote their whole attention to growing and moulting. They eat enormous quantities of food and grow large and fat. The silk worm, for example, during its thirty-day period of growth, increases its weight fifteen thousand times. At the end of its larval stage the silk worm spins for itself a cocoon by which it protects itself in the pupa stage. There emerges from the cocoon, not a worm, but a silkfly. The caterpillar of the butterfly changes to a chrysalis. The outer covering of the chrysalis is a hardened shell, usually brown in color. There emerges from this, not a worm, but a butterfly. Whereas, the worm-like larva enters the cocoon or chrysalis, it emerges an adult butterfly or moth, totally changed, both in internal and external structures, with different functions to perform and a different life to lead.

"It is during the stage of pupal sleep that the entire organism of the insect undergoes a complete and radical metamorphosis, there is a tearing down of old structures, a reshuffling of materials, the creation and re-aggregation of parts, so that what emerges from the pupa, when the transformation is complete, is an organism so unlike either the pupa or the larva that it may easily be mistaken for a totally new and distinct species.

"It is interesting to note that during the pupal stage of insect life, no food is taken. During this period of outward quiescence, all of the material stored up by the gluttonous larva is used out of which to construct a totally new and different organism. By autolysis old structures are torn down, stored materials are digested and prepared for new use, the materials are shifted from one part of the organism to another. All of this marvelous process of metamorphosis takes place while the animal is fasting. Here is a striking example of the constructive work that the organism may carry on while abstaining from food. But it should be understood that materials could not be shifted from one part of the body to another and no-longer-needed structures could not be torn down and the materials of which they are composed could not be used out of which to construct new structures, except that they are first digested. Autolysis is as essential at this stage of the insect's life as the ability to construct new parts.

"Metamorphosis in insects supplies us with one of the most remarkable examples of both autolysis and the distribution and reorganization of materials that go on in living organisms as regular parts of the process of living. The maggot of the common housefly dissolves into a creamy liquid seemingly as structureless as the yolk of an egg. The original organs are destroyed and new ones are fashioned. No new materials, except, perhaps, air and moisture, are employed in this creation of the new form. During fifteen days of fasting, the pupa of the honey bee metamorphoses into a full-grown bee, the changes undergone amounting to a transformation of one form of life into another form, with different organs, different functions, and a radically different way of life.

"The overfed caterpillar wraps itself in a hermetically sealed cocoon and goes to sleep and, during its sleep, it transforms itself into a gorgeous butterfly with bright wings that flash in the sun. As it undergoes metamorphosis, its muscles and its organs undergo dissolution into a substance that resembles a sort of pus. All of its internal structures are torn down by autolytic processes and are distributed to different parts to be completely reorganized. The metamorphosis of chrysalis into butterfly is as though some fairy with a magic wand stood by and directed operations. Here we observe no mere chemical process; here is organization and prevision; here is controlled tearing down and rebuilding; here is no mere turning out of compounds, but the construction of complex organs that are to function in the future.

"The cocoon takes no food during this period of metamorphosis; the whole reorganization process is done while fasting and the materials that are stored in the body of the caterpillar, while it is eating its way through the world, are used for the transformation of the 'worm' into a butterfly. As remarkable as is the process of metamorphosis itself, is the fact that practically no material is left over. The material in one caterpillar is just sufficient to make one butterfly.

"*DISTRIBUTION OF MATERIALS*

"The severely wounded animal refuses to eat, yet its wound heals. Great quantities of blood are sent to the site of the wound. This represents a great quantity of food taken to the part. The blood is the distributing agent in all higher forms of life. The fasting animal draws upon its reserves of food materials out of which to repair its torn, cut or broken tissues. These are first autolyzed and then carried to the part of the body where they are needed. The body cannot only distribute its nutritive supplies; it can also re-distribute them. It possesses the ability to shift its chemicals and fasting supplies many examples of this. Autolysis makes re-distribution possible.

"The ability to re-distribute substances and supplies is common to all forms of life. This ability is an ever-present protection against injury, except under the most prolonged deprivation. The digestion and re-organization of parts seen in worms and other animals, when deprived of food, the digestion and re-distribution of reserves, surpluses and non-vital tissues, as seen in all animals, when forced to go without food, constitute, for the writer, some of the most marvelous phenomena in the whole realm of biology.

"*AUTOLYSIS IS CONTROLLED*

"Autolysis is a rigidly controlled process; it is no blind, undirected bull-in-a-china-shop affair. Not only throughout the fasting period, but also throughout the starvation process, as well, the body exercises control over autolysis. The most rigid economy is exercised throughout both periods in the digestion and utilization, not only of the vital and most vital tissues, but of the dispensable and expendable tissues. Here I wish to call attention to the fact that in starvation there is no indiscriminate wasting of the body, but rather the same safeguarding of the more vital tissues and a slow sacrifice of the less vital tissues that is seen in the fasting period.

"When the frog fasts during the time it is consuming its tail, only the tail disappears. Never does one of the legs of the frog undergo autolytic disintegration. No needed structure is digested and absorbed. If planaria or flat worms, are cut in small pieces and placed where they can absorb nourishment, each piece will grow into a small worm. If they cannot get nourishment, they cannot grow. Each piece, therefore, completely re-arranges its materials and becomes a perfect, but very minute, worm. The piece that contains the pharynx, finding this too large for its diminished size, will dissolve it and make a new one that fits its new size. We have here a process similar to the metamorphosis of insects that goes on in the pupal stage. Here is manifest the ability to tear down a part and shift its constituent materials. The same thing is seen in the softening and absorption of the bone-ring support around a point of fracture. Only part of the bone-ring is digested, the remainder is retained to reinforce the weakened structure.

"Zoethout and Tuttle point out that autolysis is a controlled process and mention the following examples of carefully controlled autolysis that normally occur at certain periods of life: 'atrophy of the mammary glands at the close of lactation, of the uterus after parturition, the general atrophy of old age, and the resolution (dissolution) of the exudate formed in the lungs during pneumonia.' The atrophy of the thymus gland at puberty should also be included in this list.

"These authors offer other examples of controlled autolysis, saying: 'During starvation some organs (heart and brain) are absolutely necessary and their activity cannot be dispensed with; hence they must be supplied with proteins. These proteins are obtained from the skeletal muscles, which must be looked upon not only as organs of contraction but also as storehouses for proteins. The proteins of the muscles and other organs are digested by the intracellular proteases (enzymes) into soluble proteins, amino acids, which are then carried by the blood stream to the vital organs. Another striking illustration of the transfer of protein from one organ to another is seen in the tremendous development, in the spawning and fasting salmon, of the ovaries at the expense of the muscles, which lose as much as 30 percent of their weight.'

"Neither the ovaries, nor the heart, nor the brain can live, grow and function on a diet of amino acids. They need minerals, carbohydrates, fats and vitamins. Fasting salmon lose more than weight of muscle; they also lose fat and glycogen. There is great accumulation of phosphorus in the gonads of fasting salmon.

"It is interesting to note that this control of autolysis extends also to pathological tissues, such as tumors, deposits, effusions, etc., and is not confined to the normal tissues of the body. Examples of this will be given later.

"The fact that autolysis is a rigidly controlled and not a haphazard process, is our guarantee that the vital tissues of the body will not be sacrificed during even prolonged abstinence from food. It guarantees us that only the non-vital tissues will be digested and their constituents carried throughout the body to nourish the vital tissues.

"Three important facts stand out clearly in what has gone before:

"1. By reason of its possession of intracellular enzymes the body is capable of digesting its own proteins, fats and carbohydrates.

"2. It is fully capable of controlling the self-digesting process and rigidly limits it to the non-essential and less-essential tissues. Even in starvation, when vital tissues are destroyed, there is rigid control of the proçess and the tissues continue to be drawn upon according to their relative importance.

"3. The body is capable of utilizing the end-products of autolytic disintegration of its own tissues to nourish its most vital and most essential parts.

"THE AUTOLYTIC DISINTEGRATION OF TUMORS

"Trall asserted that all abnormal growths possess a lower grade of vitality than normal growths, hence are easier to destroy. I think it may be equally true that they do not command the support of the organism as do normal growths, as they are deficient in nerve and blood supply. This lack of support makes them the ready victims of the autolytic processes of the body. It is generally held by men with wide experience with the fast that abnormal tissues are broken down and eliminated more rapidly than normal tissue during periods of abstinence. Physiologists have studied the process of autolysis, although they have suggested no practical use that may be made of it save that of employing it to reduce weight. It now remains for physiologists to learn that by means of rigidly controlled autolysis, the body is able to digest tumors and utilize the proteins and other food elements contained in them to nourish its vital tissues. Why have they not investigated this vitally important subject? The facts have been before the world for more than a hundred years.

"Over a hundred and thirty years ago Sylvester Graham wrote: 'It is a general law of the vital economy, that when, by any means, the general function of decomposition exceeds that of composition or nutrition, the decomposing absorbents always first lay hold of and remove those substances which are of least use to the economy; and hence, all morbid accumulations such as wens, tumors, abscesses, etc., are rapidly diminished and often wholly removed under severe and protracted abstinence or fasting.'—*Science of Life,* pp. 194-195.

"The process of autolysis may be put to great practical use and may be made to serve in getting rid of tumors and other growths. To fully understand this, it is necessary for the reader to know that tumors are made up of flesh and blood and bone. There are many names for the different kinds of tumors, but the names all indicate the kind of tissue of which the tumor is composed. For example, an osteoma is made up of bone tissue; a myoma is composed of muscular tissue; a neuroma is constituted of nerve tissue; a lipoma consists of fatty tissue; a fibroma is composed of fibrous tissues; an epithelioma is composed of epithelial tissue, etc. Growths of this nature are known, technically, as neoplasms (new growth) to distinguish them from mere swellings or enlargements. A large lump in the breast may be nothing more than an enlarged lymphatic gland or an enlarged mammary gland. Such an enlarged gland may be very painful, but it is no neoplasm.

"Tumors being composed of tissues, the same kind of tissues as the other structures of the body, are susceptible of autolytic disintegration, the same as normal tissue, and do, as a matter of experience, undergo dissolution and absorption under a variety of circumstances, but especially during a fast. The reader who can understand how fasting reduces the amount of fat in the body and how it reduces the size of the muscles, can also understand how it will reduce the size of a tumor, or cause it to disappear altogether. He needs, then, only to realize that the process of disintegrating (autolyzing) the tumor takes place much more rapidly than it does in the normal tissues.

"In his *Notes On Tumors,* a work for students of pathology, Frances Carter Wood says: 'In a very small proportion of human malignant tumors spontaneous disappearance for longer or shorter periods has been noted. The greater number of such disappearances has followed incomplete surgical removal of the tumor; they have occurred next in order of frequency during some acute febrile process, and less frequently in connection with some profound alteration of the metabolic processes of the organism, such as extreme cachexia, artificial menopause, or the puerperium.'

"No more profound change in metabolism is possible than that produced by fasting and the change is of a character best suited to bring about the autolysis of a tumor, malignant or otherwise.

"The conditions Wood mentions as causing spontaneous disappearance of tumors are, for the most part, 'accidents' and are not within the range of voluntary control. Fasting, on the other hand, may be instituted and carried out under control and at any time desired. It is the rule that operations are followed by increased growth in the tumor. Spontaneous disappearance following incomplete removal is rare. The same may be said for extreme cachexia and artificial menopause. In fevers we have rapid autolysis in many tissues of the body and much reparative work going on, but we cannot develop a fever at will. Pregnancy and childbirth occasion many profound changes in the body, but they are certainly not to be recommended to sick women as cures for their tumors. Even if this were desirable, it would be a hit-or-miss process. The effects of fasting are certain. There is nothing hit-or-miss about the process. It works always in the same general direction.

"Fever is a remedial process and does help to remove the cause of the tumor. None of Wood's other causes of spontaneous disappearance assist in removing the cause of tumors. Fasting does assist greatly in the removal of such cause.

"During a fast the accumulations of superfluous tissues are overhauled and analyzed; the available component parts are turned over to the department of nutrition to be utilized in nourishing the essential tissues; the refuse is thoroughly and permanently removed.

"Due to a variety of circumstances, some known, others unknown, the rate of absorption of tumors in fasting individuals varies. The general condition of the patient, the amount of surplus contained in his body, the kind of tumor, the hardness or softness of the tumor, the location of the tumor, and the age of the patient are all known to influence the rate of tumor absorption. Let me cite two extreme cases to show the wide range of variation in this respect.

"A woman, under forty, had a uterine fibroid about the size of an average grapefruit. It was completely absorbed in twenty-eight days of total abstinence from all food but water. This was an unusually rapid rate of absorption. Another case is that of a similar tumor in a woman of about the same age. In this case the growth was about the size of a goose egg. One fast of twenty-one days reduced the tumor to the size of an English walnut. The fast was broken due to the return of hunger. Another fast a few weeks subsequent, of seventeen days, was required to complete the absorption of the tumor. This was an unusually slow rate of tumor-absorption.

"Tumor-like lumps in female breasts ranging from the size of a pea to that of a goose egg will disappear in from three days to as many weeks. Here is a remarkable case of this kind that will prove both interesting and instructive to the reader. A young lady, age twenty-one, had a large, hard lump – a little smaller than a billiard ball – in her right breast. For four months it had caused her considerable pain. Finally she consulted a physician who diagnosed the condition, cancer, and urged immediate removal. She went to another, and another, and still another physician, and each made the same diagnosis and each urged immediate removal. Instead of resorting to surgery the young lady resorted to fasting and in exactly three days without food, the 'cancer' and all its attendant pain were gone. There had been no recurrence after thirteen years and I think that we are justified in considering the condition remedied.

"Hundreds of such occurrences under fasting have convinced me that many 'tumors' and 'cancers' are removed by surgeons that are not tumors or cancers. They cause me to be very skeptical of the statistics issued to show that early operation prevents or cures cancer.

"Let me cite a comparatively recent instance from my own practice. A manufacturer brought his wife to me from Los Angeles. A growth in one of her breasts had caused her to consult two or three physicians in that city. Each of them had insisted upon the immediate removal of her breast. I placed her upon a fast which was continued for thirty days. At the end of the fast, the tumor, which was about the size of an English walnut at its beginning, had been reduced to the size of a pea. In less than a month on a vegetable and fruit diet, this small remainder disappeared.

"Subsequently the woman gave birth to five children at about two-year intervals. She nursed each of the first three children for two years and the last two for eighteen months each and during each of these nursing periods, the formerly tumorous breast functioned well. The health and vigor of the children presented unequivocal evidence of the quality of the mother's milk. Was this not better than removal of the breast? Was this an exceptional case? By no means. I see them regularly. Such cases are seen daily in institutions in various parts of the world where fasting is employed.

"The removal of tumors by autolysis has several advantages over their surgical removal. Surgery is always dangerous; autolysis is a physiological process and carries no danger. Surgery always lowers vitality and thus adds to the metabolic perversion that is back of the tumor. Fasting, by which autolysis of tumors is accelerated, normalizes nutrition and permits the elimination of accumulated toxins, thus helping to remove the cause of the tumor. After surgical removal tumors tend to recur. After their autolytic removal, there is little tendency to recurrence. Tumors often recur in malignant form after their operative removal. The tendency to malignancy is removed by fasting.

"John W. Armstrong (England) says: 'I have seen lumps in female breasts treated to fast, some of them after diagnosis by "experts," the bulk after self-diagnosis and to disappear, on water only, in from four to twenty days.'

"Bernarr Macfadden says: 'My experience of fasting has shown me beyond all possible doubt that a foreign growth of any kind can be absorbed into the circulation by simply compelling the body to use every unnecessary element contained within it for food. When a foreign growth has become hardened, sometimes one long fast will not accomplish the result, but where they are soft, the fast will usually cause them to be absorbed.'

"A small tumorous growth which had existed for more than twenty years was absorbed during Mr. Pearson's longest fast and did not return thereafter. Dr. Hazzard records the recovery, during a fifty-five days' fast, of a case diagnosed by physicians as cancer of the stomach. Tilden, Weger, Rabagliati, and many others record many such cases.

"I have seen repeated instances of the absorption of tumors in my own patients. I had one complete recovery in the case of a uterine 'cancer' during a thirty-days' fast. I have seen numerous small tumors completely absorbed and large ones greatly reduced in size.

"In Europe and America, literally thousands of tumors have been autolyzed during the past fifty years, and the effectiveness of the method is beyond doubt. I can give no definite information about bone tumors and nerve tumors; but, since these are subject to the same laws of nutrition as all other tumors, I am disposed to think that they may be autolyzed as effectively as other tumors.

"In my own experience I have seen numerous fibroid tumors of the uterus and breast, lipomas in various parts of the body, a few epitheliomas, a whole group of myomas and a number of tumors that were apparently early cancer autolyzed and absorbed while the patient fasted. I have seen many warts disappear during fasting and I have seen many warts on which the fasting process seemed to have no effect. I have never seen a mole affected by the fasting process. I have seen a number of cysts completely destroyed by fasting and others that were merely reduced in size. It will be recalled that Graham mentions having seen cysts (wens) absorbed during fasting.

LIMITATIONS

"It is certain that the autolyzing process has its limitations, for example, a tumor that has been permitted to grow to such enormous size that several long fasts during the course of two years or more, with a rigid feeding schedule between fasts, would be required to break it down and absorb it, if, indeed, it could be done. There was a school in Chicago some years ago that taught that 'the normal tissue may be consumed before the morbid tissues are used up,' in fasting. While this school did not confine this statement to tumors, there are a few conditions in which this can be a fact, and in large tumors it may be so. Aside from large tumors, it is hardly probable that this is so in any recoverable cases. Only in rare instances, where the amount of morbid tissue is very great, and these are probably all irremediable, can this occur.

"In general, good tissue is not used up as fast as bad and the tumor will 'starve' before the body. Except where it is very large, we may be sure that in all cases, hunger will return before any damage is done to the vital tissues. In more than one case of cancer, where opiates had been used to relieve pain, I have seen three or four days' fasting bring relief.

"One other limitation must be noted: namely, tumors that are so situated that they dam-up the lymph stream will continue to grow (feeding upon the excess of lymph behind them) despite fasting. In cases where complete absorption is not obtained, the tumor is sufficiently reduced in size not to constitute a menace. Thereafter proper living will prevent added growth. Indeed, we have seen a number of cases where a further decrease in size followed right living subsequent to fasting.

OBJECTION

"Dr. James C. Thomson, a prominent Natural Therapist, of Edinburgh, Scotland, has offered an objection to the use of the fast to cause the autolytic disintegration of tumors. He says that 'if the autolysis is being carried forward in a satisfactory manner, i.e., with vigor and completeness, then during a fasting period the patient will be living on bad meat, that is, on his own long-established tumor which is made up of unwholesome materials, otherwise they would not have been built into a tumor. Accordingly the better work that is being done during a fast the more certain it is that during that phase the person will be irritable, restless and at times depressed.'

"While I doubt that the flesh that makes up most human tumors is as bad as much of the flesh foods that are regularly taken by flesh-eaters, there is a small modicum of truth in what Dr. Thomson says. It should be pointed out, however, that most tumors are small and that days and weeks are often involved in their absorption, so that the amount of material they supply for any single day is very small. A few grams a day would be all that they would yield. The bad portions of this would be excreted. The food upon which the vital tissues are nourished during this period is derived from the stored food reserves and not from the tissues of the tumor — the amount the tumor supplying being so small as to be negligible.

"I doubt that the irritableness, restlessness and depression that only occasionally accompany the process of autolytic disintegration of a tumor, are due to the exceedingly small amount of unsuitable food material derived from the tumor. These states are most likely to be due to the toxins the autolytic process releases from the tumorous and other tissues, for, not only is the tumor unsuitable for food, but much of the other tissues of the body have been requisitioned as storage places for unexcreted waste and drugs. One of the most important processes that the body carries out during a fast is that of clearing out all this general unsuitability. The tumorous tissue is not the only tissue that is autolyzed and disposed of. If the process results in some discomfort, even actual pain, it is certainly worth going through for the benefits that accrue.

"PHYSIOLOGICAL REST

"An important object secured by the fast is the rest of the organs of the body. The overworking of the physiological functions, which results from over-eating, weakens and impairs them. Fasting reverses this and permits them to recuperate. During the rest thus afforded, these organs are enabled to repair their damaged structures and restore their fagging energies, thus they are prepared for renewed function and are given a new lease on life. A fast is to the organs of the body what a night of restful repose is to the tired laborer."

CHAPTER 15

UNCOOKED FOOD – DOES HEATING HELP OR HURT FOOD?

We now turn to Dr. Herbert M. Shelton's *Hygienic System,* Vol. II, Fifth Edition, 1969, published by Dr. Shelton's Health School, San Antonio, Texas, Chapter XXVIII, page 344, "Uncooked Foods."

"The *Journal of Health* in its issue of May 1833 and the *Moral Reformer,* June 1835, affirmed as a general principle that no person, whether gentleman, farmer or tradesman, woman or child, could eat to advantage, or even with impunity, vegetable matter which had not been softened and changed by cooking processes.

"People were not only afraid of plant foods in those days, but they were especially afraid of them in their uncooked or natural state. It was a day of much cooking – vegetables were par-boiled and then boiled again. The water in which they were par-boiled was thrown away. Little was left for the eater but an almost foodless husk which had been reduced to a mush that required practically no chewing.

"Graham on the other hand, laid down the principle that man's 'physiological interests would be best sustained by those vegetable products which require no culinary change, or cooking.' He thought that cooking not only reduces the value of the foods, but that it actually reduces the digestive powers of those who eat cooked foods. Then he said: 'It may therefore, be laid down as a general law, that all processes of cooking, or artificial preparations of food by fire, are, in themselves, considered with reference to the very highest and best condition of human nature, in some degree detrimental to the physiological and psychological interests of man.'

"Cooking, the most universally employed process of denaturing our foods, is in every way injurious to foods and to man. Whether we cook plant substances or animal products, cooking is ruinous to the properties of the food. The fluids of the plant are, in great part, lost in cooking. With these go the minerals and vitamins of the plant. With them also go the natural flavors and aromas of the food. The nutritive value of foods are impaired or destroyed by cooking and their digestibility is lowered.

"We must tap the richest sources of vitality which Nature possesses and turn them to valuable account. We must supply ourselves and our children with superior nutritive substances and these can only come from nature. Not to the chemist, nor to the food manufacturer, must we go for superior nutrition; but to the original source of nutrition. In nature's products are the requisites of superior nutrition. All the sources of vigor and all the means of resisting pathogenetic ('disease' producing) causes are found in natural products as these come from the hands of nature.

"In fresh fruits and green vegetables and nuts, or the juices of these, are all the minerals and vitamins and high-grade proteins, and other substances needed by the growing, developing human body to bring it to a state of physical, mental or moral perfection and to maintain it in this state indefinitely.

"All the virtues of foods are retained when they are eaten uncooked and they not only protect against the causes of disease, but they add to the joys of life, enhance bodily vigor, and give that strength to the sexual powers that means better offspring.

"Fresh foods, green foods, whole, natural foods, unprocessed foods, unrefined foods, foods that have not lost their substances nor had their values deteriorated by heating, drying, cooking, canning, and refining processes are full of the elements of superior nutrition.

"Graham wrote: 'It is nearly certain, as I have already stated, that the primitive inhabitants of the earth ate their food with very little if any artificial preparations. The various fruits, nuts, seeds, roots, and other vegetable substances on which they subsisted, were eaten by them in their natural state, with no other grinding than that which was done by the teeth.'

"It is obvious to even the least intelligent that animals in a state of nature subsist exclusively and entirely on an uncooked dietary. It is equally as obvious that man subsisted entirely and wholly on uncooked foods before he learned the use of fire. We have no means of knowing how long man lived on the earth before some enterprising young genius learned to make fire, nor how long it was thereafter before he began to apply fire to his foods. I think that we will not go wrong in assuming that the use of fire has persisted but a moment in his history.

"Prof. Jordon, of the University of Chicago, says that the people of the Stone Age were unacquainted with the art of cooking, but ate their foods in their natural state. Animals and, to a large extent, so-called primitive peoples, take their food directly from the hands of nature and eat it unchanged.

"The so-called primitive tribes live largely or wholly upon uncooked foods. The Esquamaux will catch a fish and eat him without taking the trouble to first put him to death. He will kill a walrus and feast off his fresh warm flesh at once. The Hawaiian will wade out into the sea with his harpoon or spear and dive down and spear a fish or catch some other sea creature, come up and eat him without troubling to first get onto the shore. Some African tribes will catch a grasshopper or beetle off a tree and eat it whole on the spot.

"The fact that primitive man ate his foods uncooked is evidence that raw foods are adequate to support life. Indeed there is much evidence to show that certain qualities possessed by raw foods are indispensible to life. It is quite probable that the enzymes of raw foods are of use to the body. Research may show that plant enzymes are the sources of animal enzymes.

"My esteemed friend and erstwhile co-worker, Dr. B. S. Claunch, said in an excellent talk on *How Disease is Built*, delivered at Sorosis Hall, San Francisco, December 10, 1922: 'There are nearly 700,000 species of animal life, and every-one of these species except man — the highest — lives exclusively on live, uncooked, organic food. No other animal except man eats devitalized foods that have been rendered inorganic — reduced from their organic structure to dead, inorganic substances . . .' 'As I stated before, animals of every kind live on uncooked food with the exception of man. Incidentally, man is the only species in the entire animal kingdom that is sick, with the exception of a few that have their diet prescribed for them by man — domesticated animals. They are sick the same as man, because man supplies their food and directs their eating habits instead of permitting them to select their own foods.

"He continues: 'Cooking foods and processing them — refining, sterilizing, preserving, pickling, flavoring and coloring — all tend to devitalize them. When such substances are eaten — these are practically the only kinds obtainable today in the modern eating places — about one-fourth is unchanged. The nourishment obtained from the one-fourth keeps you alive for a few years; the poison you get from the other three-fourths keeps you sick most of the time.'

"Not a single truth in these statements of Dr. Claunch's is injured in any way by the fact that he has repudiated them. No truth is impaired by the desertion of its advocates. The fact that Dr. Claunch now advocates, or did, for a while, advocate an almost exclusive meat diet, and this well-cooked, does not alter the fact that homo (SAP) iens is the only species on earth which eats cooked food. Nor does it change the fact that cooking and processing foods injures and impairs them. When a man changes his mind it does not change the facts.

"Cooking utensils only made their appearance a few thousand years ago and for a long time only some foods were cooked. During the Dark Ages the Black Art of Cooking was 'improved' and popularized and the custom of cooking spread to such an extent that those who ate uncooked foods came to be looked upon as savages, but little above cattle. Cooking became popular during the thousand-year reign of anti-naturalism, which cost the human race so much and yielded so little, and was popularized by the anti-natural dogmas of that time. The germ theory gave an added reason for thoroughly cooking everything we eat, for it taught us to thus kill the 'pathogenic microbes' in and on our foods.

"Graham declares: 'If man subsisted wholly on uncooked food, the undepraved integrity of his appetite, his thorough mastication and slow swallowing, and his simple meal, would greatly serve to prevent over-eating, and thus save him from the mischievous effects of one of the most destructive causes operating in civic life. . . . Whatever may be the kind of food on which man subsists when the artificial preparation is made as far as possible in accordance with the physiological laws of constitution and relation established in his nature, and is of simple character which leaves the proportions of nutritious and innutritious properties as nature combined them, or in the general average conforms in this respect to nature, and effects little change in the nutritious principles, and retains the natural requisition for the function of the teeth, and thus secures the proper chewing of the food, and the mixing of it with the solvent fluid of the mouth, and the swallowing of it slowly, the artificial process of preparation militates very little, if at all, against any of the physiological interests of the body. But if the preparation concentrates the nutriment properties, and destroys the true proportion between the bulk and nourishment, and effects improper changes and combinations in the nutriment elements, and does away with the necessity for mastication, and presents the food in too elevated temperature and enables us to swallow it too rapidly with little or no exercise of the teeth, and without properly mixing it with the saliva, the artificial process of cooking is decidedly and often exceedingly inimical, not only to the physiological interests of the alimentary organs, but the whole human system. And let it ever be remembered, that, as a general rule, the process of cooking, when regulated in the very best manner, cannot so perfectly adapt the substances which it is necessary to cook, to the physiological properties and powers of the human body, as to render them equally conducive to the highest and best conditions of man, with those substances which are naturally adapted to the alimentary wants. And, therefore, as already stated, all processes of cooking, or artificial preparation of food by fire – considered in reference to the very highest capabilities of human nature – must be regarded as in some measure an evil.'

"Inherent in Graham's views and principles, though in the very nature of things, this could not have been known at that time, was the saving of the minerals and vitamins of foods by eating them as nature produced them without, first, processing, refining and cooking them. No doubt it was this fact that led Prof. Stiles to declare, when the discovery of vitamins was first announced, that it was merely a re-statement of Graham's views.

"We do well to remember that chemistry was a young science or hoped-to-be-a-science, and food chemistry was not yet born when Graham penned these lines. He covered all the ground in a general, and in some particulars, a vague way, which we of today, with greater knowledge, are permitted to cover more in detail. But it is a standing monument to the genius of the man that, with all our increased knowledge of foods and their relation to the body, we can only bow to him and say, 'Yes, Mr. Graham, you are right.' For Graham's book, now nearly a hundred years old, is up-to-date, and in some respects, he is ahead of us yet. If you want to know nature cure, read Graham. If you want to know natural hygiene, read Graham. If you want the newer knowledge of nutrition, read Graham. His was a master mind. He saw clearly then what the orthodox world is just beginning to see.

"Graham said: 'If man were to subsist wholly on alimentary substances in their natural state, or without any artificial preparation, by cooking, he would be obliged to use his teeth freely, and by so doing not only preserve his teeth from decay; but at the same time and by the same means, he would thoroughly mix his food with the solvent fluid of his mouth.... Again, if man were to subsist wholly on uncooked food, he would never suffer from the improper temperature of his ailment.... If man were to subsist entirely on food in a natural state, he would never suffer from concentrated aliment.... If man subsisted wholly on uncooked food, he would not only be preserved from improper concentrations, but also from pernicious combinations of alimentary substances.... it is uncontrovertable that the alimentary organs of man and of all other animals can digest one kind of food at a time, better than a mixture of different kinds....'

"If we cut this up we find that:

"(1) Uncooked food, requiring more chewing, supply the teeth with much needed exercise.

"(2) The necessary chewing insures proper insalivation.

"(3) Uncooked food would preserve the teeth and stomach from the injury produced by hot foods.

"(4) Uncooked foods would possess the proper proportion of 'nutritious and innutritious (bulk) matter' to which 'the anatomical construction and physiological powers of the alimentary organs of the human body are constitutionally adapted.'

"(5) Uncooked foods tend to prevent 'pernicious combinations.'

"(6) Mono-trophic meals are the most easily digested.

"Today we may add the following other virtues of the uncooked diet:

"(7) Uncooked foods possess their vitamins and complettins, enzymes, salts, acids, carbohydrates, proteins and fats in the organic and unimpaired state in which nature produces them.

"(8) The necessity for chewing them insures tasting them to the fullest, and this assures proper adaptation of digestive juices to the character of the food.

"(9) Chewing and tasting the food tends also to prevent over-eating.

"(10) Uncooked foods are not so easily adulterated as are the canned, pickled, embalmed foods so largely eaten today.

"(11) Uncooked foods do not ferment so rapidly.

"(12) Uncooked foods, if spoiled, cannot be 'camouflaged' and passed off on us as good food, as cooked foods can be.

"(13) The uncooked diet saves time, food and labor in preparation.

"Graham and his co-workers had placed great emphasis upon the value of fruits, vegetables and whole grains in their natural, i.e., unprocessed and uncooked, state. The 'raw food movement' may rightly be said to have been started by Graham. Though it never made great headway until after the discovery of the value of minerals in food and, later, the discovery of vitamins. There were three thousand 'raw fooders' in Chicago alone in 1900.

"Uncooked fruits, nuts, vegetables and whole grains were not merely 'protective' foods to Graham, Trall, Allcott, Densmore, Page, and others; they were nutritive; indeed they represented the best and highest form of nutritive material. Dr. Trall proclaimed (1860) all fruits and vegetables to be protective, by which he did not intend to detract from their nutritive qualities. The world has been a long time discovering what Graham knew – namely, that cooking impairs or destroys the protective and nutritive values of food.

"It is almost axiomatic that fruits, nuts and vegetables are the only foods that can be relished raw. Other foods hardly belong to man's natural diet. Buying fruits and vegetables to provide minerals and vitamins for yourself and your family and then destroying the vitamins and extracting the minerals and throwing these away in the process of preparing them fails of its purpose. Only when you eat your fruit uncooked and consume big salads of uncooked vegetables can you be sure of obtaining a sufficient supply of minerals and vitamins.

"The 'orthodox' medical world became so frightened over germs a few years after Graham's death that they insisted on thoroughly cooking everything, to destroy germs; while their preoccupation with the calorie value of foods caused them to deny that fruits and vegetables have any food value. No wonder Prof. Stiles saw in the vitamin announcement, a re-statement of Graham's principles.

"The nearer their natural and unchanged state our foods are eaten the better for us. The natural 'affinity' existing between the needs of our cells and the nutritional elements in natural foods supplies us with an infallible guarantee that we will get the needed salts, vitamins, and other food elements from natural foods. All true foods are more tasty 'raw' than cooked. Cooked food, sans seasoning, are flat and insipid, as well as less nutritive.

"Eugene Christian says: 'We have in this country hundreds of articles of food which can be most advantageously used without cooking; yet the cook intrudes his art, bakes, boils, stews, broils, and heats these things, until their original elements are wholly changed, until many of them are rendered almost totally valueless.

" 'Thus robbed of their elementary and delicious flavors,

the cook endeavors to make them appeal to the sense of taste by mixing, jumbling together, spicing, and using decoctions called extracts, the properties of which he knows absolutely nothing, until the original substance is so disguised that it cannot be recognized in taste, color and flavor.'

"In one of his splendid *Health and Diet Bulletins,* Ralph E. Sunderland says: 'These are true foods because their original organic nature has not been changed, by oxidation, to inorganic status. Only organic substance is food. No inorganic substance is food because it is not assimilable in the body. This is a law. Every cooking process which involves exposure of the original organic food substance to the oxygen of the air fosters oxidation. This is true whether the cooking is done at home or in some factory. There must be life in food. Life in food is expressed only by its organic nature or condition. There is no life in oxidized (inorganic) substance. Upon this foundation all scientific diet teaching must rest.'

"RAW OR UNCOOKED?

"In its original sense 'raw' meant 'unfinished.' We speak of 'raw materials' and the 'finished product.' It originally had no reference to cooked or uncooked foods. Custom, however, or usage makes language and since usage now sanctifies the use of the word 'raw' in the sense of 'uncooked' we shall accept this usage and so emply the word in this book. But let us keep ever in our minds that nature finishes or perfects her foods and they require no fixing to complete them.

"'Foods that have been ripened and brought to a state of maturity by nature cannot consistently be called "raw,"' says Eugene Christian. 'Think of applying this ugly word to a luscious bunch of purple grapes swinging to and fro in bowers of green. Or to a hickory nut that has ripened in the top of a mountain tree, whose life-giving properties have been filtered through a hundred feet of clean, white wood. Or to a delicious apple, or peach, reddened, ripened and finished — nursed in the lap of nature, rocked in her ethereal cradle, and kissed from the odorous blossoms of infancy on to maturity by the soft beams of the life-giving sun, ready for use; they are perfect, they are not raw, they are done; and when they are cooked they are undone. They are as far removed from their finished condition as if they were green or but half grown.'

"DEFENSE OF COOKING

"Cooking is claimed to be a predigesting process; it renders foods more digestible and thus saves the energies of the body. We are advised to avail ourselves of the advantages of this 'pre-digesting' process. Invalids are especially admonished to eat well-cooked, toasted, dextrinized, etc., foods.

"It has been previously shown that cooking does not pre-digest our foods. With rare exceptions, such as that of egg white, foods are rendered less digestible by cooking and all of them rendered less nutritious.

"But if this claim were true, there still seems to be no reason why we should cook our foods. Why we should substitute the wasteful processes of cooking for the conserving processes of digestion.

"We should certainly avoid 'pre-digested' foods. Our organs of digestion are made to perform the work of digestion and we should look with much suspicion upon all substitutes for these. If we do the work of the digestive organs for them, we weaken them and their functions. I do not believe that we can strengthen a weak digestion by eating so-called pre-digested foods, any more than we can strengthen a weak arm by refusing to use it.

"The digestive juices are the natural food solvents and instead of weakening these by resort to half-foods, so-called pre-digested foods, and by resort to drugs and various 'aids to digestion,' we should correct the causes of impaired digestion and feed naturally.

"If there is a need for rest of these organs and functions, give them a rest; but do not try to do their work for them. To 'nourish' a sick body on 'pre-digested,' denatured products will not produce health and strength.

"ECONOMY OF UNCOOKED FOODS

"A raw food diet saves time, labor and money. It is estimated, and the estimate is probably approximately correct, that 'as compared with cooked, it only takes about half the quantity of uncooked food to sustain life.' The digestibility of foods is not increased by cooking; but their food values are greatly reduced. Cooked foods do not nourish the body as well as uncooked foods. It is impossible to nourish the body on a diet consisting exclusively of thoroughly cooked foods. We subsist largely on the uncooked foods in our diet and on the uncooked or but partially cooked portions of our cooked foods. Cooking renders a large part of food valueless as food. He who lives on uncooked foods may, therefore, live cheaper at the same time he lives better.

"The Esquimaux, in his remote haunts, lives largely on a flesh diet. He eats practically the whole of the animal and eats it raw. He catches up a fish out of the water and eats it 'blood-raw' with as much relish as his civilized brother eats a piece of candy. But where he attempts to live on a diet of cooked meat, his health and strength fail and he becomes diseased.

"The un-fired diet eliminates entirely the fuel bill in as far as this relates to cooking. But of greater importance than this is the saving of the time and energy of women. 'When the house is provided,' says Dr. Christian, 'and the woman who has dreamed of a true home is settled therein, it gradually dawns upon her that instead of being a queen, she is an imprisoned vassal. She finds she must stand over a miniature furnace for an hour in the morning and breathe the poisonous odor of broiling flesh, and spend another hour among the grease and slime of pots and dishes, instead of occupying that time walking in the life-giving sunlight and drinking in nature's purifying air.

" 'She soon realizes that the fires of the morning are hardly out until those of the noon are kindled and the labors from luncheon often lap into the evening, and those of evening far into the night. The throne over which she dreamed of wielding the queenly sceptre has been transformed into a fiery furnace, gilded with greasy pots and plates, blood and bones, over which she has unfurled the dishrag, and by the common custom of her country, it waves over her helpless head as an ensign of her rank and profession, under which she is really a slave.'

"She is forever washing dishes, greasy dishes, in the sink. She spends six to eight hours a day preparing meals and washing dishes. The realization of this great waste of human time and labor was forcibly brought home to me during World War I. I served for seven months in a kitchen where we fed over two hundred men three times a day. We had a mess sergeant, several cooks, a dining room orderly and several kitchen police. The work started before dawn when the other soldiers were all asleep and ended late in the evening about the time the other men were ready to retire. We spent our time spoiling good food or further spoiling foods that had already been greatly spoiled at the factory or cannery, and in washing greasy pots, pans, dishes, etc. An army of men was required to feed the army.

"Hotels, restaurants, and housewives have spent ages in competition with each other to see which could prepare the greatest variety of tempting, but foodless dishes, with which to tickle the palates, usually the perverted palates, of the eating world. I am not alone, however, when I say that experience has shown that men are usually more willing to accept a dietary reform than women. Women want to 'fix' things and mix things and prepare that which appeals to the eye. For ages the kitchen has been the chief medium of expression for her and it was through the art of cooking that she expressed herself. She finds it hard to break away from her traditional channels of expression. Dietary reform is greatly handicapped by the opposition of those who would profit most by it.

"OBJECTIONS TO THE UNFIRED DIET

"It is frequently objected that 'prolonged maintenance of the body in a state of health and fitness on a diet of raw foods is possible only when the foods are judiciously chosen.' The same is true, but to a greater extent, of cooked foods.

"Dr. Kellogg says: 'A person who desires to live upon a raw diet, in arranging his bill of fare cannot base his selection upon the supposition that all raw foods are complete nutriments, but must possess a sufficient knowledge of the newer facts pertaining to nutrition to enable him to make such combinations of food stuffs as will constitute an aggregate complete in all the elements required for perfect nutrition and in adequate quantities.'

"This fact is equally true if one is going to eat a diet of cooked foods. The cooked diet must also be made up of 'such combinations of food stuffs as will constitute an aggregate complete in all the elements required for perfect nutrition and in adequate quantities.' I know of no one who claims or supposes that 'all raw foods are complete nutriments.' But the newer facts of nutrition prove beyond a doubt that it is much easier to be properly nourished on a raw than on a cooked diet.

"There never was a time when any portion of the

human race lived almost entirely on cooked foods, nor was there ever a time, until within very recent times, when a large part of the race subsisted chiefly on cooked foods.

"Well does Adolph Just say in his *Return to Nature,* 'If you are well and would keep well, why not listen to Nature's appeal? Think you; were there no fine men and women roaming about the earth thousands and thousands of years even before the discovery of fire, and before either the first chef or medico was evolved? Will you believe that nature, at the outset, overlooked the matter of man's health, and that he remained an outcast in the plan of things, until, by his own wit, pills, drug-lists, and patent foods had brought him his salvation? Man's food was sun-cooked in those ancient days, and the sun cooks our food at the present time. Artificial cooking is no blessing to mankind. It may be accepted as an axiom that cooking kills; and there is a vast variety of natural foods — beautiful sweet-scented, and delicious — on which we may draw both for our sustenance and for the mere pleasure of the palate.'

"An objection has been raised to the use of uncooked foods in Northern climates because the 'shipped-in green-picked fruits and sprayed vegetables come devitalized during the winter season.' That the people of the North do not always have access to the best of green or fresh foods in the winter months is true enough, but this is all the more reason why they should consume them in the uncooked state. Cooking these fruits and vegetables wilts and devitalizes them still more. Cooking them renders them less nourishing than they are when purchased. The less suited are these foods for nutritive purposes the greater is the need to avoid further reduction of their nutritive values. It is necessary to preserve to the utmost, all the food values they possess and not destroy them in any manner whatsoever.

"Rather than a 'good five cent cigar,' what this country needs is a great teacher, one who, with the eyes of a superior being, can see the roots of our troubles, the causes of men's perennial lassitude, constant seeking after stimulants, the causes of their deterioration, weakness, decrepitude, impotency and suffering; one who possesses a deep knowledge of the secrets of nature, who knows the almost magic virtues of fresh fruits, uncooked vegetables and nuts, and who can stir our people as no man ever stirred them before.

"Piles of shattered pottery, superfluous stew pans, crushed baking ovens, and the ash-heaps left from the burning of 'food' factories, refineries, etc., would be found in the wake of such a saviour of our nation. Our people must be made drunk with enthusiasm and wild with eagerness for a new life based on a new and superior nutrition. The man who can stir this nation to its roots and bring it back to a pristine state of health and perfection will deserve to rank among the world's greatest men.

CHAPTER 16

A RAW FOOD DIET USED WITH CANCER

"*Raw Food Treatment of Cancer* was written by Dr. Kirstine Nolfi (Denmark). Dr. Nolfi passed her medical examinations in 1907, after which she spent twelve years at various hospitals in Denmark, including the Communal Hospital in Copenhagen (Departments of Surgery, Medicine, Dermatology and Psychiatry), the State Hospital, Copenhagen (Departments of Pediatrics, Ophthalmology, and Psychiatry), and in various Children's Hospitals.

"From 1919 to 1945 she was in private practice in Copenhagen, and acknowledged as a specialist in diseases of children. From 1945 to 1958 she was in charge of the Humlegarden Rawcost Sanatorium, Denmark.

"The following was published by The Shangri-La Health Resort, Bonita Springs, Florida, First Edition, July 1969.

"'Before I realized the actual importance of raw vegetable food, my attitude was exactly the same as that of other doctors — to treat the symptoms of the disease without thinking of preventing it. It *ought* to be the duty of the medical profession in future to find means of preventing to a much higher degree than now, instead of having to cure later on.

"'That I, as a doctor, went in for *exclusively* raw vegetable food is due to the fact that I became ill, even seriously ill, myself. I developed cancer of the breast. The disease had, of course, been preceded by *wrong nourishment and wrong habits* in the course of my twelve years of hospital training, when I suffered from sluggish digestion and catarrh of the stomach all the time, disorders which are still of quite common occurrence among hospital staff members. Since that time no change of the hospital diet has taken place in Denmark in this very important domain.

" 'On one occasion I was in a dying condition because of a bleeding gastric ulcer. This made me abandon meat and fish, and I became a *vegetarian.* Later, I took to eating a good deal of raw vegetable food. In this manner my digestion became regulated, and I felt better, though not completely well. In the winter of 1940 to 1941 I was exceptionally *tired and dull,* but I was unable to ascertain any specific disease. At that time I did not understand what was wrong with me, but in the course of the Spring I discovered a small node in my right breast.

" 'Tired and dull as I was, I did not pay any attention to it until, five weeks later, I discovered that the node was the size of a hen's egg. It had grown into the skin — a thing only cancer does. As a doctor I had seen enough to be unwilling to submit to the treatment of cancer generally employed. I consulted my good friend, Dr. M. Hindhede, who dissuaded a trial microscopy. It would open up the blood-streams and the cancer would spread; so I gave it up. And then I felt it as quite a natural thing that I would have to carry through a *one hundred per cent, raw vegetable diet.*

" 'I went in search of nature, lived for some time on a small island in the Kattegat, took sun-baths from four to five hours daily, slept in a tent, bathed several times a day, and lived exclusively on a raw vegetable diet. Later I introduced this habit of life at the sanatorium "Humlegarden."

" 'But I was still tired and continued to be so for the first two months, and during that period the node in the breast did not diminish; it remained unchanged.

" '*But then the improvement came.* The node diminished, my strength returned, apparently I recovered and felt better than I had done for many years. When I had experienced good health in this manner for about a year, I tried by way of experiment (and urged to do so by Dr. Hindhede) to revert to a vegetarian diet supplemented by fifty per cent of raw vegetable food.

" 'But it was no good. In three or four months I began to feel a stinging pain in the breast, in the sore-like tissue which the cancer had left where it had originally adhered to the skin. This pain increased much during the weeks that followed, and I realized that the cancer had begun to develop again.

" 'Once more I reverted to pure, raw food, which caused the pain to subside rapidly and the fatigue to become less pronounced. But, being a doctor, I realized that I would have to use the experience I had gained to help my sick fellow creatures. So I set up my home so that I could have four or five patients staying with me the next summer. We took a hundred per cent raw vegetable diet, and all went well; but it was not satisfactory with so few patients. I understood that this cause would have to be advocated under quite different and larger conditions if any proofs were to be given. On my initiative a joint stock company was then formed which bought a property, "Humlegarden," well suited for the purpose; it was set up as a sanatorium, where I became the chief physician. Here, we eat *only* raw vegetable food, patients as well as employees, and the establishment is now in its sixth year.

" 'Now, what is the reason why a one hundred per cent, raw vegetable diet exerts such a beneficial effect on civilized individuals? First and foremost, because the raw food is *live food as it is handed to us by nature.* We all know that life on earth is completely dependent on our sun. If we had no sun the earth would be without any life, dark and icy cold. Vital force is therefore identical with sun energy!

" 'According to Dr. Hesselink, it is, however, only the plant with its widely unfolded thin green leaves, that is able to catch the sunlight and to deposit it in the form of roots and tubers, fruit and seeds. We human beings and the animals, with massive bodies, are not able to utilize it to a sufficiently high degree. Therefore, both man and beast use plants as carriers between the sun and themselves. A *fresh, raw vegetable diet is sunlight nourishment!*

" 'Dr. Bircher-Benner, of Zurich, realized this long ago. Dr. Hesselink, from Holland, believes that it is the atoms which are the carriers of the solar energy.

" '*Fresh, raw vegetable food possesses the highest nutritive value,* and this cannot be *increased* or improved; anything else, such as heating, drying, storing, fermentation or preservation, will tend to reduce and destroy its value. Boiled vegetables taste of nothing, so something must be done to make them palatable. We mix many different things together; we add salt, sugar, spices and butter. We remove the germ and the husk from the wheat to use the flour for baking. We polish the rice, we refine the sugar; we remove the skin, seeds, and cores of apples and pears, we peel the potatoes and scrape the carrots. Meat, fish, eggs and cheese supply us with an enormous surplus of animal protein. We make beverages of coffee and cocoa beans, and tea, which contain stimulating poisons.

" 'We use the grapes for wine and brandy – intoxicating poisons – which *first stimulate* the grey cortex of the brain, and later paralyze it. We preserve food with chemicals, such as benzoic acid, salicylic acid, nitre, boric acid and sulphurous acid in order that it may keep well, and look attractive. Further, we take anodynes, hypnotics, sedatives, and aperients – all strong chemical poisons – or at any rate substances that are foreign to the organism. Among drugs which are misused to a great extent tablets for headache, hypnotics, and aperients are much too predominant. In a small country like Denmark the adviser on pharmacological matters of the Public Health Authorities is able to give us the following figures: consumption of drugs for headache 150 tons, aperients 15 tons, hypnotics 9 tons – annually.

" 'Nicotine, too, is a ruinous stimulant, a still stronger poison than spirits; it causes sclerosis of the heart and the cardiac musculature to become undernourished. The heart becomes a flaccid bag instead of a firm muscle. Many busy men who die about the age of fifty years die of heart failure caused by chronic nicotine poisoning. Here, too, I have experienced that patients on a pure, raw vegetable diet *gradually* lose their taste for tobacco completely.

" 'The ground, too, is wrongly cultivated when it is fertilized too much and too uniformly with chemical manure. We may run the risk that the ground becomes just as diseased as man — overacidified, over-nourished, and that it yields sick plants which are not fit for human food.

" '*Raw* food is termed *live* food by me, in contrast with such food as has been treated by heating, which I consider dead food. Care should be taken that the food does not include substances which counteract the chemistry of the organism, so that the waste products are not retained too long and putrefy in the large intestine. The *best food is therefore completely natural food which has not been subjected to denaturation of any kind.* To this must be added that live food is much easier to digest; it helps in the digestion itself just as the living baby cooperates in its delivery.

" 'Raw vegetables have been digested in the stomach and the intestines *in an hour;* boiled vegetables require almost three hours and leave more waste products, also offensive stools, impure blood, and poisoned and gradually impaired organs, whereas the raw food — live food — the sunlight nourishment, dissolves and excretes these poisons. Raw food is easy to digest, it spares and strengthens the organism in every respect because of its content of *life, bases, and vitamins* in their natural, living combination and relationship to one another.

" 'Everybody who can think must be able to understand that our present nutrition is highly destructive — and is the most common and most serious cause of physical and pyschic diseases and constitutional degeneration. We must seek more wholesome nourishment and more wholesome habits of life if we are to live better now and in the future. We *cannot afford to compromise when life and health* are concerned. We must follow the only right way – the one hundred per cent raw vegetable diet.

" 'Let us consider for a moment how it influences our many different diseases. In the individual case it will always, on the one hand, depend on how good a *constitution* the patient has and how *old* he is, and on the other hand, how *poisoned, weakened and broken this constitution has gradually become because of preceding wrong nutrition and wrong habits.* But it may be said, largely, that if, in spite hereof, the organism is fairly fit for work and able to utilize the exclusively raw diet, the latter will exert a curative effect on almost all our diseases, both those we have acquired during our span of life and those determined by hereditary predispositions.

" 'Even the baby unborn may be injured in various ways. The impaired germ may determine both physical and psychic diseases. The baby may be injured by the wrong nutrition of the mother, because it is nourished through the impure blood of the mother. This may pave the way to disease so that the baby is born ill. After its birth the condition is aggravated, mostly because the mother's milk is not as good, both qualitatively and quantitatively.

" 'Children all over the civilized world are born weaklings in a mild or severer degree, and who can estimate the future consequence thereof? Therefore, the sooner we go in for exclusively raw vegetable food, the sooner and better it will exert its effect.

" 'Children are *assisted* by nature, older individuals are rather *opposed* by nature. When a mother goes in for pure raw food, her milk secretion is immediately increased, the child thrives in all respects, the vitality is increased, and the mother can soon begin to give even young babies an addition of finely chopped fruit and vegetables; never, however, fruit and vegetables at the same time – always separately. It borders on the incomprehensible that a change can be effected so rapidly, just by giving the child *wholesome mother's milk,* as much as it requires, and afterwards fruit and vegetables.

"'I have often experienced how a large family of brothers and sisters living exclusively on a raw vegetable diet became healthy, happy, lively and nice children in the course of a few months, so good is the effect of the exclusively raw vegetable diet in childhood, which is still assisted by nature and has not yet been ruined. The effect does not appear quite as soon in adults, but it is indisputable that raw vegetable food exerts a good effect on adults too, even physically – it brings about *equanimity and harmony, kindness and sympathy.*

"'But what of the *elderly sick or the very sick people* who have gone in for this diet *too late?* How about them?

"'Well, they have to be *patient,* energetic, and *very interested,* and they must be able to *rest much,* at any rate to begin with. The first few days may be troublesome until they have become accustomed to this different food and habit of life. But they will soon do better; the bowels open regularly – two or three times daily – and this is a great encouragement to many. At the "Humlegarden" garlic has its great share in this improvement. Just one clove with every fruit meal is of effect, but it is, of course, better to eat a medium-sized garlic (from five to ten cloves) with the fruit meals. A number of works by various investigators have been published, dealing with the bactericidal effect of garlic, which people of former times guessed. According to investigations reported in the *Journal of the American Chemical Society,* 1944, a substance known as allicin, which exerts a great inhibitory effect on bacteria, has been found in garlic. This substance has been compared with penicillin in a number of experiments, and it appeared that allicin exerts its effects on practically all bacteria, in contrast with penicillin, the effect of which is certainly stronger but much more limited. The use of garlic is rendered difficult because of its peculiar odor; therefore, people in Denmark often return to the "Humlegarden" to undergo a course of treatment with garlic. In the company of others who eat garlic themselves the odor cannot be smelt at all.

"'Raw vegetable food, and in particular raw potatoes, exert an excellent effect on all forms of *rheumatism and rheumatic arthritis* when these diseases have not progressed too far. A good effect is also seen on the diseases related to those just mentioned and of the same causation, namely, loading with uric acid; it applies to psoriasis, hemicrania, stone-formation in the gall bladder, the renal pelvis and the urinary bladder. Almost all diseases of the skin are cured, in many cases even rapidly. Loss of hair, fat formation, and dandruff cease. All infectious diseases are *cured or improve.*

"'The garlic we eat exerts an excellent effect on putrefaction in the large intestine, and a clove of garlic in either side of the mouth, placed between the cheek and the teeth, will greatly accelerate the expurgation and cure of diseases in the upper respiratory tract, first and foremost ordinary colds if dealt with in time. Diseases such as catarrh of the nose, the throat and the larynx, bronchitus and tuberculosis of the lungs, inflammation of the frontal sinus or the maxillary sinus, *chronic inflammation of tonsils and gums,* inflammation of the middle ear, and others, are cured completely in most cases. *Gastric catarrh, gastric ulcer, duodenal ulcer, catarrh of the large intestine, and hemorrhoids, too.*

"'Women who carry through the raw diet during pregnancy feel well — *delivery takes place readily and rapidly and almost without pain,* the *slender, healthy, strong baby cooperates.* The raw food produces *copious and good milk for the child* during the first year if the mother continues with this diet.

" 'When a person is on an exclusively raw vegetable diet it will, as a rule, be easy to stop *smoking and drinking.* Liquor does not taste well with raw vegetables. Smoking does not agree with garlic. On an exclusively raw vegetable diet no stimulants of any kind will be needed any more.

" 'When cancer occurs, the organism, is, as a rule, thoroughly destroyed. Cancer is the terminal stage. Here a one hundred per cent raw vegetable diet may prove *helpful,* alleviate the pain, *prolong the life* to some extent, because it agrees well with the patient. In the most favorable cases, when the *cancer is dealt with in time,* it may perhaps also be checked even for many years in some cases. I am an example of this myself, but then the seat of the cancer must not be in vital organs, such as the lungs, liver or stomach. And the treatment with raw food should be commenced as soon as the cancer is discovered, and it is an absolutely necessary condition that it is carried through one hundred per cent.

" 'I want now to tell a little about my own case from 1942 to the present year. Up to 1946 I was doing well on my exclusively raw diet — the cancer of the breast was completely quiescent, and my general health was good.

" 'But in the spring of 1946 we got some *dried fruit* from Sweden (raisins, dates, prunes, and figs). I thought then that it would be all right to eat it; but it was not. These are fruits which have been treated with chemical poisons in order to preserve them and to make them look attractive. Having taken them for three or four months I suddenly developed violent pains in the scar-like tissue in the breast, and, on closer examination, I found a *small node in the right breast, in the same place as before.* Once more I reverted to the *fresh* raw food, and the node disappeared.

" 'The last and most dangerous thing for me was, however, the *trial microscopy against which I had been dissuaded* by Dr. M. Hindhede. I *had* to let it be done because so many

— doctors in particular — maintained that I had never been suffering from cancer. It was made at the Radium Centre in Copenhagen, in January, 1948. This trial microscopy was positive; there were cancer cells in the scar-like tissue in the skin of the right breast, but it was a benign form called scirrhus. *My originally malignant, rapidly growing form of cancer had thus, under the influence of raw food, been converted into a benign form of cancer, which remains quiescent.*

"'But still this interference was just on the point of stirring up the cancer so much as to frighten me seriously. For the first time I developed metastases (two small nodules) in the armpit; and about six months — on the exclusively raw diet — were required to make them subside again. But it went well this time. Since then I have been in excellent health — all through last summer I was up at sunrise, and in my garden where I have been working hard several hours daily. This was far more wholesome than sitting indoors *working as a doctor.* Not only had I the patients at the "Humlegarden," but also a *large practice and correspondence* out of town; this was more than I could manage.

"'On January 1st, 1949, I stopped practicing and took up gardening again, which had always been my great interest. For this purpose I had acquired about a half a hectare (about one-and-a-quarter acres) of land near the "Humlegarden," and here I learned how right it was to grow both fruit and vegetables biologically, that is according to *the laws of life.* For manure I use only *compost, seaweed, straw or hay; no chemical manure, no dung.*

"'In conclusion, just a few words about the practical conditions and the everyday use of raw vegetable food. I am glad to be able to refer to my book *Live Food,* which has just been brought out by a Dutch publishing house and which gives a detailed picture of the procedure to be followed when changing to a pure raw vegetable diet. It would be of great consequence if the medical profession would acquire greater knowledge in this field to a higher degree than is actually the case. Doctors from Denmark and from foreign countries have visited the "Humlegarden" for shorter or longer periods and have utilized their experience in their practice.

"'The "Humlegarden" is visited by about one thousand patients annually. Here the patients, as well as the members of the staff, live exclusively on *food that has not been treated by heating,* and our experience is that a transition diet is quite superfluous. The raw vegetable diet can *only* be varied according to the seasons, and consists of three meals daily. We get a fruit meal in the morning and in the evening and a vegetable meal in the middle of the day. Fruit and vegetables are never mixed. If the condition of the teeth permits it, the raw food is taken *whole,* otherwise it must be grated and reduced to small particles *immediately* before the meal. Once the raw food has been grated or chopped, it will not keep because it loses its *content of vitamins.*

"'The raw food should be carefully chewed, preferably so well that it passes down all by itself, and even the grated raw food should at any rate be mixed well with saliva. We drink raw whole milk with all our meals, from half a litre to one litre daily (one litre equals one-and-three-quarter pints approximately). Germinating corn, or dried corn, crushed or ground immediately before the meal, is taken with the fruit. Garlic is medicine and is eaten with fruit and milk, cut into small pieces in varying quantities.

"'All kinds of nuts provide a good supplement. The vegetable meal consists of green *leaves, roots and tubers,* with an admixture of a spoonful of honey.

"'Potatoes are eaten with the peel because of the presence of an element – fluorine – which preserves the enamel of the teeth. Similarly, all fruit is eaten with the peel. In the cases of diseases such as gastric catarrh, gastric ulcer, and the like, care should, however, be taken during the initial stages.

"'If the exclusively raw food with its associated sound

habits of life prevails, a variety of things will improve. Diseases will gradually be obviated. Obesity, the most dangerous of all diseases, will become a rarity.

" 'The housewife's work will be reduced to half the time — and the leisure hours thus gained will be an invaluable advantage and joy for husband, children and home. The slender build, the erect carriage, the supple gait, the fresh complexion, the white, sound teeth and the vigorous hair, will dominate the picture. When the body is healthy, the result will invariably be a sound mind. Our negative thoughts will be changed into positive ones, and develop the great cultural progress which the world is waiting for. *Only then will life be worth living'*

"Published by the Shangri-La Health Resort, Bonita Springs, Florida 33923.

Publisher's Note:

"This booklet has been reprinted exactly as Dr. Nolfi wrote it. However, from a hygienic point of view, we do not approve the idea of 'curing' cancer which Dr. Nolfi indicates by advocating the use of garlic and onions as medicine, nor her general attitude toward the use of raw food as a 'treatment.'

"Food is only one of the factors of health. Equally important is the use of fresh pure air, sunshine, rest, exercise, mental poise and fasting.

"Healing is a physiological or biological process, from the inside, and is not something that can be brought about by treatments or cures. If we provide the conditions for disease, we must have disease. However, if we provide the conditions for health, we must have health. The important thing is to learn and put into practice the natural laws of health.

"We do not recommend the use of honey or milk which Dr. Nolfi mentions in the booklet. These are second-rate substances and do not qualify as *live foods.* They are also objectionable for many other reasons. Neither do we approve the use of such irritating foods as garlic, onions, radishes, endive, parsley, etc.

"We also believe that the program advocated by Dr. Nolfi can be improved by observing the rules for proper food combining, as explained in Dr. Shelton's book *Food Combining Made Easy,* and as illustrated on our 'Correct Food Combining Chart.'

"The primary value of this booklet by Dr. Nolfi is that it brings out the importance of raw foods for human nutrition.

"For other books and pamphlets on healthful living —

SUGGESTED READING

HS-66	Vol. II, *The Hygienic System — Foods & Feeding.* Herbert M. Shelton, N.D.
HS-68	*Food Combining Made Easy.* Herbert M. Shelton, N.D.
HS-69	*Superior Nutrition.* Herbert M. Shelton, N.D.
RC-102	Correct Food Combining Chart
RC-104	Shangri-La Food Program with Recipes
AD-61	*The Hygienic Way of Life — The Argument for Vegetarianism.* Hereward Carrington, Ph.D.
HS-61	*Introduction to Natural Hygiene.* Herbert M. Shelton, N.D.
HD-62	*Health Can Be Harmless.* H. Jay Dinshah
HS-71	*Getting Well.* Herbert M. Shelton, N.D.
HS-76	*Health For All.* Herbert M. Shelton, N.D.
JT-61	*Toxemia Explained.* John M. Tilden, M.D.
HS-104	*Animal Foods.* Herbert M. Shelton, N.D.
HS-106	*A Month of Menus.* Herbert M. Shelton, N.D.
HS-108	*Lumps in the Breast.* Herbert M. Shelton, N.D.
VV-101	*Can the Cancer Problem Be Solved?* Virginia Vetrano, D.O.

LC-61 *Discourses on the Sober Life – How to Live 100 Years.* Luigi Cornaro
GR-101 *The Case for Vegetarianism.* Geoffrey L. Rudd

CHAPTER 17

NEWS RELEASES

This book may not be as nearly complete as I would like, even though I have spent many months in its preparation. Unfortunately, anyone wishing to make the kind of study I made would necessarily spend months at the project. Otherwise, the seeker after knowledge must limit his information to that of whomever he might ask, or to the viewpoint of a group enthusiastically espousing one approach to cancer, while refusing to look at any other.

I cannot even tell you all I know, because those who sell books at double digit cost stake out their claims to territory. Thus some with a life-and-death problem may feel they cannot even afford to look.

Many who find they have cancer may reconcile themselves to death and refuse to look up again. They feel they cannot endure such anguish twice. Moreover, such may be denied the right to look up.

Speciously, those with copyrights may say that permission may be obtained to use material. What this means is that the owner of the copyright wishes to reserve the right to censor and censure any material containing anything of his.

With such requirements, writing for all releases would take more time than I might expect to live. I might well die from cancer myself, while waiting for releases necessary for an epistemological review, or a review, in terms of accumulated knowledge, rather than viewpoint.

I know how people may be affected by the kind of cultural cancer I describe, because of involvement locally through the International Association of Cancer Victims and Friends, and through involvement long before acquaintanceship with this organization, through relationship with research.

For those who use copyright laws against the public interest, for other than protection from exploitation through advertising or out-and-out plagiarism, I feel sorrow over what these people are doing to others.

I take no responsibility for all the viewpoints offered, however.

With this apology and explanation, I will provide some news stories. Out of tons of information, ultimately must come a meaningful program which may be followed by the public to prevent, and hopefully, to arrest cancer.

At the conclusion shall be offered a program intended to wipe out cancer, within ten years, hopefully. Should cancer prove to be essentially a nutritional illness, it could be wiped out in ten years.

CHAPTER 18

MICROORGANISMS

National Dairy Council

6300 North River Road, Rosemont, Illinois 60018 Telephone (312) 696-1020

Mr. J. Gordon Roberts
161 Flamingo Drive
Clearwater, FL 33516

Dear Mr. Roberts:

Your August 3 letter to National Dairy Council has been forwarded by the Dairy and Food Nutrition Council of Florida. We regret that prior deadlines prevented our answering sooner.

The periodical from which you wish to quote is "Nutrition, Diet, and Cancer," Dairy Council Digest, Vol. 46, No. 5, September-October 1975.* True, the Digest may be reproduced in whole or in part only with full citation and credit to National Dairy Council. Consequently, we request your use of the following: "Courtesy, Dairy Council Digest, National Dairy Council. National Dairy Council assumes no responsibility for the contents of this book other than the portion(s) excerpted from the Dairy Council Digest."

We would appreciate your sending a copy of the book upon its completion.

Sincerely,

Elwood W. Speckmann, Ph.D.
Director
Division of Nutrition Research

Since 1915—A Nonprofit Organization for Nutrition Research and Nutrition Education in the Use of Dairy Foods

The following article appeared in the *Nutrition News*, December, 1975, Vol. 38, No. 4, published by the National Dairy Council, 111 North Canal Street, Chicago, Illinois 60606. The author is Marvin L. Speck, Ph.D., William Neal Reynolds Professor of Food Science and Microbiology, North Carolina State University.

"Contributions of Microorganisms to Foods and Nutrition

"Roles of Microorganisms

"Microorganisms perform essential roles in aspects of man's existence, such as the fixation of atmospheric nitrogen for the growth of plants, the production of foods for direct human consumption, the production of antibiotics, and the disposal of organic waste materials.

"For the preservation and processing of foods, man has used various microorganisms for centuries. Cheeses, wines, fermented vegetables, etc., were the result of natural interactions between raw foods and microorganisms which allowed man to preserve the raw food for extended periods of time.

"Acids undoubtedly are among the most important preservative compounds produced when microorganisms bioconvert foods into fermented or cultured products.[1] Lactic acid is the primary acid produced by most of these cultures.

"As man has used cultured foods in his diet he has consumed vast quantities of the lactic acid bacteria in foods such as buttermilk, yogurt, cheeses of various types, sauerkraut, pickles, cured meats, and other foods that depend on the controlled actions of various microorganisms for their production. Lactobacilli have been reported to produce various antibiotics.

"Lactobacillus in Digestive Tract

"Certain lactic acid bacteria have established a beneficial ecological relationship with humans which begins at the time of birth and persists throughout life. Especially important among these microorganisms are the lactobacilli. Soon after birth the digestive tract is colonized by a variety of microorganisms.[2] Among the first present are the lactobacilli which originate in the maternal vagina during birth of the child. During puberty Doderlein's bacillus, which is considered to be identical with *Lactobacillus acidophilus,* establishes itself as a predominant vaginal microorganism. In addition to its microbial interactions, it provides inoculum to the infant during birth.

"As a consequence of breast feeding a stable microflora develops in the intestinal tract within several days. The microflora of the infant's fecal contents consists mostly of Lactobacillus bifidus (bifidobacteria). There is a drastic reduction or even absence of putrefactive bacteria which had colonized the intestinal tract before breast feeding began. In infants being bottle fed, the fecal microflora is more typical of that of the adult.

"The stomach contains only a few indigenous microorganisms. The predominant flora in the small intestine has recently been reported to be *Lactobacillus acidophilus.* The ileum (last section of small intestine) is colonized with bacteria that are representative of those in the colon but in fewer numbers. The largest number of microorganisms in the intestinal tract occurs in the colon. There is some variation in the microflora of different age groups; that of adults is the most stable.

"Need for Research

"The needs for information on various activities of the intestinal microflora outweigh existing knowledge of specific roles. Relatively little is known about changes in the microflora resulting from changes in dietary intakes. Metabolic activities of intestinal bacteria have been associated with cancer of the colon. It has been hypothesized that carcinogens were produced from dietary components, or from intestinal secretions produced in response to the diet. However, much research is needed to establish actual causal mechanisms of cancer in spite of suggestive evidence linking the intestinal microflora with cancer.

"Fermented Milk and Cholesteremia

"A very interesting study has recently been reported on the relationship between fermented milk in the diet and cholesteremia in a Maasai tribe. After a diet, primarily of meat for two days, 24 warriors, aged 16 to 23 years,[3] ate only fermented milk made with a wild culture of a Lactobacillus for three weeks. Half consumed milk to which a surfactant (emulsifier) had been added. The study was designed primarily to determine the effect of a dietary surfactant on cholesteremia, but the greatest impact from the study was that serum cholesterol was reduced. The surfactant had only a minor, if any, influence on cholesteremia in the men. Average daily fermented milk consumption was 8.33 liters. Eight of the men increased their weight by six or more pounds, and their cholesterol decreased an average of 28 mg per 100 ml; 16 men gained five or less pounds and showed a cholesterol decrease of 8.19 mg per 100 ml. The authors concluded that the fermented milk furnished a factor(s) that impaired the synthesis of cholesterol and thus led to a lowering of serum cholesterol level. It would appear possible, however, that with such a massive intake of lactobacilli the intestinal microflora could have been very drastically altered which degraded bile acids or cholesterol and promoted their excretion in the feces. Obviously more information is needed on the relationship of the intestinal microflora to functions that may affect cholesterol levels.

"Increasing Dietary L. acidophilus

"At the turn of the present century, a theory was proposed by Metchnikoff that inhabitants of the Balkan countries had an unusually long life span because of the large quantities of lactobacillus fermented milk that they drank. This sparked much interest in using *Lactobacillus acidophilus* to alter the microflora of the intestinal tract to contain primarily this microorganism. Not all of the reports agreed on the merits of acidophilus milk, but the majority indicated beneficial results when the L. acidophilus was fed.[4] This product had a demise, however, owing to difficulties in its manufacture and its unsavory flavor. In more recent years, impetus to the feeding of lactobacilli has resulted from the increased use of antibiotics. Antibiotics alter the intestinal microflora and intestinal discomfort results caused by flatulence and diarrhea. Replenishing the intestinal tract with L. acidophilus results in an accelerated return to normalcy in the intestinal microflora and body comfort.

"Contrary to the beliefs by earlier workers that beneficial effects from feeding lactobacilli depend on replacing other types of bacteria in the intestinal tract, evidence now indicates that the maintenance of a proper balance among the various normal inhabitants of the intestinal tract is needed.

"In Europe various products have been developed which have taken advantage of the increased consumption of yogurt for use as a carrier for *Lactobacillus acidophilus.* The usual cultures involved in yogurt manufacture (*L. bulgaricus and S. thermophilus*) are not microorganisms that establish in the intestinal tract. However, efforts have been made to add *Lactobacillus acidophilus* as one of the component strains for yogurt manufacture. This seems to have met with little if any success because the *L. acidophilus* is too easily overgrown by the other two strains. However, different yogurt products have been marketed which are made by adding a preparation of *L. acidophilus.*

"The most recent product introduced in the United States is a lowfat milk to which *Lactobacillus acidophilus* has been added. Unpublished results have indicated that this acidophilus product does result in the increased numbers of *L. acidophilus* in feces.

"Evidence is increasing that there is a definite place in the American diet for products containing lactobacilli. While a number of foods can be used to carry the *L. acidophilus,* milk has many of the preferred characteristics for such purposes.

"There is an interesting and close relationship between microorganisms used in preservative food fermentation and those inhabiting different parts of the human body. Many metabolic interactions of the microorganism involved in food bioconversions have been clarified; extended and new applications now appear possible for their use in prolonging the safety and shelf-life of modern foods. While basic information on the role of the intestinal microflora still is in its infancy, information is developing rapidly on the metabolic functions of the intestinal microflora and should provide a guide for its more judicious control.

"References

"[1] Speck, M. L. 1972. Control of food-borne pathogens by starter cultures. J. Dairy Sci. 55:1019-1022

"[2] Haenel, H. 1970 Human normal and abnormal gastrointestinal flora. Am. J. Clin. Nutr. 23:1422-1439

"[3] Mann, G. V., and Spoerry, A. 1974. Studies of a surfactant and cholesteremia in the Maasai. Am. J. Clin. Nutr. 27:464-469

"[4] Sandine, W. E., Muralidhara, K. S., Elliker, P. R. and England, D.C. 1972. Lactic acid bacteria in food and health: A review with special reference to enteropathogenic Escherichia coli as well as certain enteric diseases and their treatment with antibiotics and lactobacilli. I. Milk and Food Tech. 35:691-702.

"About the Author

"Marvin L. Speck, Ph.D.

"The awards of Dr. Speck, William Neal Reynolds Professor of Food Science and Microbiology, North Carolina State University, include the Borden Award in Dairy Manufacturing, the Pfizer-Lewis Award in Cheese Research, and being a World Health Organization Fellow.

"He is Chairman of the Inter-Society Committee for the Development of Compendium of Methods for the Microbiological Examination of Foods, American Public Health Association; a special consultant for the U.S. Public Health Service, and the Pan American Health Organization.

"Many of Dr. Neal's 133 publications have been on his research in nutrition and metabolism of starter bacteria, concentrated starter bacteria, intestinal microflora, and bacterial injury by environmental stresses.

"The Vitamin Conspiracy, 1975

"By John J. Fried, New York: E. J. Dutton, *Saturday Review* Press

"Mr. Fried thoroughly reports his review of the literature and his interviews with proponents and opponents of megavitamin therapy in answering the question, 'Is vitamin therapy beneficial or harmful and dangerous?'

"The author traces the development of megavitamin therapy and gives the reasoning of its proponents, emphasizing the claims and counterclaims about vitamin E for the treatment of heart disease, niacin for the control of schizophrenia, and vitamin C for resistance to colds. He points out that vitamin therapy enthusiasts believe there is no reason why their theories should not work, but that scientifically designed investigations by leading medical researchers have not proved the theories. If vitamin therapy was only ineffective and a waste of money ($700 million annually), he says it would not be disturbing, but there can be dangerous consequences of megavitamin therapy and of self-prescribed daily vitamin supplementation.

"The author challenges the scientific nutrition community to communicate more effectively with the public; and he blasts the mass media for helping spread unscientific claims.

"The Vitamin Conspiracy suggests that a massive new program to educate physicians and the public is the logical answer to the vitamin dilemma, to assist Americans to be well nourished, and free them from the influence of faddists.

"The Vitamin Conspiracy is an impartial book recommended for fascinating, factual reading by professionals and laymen alike.

"From National Dairy Council, 6300 River Road, Rosemont, Illinois 60018.

"Sour Cream . . . Convenience Food with a Gourmet Touch. 7¢

"A sheet covering sour cream's new standards; processing; role in the diet; shopping, storage, ad serving tips.

"Yogurt . . . Ancient Food with Modern Ways. 5¢

"A sheet presenting yogurt's history; shopping, storage, and serving; tips; and the nutrient content of different types of yogurt.

"Opinions expressed in *Nutrition News* articles are those of the authors."

CHAPTER 19

NATURAL HYGIENE NEWS

The *Natural Hygiene's,* which is the membership publication of the American Natural Hygiene Society, Inc., Winter 1976, Special Edition, contained an article from the *St. Petersburg Times,* Monday, December 1, 1975, 5A. "(Natural Hygiene is a way of life, the only normal way of life. It is not a branch of the healing arts. No physician, doctor, drug, or any medication or treatment of any kind can curé anything. The body is self healing when the basic needs of life are supplied. Our organization is, therefore, devoted to the primary principle of teaching people how to live healthfully.)" The article is as follows:

"Cancer may get start in the diet

By Al Rossiter, Jr., United Press International
"Washington

"Diet may have a role in half of all cancers in women and in a third of those affecting men, a public health authority said in a report published Sunday.

"Dr. Ernst L. Wynder said that studies made around the world suggest that cancers of the stomach, colon, breast, kidney, bladder, pancreas and prostate and possibly leukemia may be directly or indirectly related to nutrition. He said some of the research leads appear especially promising and should be actively pursued.

"He said diet may influence cancer genesis three ways:

"✓ In the form of nutrietns, additives or contaminants that start, promote or accelerate cancer growth.

"✓ As dietary deficiencies leading to biochemical abnormalities, which, in turn, may initiate cancer processes.

"√ In the form of nutritional excesses that may induce metabolic abnormalities that could promote cancers.

"Too much of some kinds of food may be particularly important in developing cancers. Wynder said, citing an ancient writing that 'it is the dosage that makes the poison.'

" 'As a matter of public health, it seems prudent to suggest that all individuals should lower their intake of total fat calories and cholesterol,' he said in concluding remarks at the conference."

The following article also appeared in the *St. Petersburg Times* on Monday, January 19, 1976, and was published in the same edition of *Natural Hygienews.*

"Cutting of cancer death rate hinges on risk factor knowledge: study

"By Stuart Auerbach, *Washington Post*

"Washington

"What causes cancer? From recent headlines it sometimes appears that everything does; jobs, food, worry, smoking, air pollution, family background, chemicals, viruses, alcohol, sex.

"A study released Sunday by the National Cancer Institute and the American Cancer Society shows that those factors and others play a part in causing different forms of cancer – the most feared illness and the second leading killer of Americans.

"The study shows clearly that there is probably no single cause, nor single cure for cancer. Rather the disease is caused by two, three or even more factors working together."

The *St. Petersburg Times,* Thursday, December 11, 1975, edition contained an article by Jane E. Brody (c), *New York Times,* under the heading of 'medicine,' as follows:

"Cancer

"The complexity of the diseases called cancer are overlooked in the profusion of discoveries about its possible causes.

New York

"Hardly a week goes by without a new report that some previously unsuspected substance has been found to cause cancer. Thus far, the scientists have pinpointed more than 1,000 agents as definite or suspected causes of cancer in man.

"In recent years, such agents — called carcinogens — have been discovered in the air we breathe, the water we drink, the foods we eat, the clothes we wear, the drugs we take, the jobs we hold, the habits we pursue.

"Last week three new reports were released on cancer causes — one stating that a number of common cancers may be caused, directly or indirectly, by ordinary components of the daily diet; a second linking the use of estrogens during and after menopause to an increased risk of developing uterine cancer and a third describing a high rate of skin cancer among workers who produce synthetic fuels.

"Fats in the diet do not appear to directly change cells from normal to cancerous. Rather, the fats are believed to change the metabolism in ways that render organs like the colon and breast more susceptible to cancer. Yet, even if a fatty diet is only an indirect cause of cancer, a change in that diet would lower a person's cancer risk.

"For example, at a conference last week on the genetic aspects of cancer, a survey of 5,000 persons was described. It showed that, on a routine checkup, nearly 10 per cent of those who had a parent or sibling with cancer were also found to have cancer. If two immediate relatives had cancer, risk was 16 per cent, and it jumped to 22 per cent — more than one in five — for persons with three or more cancer victims among their close relatives."

The following article appeared in the *Sunday World Herald,* Omaha, September 25, 1966 – 15 B:

"N.U. Man Says Milk May Help Stop Cancer

"A University of Nebraska scientist said Saturday that milk, the mother fluid of human life, may hold a key to saving that life from cancer.

"Dr. K. M. Shahani said he has slight indications that he is on the trail of a cancer-fighting agent.

"'But every hopeful hint of the existence of such an agent must be followed up. I believe we have such a hint here at Nebraska,' he said.

"Dr. Shahani's anti-tumor substance comes from some of the microorganisms that cause milk to sour.

"'It has long been known that fermented (sour) milk products could be used successfully in treating a variety of infectious diseases,' he said. 'However, a search of the scientific literature a few years ago revealed very little research had been done to find out if such products had any effect on cancer.'

"This sparked his study. The India-born scientist was encouraged with a grant from the Roberts Dairy Company of Omaha.

CHAPTER 20

CANCER AS A MATHEMATICAL PROBLEM

Usually the cause of cancer is considered the unknown.

In this book, what prevents cancer has been considered the unknown.

Normal life is considered a form of negative entropy, the force which somehow keeps the universe from cooling off.

Looking at cell-life as from a blimp high in the air, we observe that "cancer" cells are the normal ones in terms of all the cells on this planet. Those cells which maintain a direct, interdependent relationship are unusual and comparatively rare.

People consider wakefulness the normal condition, with some taking pills to go to sleep. But the body requires a device to induce wakefulness. Sleep is "normal."

Cancer is "normal" unless prevented.

Looking at cancer in this fashion, we may not pass over the reason that newborn babies are almost entirely free of cancer as irrelevant to the problem of prevention.

Let's look at the newborn as an example of preventing cancer. Such a look also requires looking at milk.

Milk contains carbohydrates and proteins which may produce digestive conflict.

The fat in milk may act as a mediator, forcing the antagonists to "cool off," through delaying digestion. For proteins and carbohydrates in conflict may produce poison, putrefaction.

Nature, however, does more than provide fat in the milk of those mammals requiring it. Nature provides bacteria which work against putrefaction.

Bifidus in the case of the nursing human mother.

Is bifidus present in milk as an anti-cancer agent? If not, why is it there?

This book has examined the foregoing and other questions from the premise indicated. From such a premise, in one way, cancer may be similar to alcoholism. There may be no "cure," at best a way to arrest "entropy."

Dr. Sydney Webb, in his book, *Nutrition. Time and Motion in Metabolism and Genetios,* indicates that cellular organization depends upon "time clocks." Should such be the case, how might this be possible without a wave of time of finite dimension?

Uri Geller told me there is no such thing as time, but according to this book, there is, for all practical purposes.

THE ROLE OF L. BIFIDUS

One cancer theory assumes that cancer cells and the trophoblast cells of early pregnancy are virtually the same.

Do bifidus bacteria perform any function in controlling trophoblasts?

Bifidus bacteria are virtually the same as Doderlein's bacteria. Doderlein's bacteria increase in the vaginal tract, at pregnancy, according to material I have read.

The trophoblast cells perform like cancer cells in embedding themselves at pregnancy, to be fed by the placenta.

Cancer cells, imbedded into a hamster, will be nourished by a circulatory system which develops to feed them, according to Dr. Solomon Garb.

Are all these factors coincidental? And in relation to what? I don't pretend to know. I just wonder.

You'll read more later from those who declare they have more answers.

CHAPTER 21

CREIGHTON UNIVERSITY WORK ON CANCER – THE KIND OF WORK OFFERING BASIC ANSWERS

The following article appeared in the Creighton University *Alumnews,* Omaha, Nebraska, February, 1976, by Dr. Henry T. Lynch.

"The Cancer Family: Life-and-death detective work
pays off for preventive medicine physicians
and their patients

"On this and following pages the Department of Preventive Medicine and Public Health is featured. The research and teaching efforts described here are only a part of the work being done in that School of Medicine department.

"While Dr. Henry Lynch was a resident in internal medicine at the University of Nebraska Medical Center, he encountered a patient who announced that since everyone else in his family had died of cancer, he presumed he would, too.

"The patient did die of cancer and the encounter sparked Dr. Lynch's curiosity about the possibility that some persons inherit a susceptibility to cancer.

"Now Dr. Lynch, chairman of the Department of Preventive Medicine and Public Health in Creighton's School of Medicine, is recognized as the researcher who described the Cancer Family Syndrome.

"Dr. Lynch, working with other members of Creighton's faculty and with researchers at other medical centers, is continuing his study of the Cancer Family Syndrome and his work is leading to even more discoveries about genetics and cancer as well as some other diseases.

"Syndrome

"A syndrome is a group of features which, when occuring together, add up to a disease. In the genetic system the features repeat themselves, passing from one generation to the next in much the same pattern. In this disease the mode of genetic transmission is referred to as a Mendelian dominant.

"Researchers from Creighton, working with colleagues in other parts of the U.S. and some foreign countries, have traced some 15 'cancer families' involving thousands of relatives.

"From the first description of the Cancer Family Syndrome, other discoveries have been made. Five hereditary breast cancer syndromes have been described by Dr. Lynch and his Creighton team and are currently among the discoveries being classified in the medical literature.

"The research program under Dr. Lynch's direction involved extensive travel, precise gathering of medical samples under difficult field conditions and complex record keeping.

"Groups

"'We have developed an approach to cancer genetics which is based on large groups of related persons,' Dr. Lynch said. 'It means studying the causes of morbidity and mortality of all types but particularly cancer in all available relatives. We have to document the causes with good pathology and genealogic correlation. The process involves pathologists, biostatisticians and epidemiologists working to provide a comprehensive approach to cancer genetics.'

"Members of a 'cancer family' face a greater than average risk of developing cancer but the factors that may cause the cancer to develop aren't the same in every family.

"Research conducted by the Creighton team in conjunction with the Michigan Cancer Foundation reveals that an estimated seven percent of the population are prone to develop cancer in a familial pattern, Dr. Lynch said.

"Familial

" 'But being in that seven percent category doesn't necessarily mean the cause is genetic,' Dr. Lynch said. 'It means cancer develops in a familial pattern, but the cause could involve environmental factors in concert with genetic factors. It could mean a family has a suceptibility so that members are prone to certain environmental cancer-causing agents.'

" 'We know that every one who smokes doesn't develop cancer of the lung,' Dr. Lynch said. 'But we also know there are families prone to cancer wherein no member of that family should ever smoke. Their smoking is like playing Russian roulette with two or three cartridges in the gun – Of course nobody should smoke in the first place.'

"Difference

"What is 'different' about cancer families? Laboratory research is being conducted to find out. One theory currently under investigation relates to body enzymes. An enzyme has been discovered that seems to have some association with lung cancer, for example. One of Dr. Lynch's associates, Dr. Hoda Guirgis, is experimenting with the apparent fact that the enzyme runs in families and that one form of the enzyme appears to correlate with lung cancer in smokers.

"Some observers have suggested that all of the causes of Cancer Family Syndrome can be attributed to environmental causes. To test that possibility, Dr. Lynch studied a family of 2,000 members both in the U.S. and in Western Europe. The visit to Germany by Dr. Lynch and Mrs. Lynch revealed that:

" 'It didn't make any difference whether they were migrants who settled in the U.S., whether they entered the ministry, law or farming,' Dr. Lynch said. 'Because we found the same pattern of cancer occurrences among the family members who didn't leave Germany.'

"Value

"Doubt about the existence of the syndrome has now been erased, Dr. Lynch said. It is now described in medical textbooks.

"The value of knowing about the syndrome is the ability to protect the lives of members of 'cancer families' by early detection or avoidance of certain cancer-causing agents.

"Members of families with Cancer Family Syndrome are subject to a higher than normal rate of organ-related cancers of all types but particularly those associated with the colon and lining of the uterus (endometrium). The cancers occur at an earlier age than is typical, occur at more than one primary site, and are inherited in a dominant genetic manner.

"Dr. Lynch cites this example of how knowledge of the syndrome can help prevent cancer deaths:

"In a Pennsylvania family there were 40-year-old twins. One of the identical twins developed uterine (endometrial) cancer. Since there was a well-developed history of such cancer in the family, the twin sister of the above affected patient underwent examination and the same cancer was discovered. The cancer was discovered early enough to save her life.

"When the twins' brother developed a colon cancer, the first twin to discover uterine cancer requested a proctoscopic examination. The test, a visual inspection of the colon wall, revealed an early cancer, again found in time to be removed surgically.

"Although Dr. Lynch can point to numerous cases where knowledge of the abnormally high risk of cancer led to early diagnosis, he believes a more formal system of recording cancer families and notifying them of the increased risk would be a worthwhile preventive medicine program. He proposes to center the national network at Creighton.

" 'It is my idea and I know how to do it,' Dr. Lynch said. 'I am embarassed at its simplicity but it is needed now and could save lives.'

"What Dr. Lynch proposes is a series of regional networks that would collect relevant data about cancer patients and feed the information to a national center. By use of computer programming, pedigrees would be compiled, physicians caring for persons with hereditary cancers would be notified and the nature of the increased risk outlined in detail. Dr. Lynch believes computer technology would then make it easy to spell out exact diagnostic procedures to be followed by the attending physician, directing him to cancer risk involving specific organs, and the most up-to-date recommendations for the management and therapy of patients. The Creighton team will be submitting their proposals to the National Cancer Institute.

"Skin

"In another cancer educational program designed to produce early detection, a family prone to develop skin cancers (malignant melanoma) has been provided a printed card that pictures skin conditions at very early stages to be reported if they develop. The innovation, developed by Dr. Lynch and University of Nebraska-Creighton Dr. Bert C. Frichot is now being copied by others, including colleagues at the National Cancer Institute.

"Dr. Lynch recently made national headlines by reporting that the ability to predict that certain cancers are likely to develop had led to recommendations of preventive surgery. In one case, where the risk for the patient developing cancer was approximately 50 percent, a young woman had both breasts surgically removed. 'This is not a blanket endorsement for prophylactic mastectomy,' Dr. Lynch said. 'Rather, it is a decision that must be made on the merits of risk factors in a specific family.'

"Too extreme? 'Death is extreme, too,' Dr. Lynch said. He added that seven of the nation's top cancer surgeons backed his decision with no dissent.

"Dr. Lynch's work is not restricted to cancer. A Creighton team from Preventive Medicine and Cardiology is working on a syndrome discovered in the area of cardiovascular disease. Work in that area is being partially funded through a grant from the Nebraska Division of the American Heart Association.

"Other funding for his research comes from the National Cancer Institute, National Institutes of Health and the Fraternal Order of Eagles."

CHAPTER 22

NEBRASKA METHODIST HOSPITAL RECORDS

The following article appeared in *Pulse Beat*, Volume 12, Number 1, 1976, Nebraska Methodist Hospital, Omaha, Nebraska:

"'Presently 5,867 cancer patients are being followed through the Hunt Tumor Registry'

"When statistical reports are prepared, cases in the Hunt Tumor Registry are categorized by the part of the body where the cancer was diagnosed. Showing both male and female cases, the registry indicates the extent of the disease in patients when diagnosed, and also computes the survival rate for the patients after both a three-year and five-year period.

"The Nebraska Methodist Hospital tumor program has received accreditation from the American College of Surgeons. Dr. Karrer explains that certain requirements must be met for a tumor registry program to receive accreditation. To have an accredited registry, Nebraska Methodist Hospital must have a 95 percent follow-up rate for patients and also must have an on-going cancer education program. 'The Hunt Tumor Registry is working above the 95 percent rate and our weekly tumor conferences at the hospital satisfy the other requirement,' says Dr. Karrer. The entire Tumor Registry Program is supervised by a multi-specialty physician committee that meets monthly.

"There are presently 5,867 cancer patients being followed through the Hunt Tumor Registry, says Dr. Karrer. 'I think that our use of the Hunt Tumor Registry has a reassuring effect on many of our patients,' says Dr. Karrer. The patients know that their condition is being followed and studied and they are directly helping us find new avenues in treating and curing our cancer patients in the future."

CHAPTER 23

THE FAMILY CIRCLE MAGAZINE OFFERS MEDICAL MATERIAL ON MAGNESIUM

The following article appeared in the magazine *Family Circle,* March, 1971, written by John Prutting, M.D., with Pat Curtis. Dr. Prutting, a practicing internist in New York City, serves on the medical board of Doctors Hospital, New York. He is president of the Foundation for the Advancement of Medical Knowledge, and has published numerous professional papers. Excerpts follow:

"The Miracle Mineral That Keeps You Fit
(Abridged)

"A 33-year-old woman sat in her doctor's office feeling very depressed. Her physical complaints were that she felt tired and weak. But what upset her most was that she couldn't remember things the way she used to and felt unable to cope with her household. She had what is sometimes called 'housewife blues.'

"The doctor gave her magnesium by injection and put her on a high-magnesium diet. Within two weeks her symptoms had cleared. She felt more energetic, she could handle her housework and she could remember names and appointments as well as ever.

"Magnesium is especially important as an activator of enzymes through which we use protein and vitamins. It also helps the utilization of potassium. Magnesium starts the chain reaction in the body to metabolize (make use of) food. In fact, many of the nutrients we consume do us no good unless magnesium is present in the proper amount. For example, undernourished hospitalized patients given large doses of thiamin (B_1) and other vitamins by injection remained deficient in those same vitamins till magnesium was added to the injections; then the vitamin deficiencies cleared. Similarly, doctors working with children suffering protein-calcium malnutrition have noted that vitamins and minerals do not help these children without the addition of magnesium.

"Excessive use of alcohol is often the culprit in magnesium deficiency."

CHAPTER 24

ABSENCE OF ADEQUATE INFORMATION ABOUT ENZYMES

Here is illustrated the lack of adequate information on enzymes to judge fully their role in health. The following are excerpts from Research Papers.

"Enzymes in Bovine Milk: A Review[1]

by

"K. M. Shahani, Department of Food Science, University of Nebraska, Lincoln 68503

"W. J. Harper, Department of Food Science and Nutrition, Ohio State University, Columbus 43210

"R. G. Jensen, Department of Nutritional Sciences, University of Connecticut, Storrs 06268

"R. M. Parry, Jr., and C. A. Zittle, Eastern Marketing and Nutrition Research Division, USDA, ARS, Philadelphia, Pennsylvania 19118

"Abstract"

"During the past few years the Committee on Enzyme Nomenclature of the Manufacturing Section of the American Dairy Science Association has collected data on numerous enzymes in bovine milk. At least 20 enzymes have been either purified or isolated from milk or definitely identified to be native constituents of milk. However, nomenclature is not uniform; neither does their exist any uniformity among the assay procedures, substrates used, or units expressed concerning the same enzyme by various workers."

Received for publication July 14, 1972.

"[1] Report of the committee on Enzyme Nomenclature, Manufacturing Section of the American Dairy Science Association."

CHAPTER 25

HERBS – SORRY, I CAN'T OFFER MORE BUT I CAN'T FIND PUBLISHER

The following is from *Nature's Healing Grasses,* by H. E. Kirschner, M.D., Chapter 1, entitled "Remedial Properties of Herbs."

"Visitors to my Yucaipa (California) garden have been surprised to see so many beds devoted to the growing of alfalfa, mint, spearmint, parsley, comfrey, dandelion, thyme, and other simple grasses and herbs. 'Doctor,' they ask, 'just why do you *waste* so much valuable space on all these *weeds*?"

"Perhaps *you* would wonder too; so in order to clear up the mystery of my herb garden, I am writing this little book dealing with the therapeutic value of simple herbs – including some common, everyday wayside grasses and weeds as dandelion, filaree, mustard, lamb's quarter and malva. You may be surprised as I was to learn that you have a wealth of medicinal plants at your very finger-tips – and all for *free!*

"What can herbs and grasses do for you? Scientists have discovered that they are essential to make gastric juices flow; that it is through their pleasing flavor that the 'appetite juices' start digestion. They should be freely used in place of salt, pepper and vinegar.

"The great remedial properties of herbs and juices of fruits and vegetables have been recognized and appreciated from time immemorial, especially by primitive peoples. In fact, herbal healing was the first system of healing that the world ever knew, and its effectiveness all through the centuries has never been questioned."

CHAPTER 26

SLEEP AND CANCER

Charles C. Chapple, M.D., wrote "Developmental Defects: Some Thoughts on Their Causes," under *Birth Defects*, Original Article Series, Vol. VIII, No. 6, September, 1972, published by the National Foundation - March of Dimes.

He makes what appear to me as remarkable statements. For example, on page 65, he declares estrogen and adrenaline may each cure rickets and scurvy.

"Estrogen and cortisone reduce lymph tissue similarly. But cortisone and progesterone have a relaxing effect in common. Adrenaline resembles estrogen in raising blood pressure and these hormones have some similarity in their stimulatory effect on muscular activity, but there is a difference in degree. Normally, the promptness of response to adrenaline is almost electric and its amplitude is great. Adrenaline's influence on mental attitude is not pleasant. Normally, the response to estrogen is slow in coming, never out of bounds in degree and might be described as a manifestation of an increase in efficiency."

On page 62, he declares that high levels of the hormone, progesterone, are associated with high electrical resistance of the skin, anaesthetic, and, therefore, involved with an increase in skin resistance with the onset of sleep.

"In addition, since progesterone increases the spread, it is not unexpected that high progesterone levels are associated with high electrical resistance of skin. Again, since there is every reason to believe that a similar effect would take place concurrently elsewhere, it seems logical that the nervous system would be included in the response. This may be important in the phenomenon called sleep because it is unlikely to be an accident that the hormone is an anaesthetic and that an increase in skin resistance occurs with the onset of sleep."

On page 65 he says that estrogen and progesterone are antagonists; presumably having an opposite effect on skin resistance.

What is the point of all this, in relation to cancer?

Already, a possible relationship of free radicals to cancer has been indicated.

It is just possible that rest may represent a factor in cell normalcy, and that drugs and alcohol may interfere with such normalcy.

A combination of cigarettes and alcohol may increase cancer incidence by fifteen times, according to an account in the *St. Petersburg Times*, March 30, 1976.

The figures were offered by Dr. Marvin Schneiderman of the National Cancer Institute, based upon information gathered by Dr. Kenneth Rothman of Harvard.

Gay Gaer Luce wrote *Body Time*, Pantheon Books, a division of Random House, New York, 1971.

One section is titled, "Cancer Rhythms in Rodents," and another "Human Cancer." According to this book, cancer cells appear to be arhythmic as compared to normal cells.

The book also shows that hormones may have a rhythm of activity. Even enzymes appear to have rhythms of their own.

Again, the point is made that drugs may alter rhythms. It would seem advisable for any doctor, or anyone in cancer research, to read the aforementioned book, because prescription drugs may be involved and results may occur after the conclusion of use.

Should there be any rhythm to protection against cancer, the manner of protecting the newborn during a period of extremely rapid cell proliferation might well be relative to the prevention and arrest of cancer. This thought entered into looking at bacteria in human milk, in the first place.

The material in the "Addendum" of Dr. Chapple's book on birth defects might be relevant:

"Recently an old Omaha friend, Gordon Roberts, noted that my paper propounds the thesis that physiologic laws are not inexplicably reversed, and suggested that if a low incidence of cancer existed in the unborn it would seem worthwhile to learn the factors which protect at that stage of life in order to duplicate them, if possible, as preventive or therapeutic measures for the born. Interested, but uninformed, I turned to the old reliable authority, Potter and Adair's *Fetal and Neonatal Death,*[1] and found there a literature survey of congenitally malignant tumors by H. G. Wells (not otherwise identified). In it he reported that before birth a malignancy of any nature is rare indeed, and that he had found no instance of carcinoma, not even a suspected one. If this survey is a true indication of the occurrence rate, and there is no apparent reason to doubt that it is, the resistance against carcinoma appears to be as transcendental as the fetal insusceptibility to all teratogens. The universal factor this time would seem to be the hormonal balance which maintains pregnancy. Be that as it may, this suggestion by a layman may well offer cancer research a new sector."

[1]Potter, E. L. and Adair, F. L.: *Fetal and Neonatal Death,* The University of Chicago Press, Chicago, 1949.

CHAPTER 27

ONE VERSION OF LAETRILE – THE STORM GATHERS

A review of data on the cancer remedy known as "laetrile" has been made by representatives of the Cancer Control Agency of B.C., Canadian Cancer Society, B.C. & Yukon Division, and British Columbia Medical Association. Additional data was obtained from the American Cancer Society, the Sloan-Kettering Institute and the National Cancer Institute of Canada. The following statement has been prepared for dissemination in the Province of British Columbia.

"1. *Chemistry*

"A. 'Laetrile' is a commercial product sold in several forms for oral and parenteral use. One source currently being promoted is dried apricot pits. Amygdalin, said to be the primary substance in these products, is a molecule containing 2 glucose moieties linked to mandelonitrile, a molecule containing benzaldehyde and hydrogen cyanide.

"B. It is hypothesized by the proponents of 'laetrile' that:

"(a) there is a larger amount of beta glucosidase in tumors than in normal tissues. (This hypothesis has never had any data to support it; however, experimental data show *no* differences.)

"(b) amygdalin therefore should be selectively toxic to tumor cells. (No evidence has been adduced to support this, but laboratory studies showed no effect of 'laetrile' when added directly to human or animal cancer cells.)

"(c) beta glucuronidase in human tissue splits amygdalin into active products. (This enzyme is high in some tumors, but is incapable of splitting amygdalin, which would require a glucosidase.)

"(d) hydrocyanic acid is preferentially released by tumors from amygdalin or mandelonitrite. (There is no evidence for this, and substantial evidence that any cyanide produced from dietary or other cancer is rapidly converted to non-toxic cyanates.)

"(e) hydrocyanic acid is selectively toxic to tumor cells. (There is no evidence for this and substantial studies show similar toxicity of HCN to normal and malignant tissues.)

"(f) tumors have less rhodanase than normal tissues and hence cannot protect themselves against HCN. (Assays of this enzyme have shown no such differences.)

"C. It has been stated by its promoters that laetrile is a B Vitamin, numbered 17. (A vitamin is a trace substance required for the maintenance of health; much evidence has accumulated on the growth of tissues in culture from many species of animals, including man, on purified diets containing no amygdalin, that such tissues will grow quite normally. Lacking legal restriction of the use of the word 'vitamin' any substance can be so described and sold so long as it is not claimed to be effective in the treatment of disease.) (There is no vitamin of the B complex that is recognized in human nutrition as Vitamin B^{17}," U.S. District Court, Central District of California, April 18, 1975.)

"D. The amygdalin in apricot pits could, following oral ingestion and hydrolysis by gastric juices, cause serious toxicity to infants and weakened adults.

"2. *Effectiveness: Anti-tumor activity*

"A. *In animals,* recent extensive studies have shown no evidence of shrinkage of tumors, nor prolongation of life of animals with tumors. These were conducted by: Dr. Kanematsu Sugiura - Sloan-Kettering; Dr. Daniel S. Martin - Catholic Medical Center; A. D. Little Inc. - Cambridge, Mass.; Southern Research Institute - Birmingham, Ala.

"The tumors used included spontaneous rodent breast cancers, and L1210, P388 leukemias, B16 melanomas, rat Walker tumors and mouse Lewis lung tumors.

"B. *In humans,* extensive trials at numerous centers have produced no evidence for anti-tumor effect.

"A review of cases submitted by 'laetrile' proponents to the U.S.F.D.A., to an Independent panel of U.S. experts, to the U.S.N.C.I., to the California Cancer Commission, to the Canadian F.D.A., and to the Canadian Medical Association Journal, have been determined to show *no* anti-tumor effects.

"The publications referred to by 'laetrile' proponents represent testimonial cases in non-peer-reviewed journals. Mrs. Cecile Hoffman, who promoted 'laetrile' after taking it and being 'cured' died in 1969 on July 19, of the same cancer.

"Analgesic Activity — There are standard scientific methods for the evaluation of pain-relieving and appetite-inducing remedies. No positive data using these uniform methods have been produced by the sellers of 'laetrile.'

"In many analgesic trials, the so-called 'placebo' effect can result in 25% beneficial effects. This is in the range claimed by 'laetrile' proponents.

"3. *Dangers.*

"The potential for toxicity occurs when amygdalin is taken orally. 'CAUTION, Laetrile . . . is NOT TO BE TAKEN ORALLY.' This is an exact quotation from a laetrile brochure printed by the McNaughton Foundation, Danys Press, Montreal, 1962.

" 'Due to its hydrogen cyanide content, Aprikern is unfit for food.' (U.S. District Court, Central District of California, No. CV73-2917-MML, April 18, 1975.)

"More importantly, that as 'bad money drives out good money' quack remedy proponents tend to discourage patients from taking effective drugs. There is an increasing number of effective new drugs, and for which the new Cancer Control Agency of B.C. has mounted a major new program.

"4. *Conspiracy.*

"A. The Federal Governments of Canada and the U.S.A. have always been prepared to accept for study new data presented by the developers of potentially helpful agents. (Most drug companies take losses on new cancer drugs because of the high cost of development, and low sales volumes.) These federal agencies and others have examined all data provided by 'laetrile' retailers and found no evidence of effect. To expect the taxpayers' money to be used to re-examine this material in the absence of new data from the proponents would be irresponsible.

"B. To use tax dollars to test any new agent in the absence of data from the seller would require that the government spend thousands of dollars to study 'hunches' about, for example, the possible anti-cancer effects of MacMillan-Bloedel sawdust, or of salmon by-products. Cancer care in B.C. is cost-free. Who would be the beneficiaries of a conspiracy against selling 'laetrile'?

"C. The public is not being prevented from eating apricot pits, which may be given for free distribution by 'laetrile' proponents, without hindrance. Since the material is virtually costless to produce, it could easily be given away.

"It is only when 'laetrile' is sold at a profit (and immense profits are currently being made) for an unproved medical purpose, or as a food additive, that its sale *for profit* becomes illegal. Any conspiracy, if one exists, is in the 'laetrile' sellers' efforts to convert a cheap and useless fruit waste-product into a commercially profitable item by preying on the fears and anguish of cancer victims.

"D. Many physicians, scientists and lawyers have lost loved ones to cancer, and would desperately have wanted them to live; to suggest a medical conspiracy to cause people to die is also to indict these professions as comprising persons inhuman toward their own relatives.

"5. *Characteristics of Quack Remedies*

"1. They are always cheap to produce and sold at great markups. The proponents commonly incite legal actions which reduce artificial scarcity and increase prices, thus increasing their profits.

"2. The materials are never given away, even though they are cheap to produce.

"3. They are never effective, because if so, they would receive universal acceptance, and possibly wipe out the disease involved.

"4. They are never toxic at the suggested doses, for if so, they would discourage their own use.

"5. They are sold and used in a milieu of mistrust of the medical and legal systems of the country.

"6. They are used by people who lack a knowledge of the natural history of disease, and who attribute painfree long survival to indicate drug effects, not realizing the chronic nature of cancer, e.g. that the average untreated survival time of breast cancer patients exceeds 2 years.

"7. They thrive in countries such as Mexico and the Philippines which lack high quality cancer diagnostic facilities, so that the frequency of cancer misdiagnosis is high, and some people are treated for a non-existent diagnosis of cancer.

"8. Tragically, those who fail on the 'drug' are not around to tell their side of the story.

"9. They are claimed to be uniformly effective; conventional drugs are effective at best against a fraction of human tumors, but 'laetrile' and other 'quack' remedies are proposed as cure-alls.

"6. *Specific Suggestions to Cancer Patients.*

"A. Inform yourself of the entire problem; balance a flashy editorialized news item against a quiet perusal of the extensive scientific factual files on 'laetrile' at the Canadian Cancer Society, the Cancer Control Agency, or the B.C. Medical Association.

B. If you must try 'laetrile' ask for it free. It is

essentially costless to produce and can be distributed free. It is not illegal for the pushers to give it away. Their literature states that they collect money and support laboratories, so they do not need your purchase price. All effective cancer drugs in B.C. are distributed free through the Cancer Control Agency and the Canadian Cancer Society. Why should 'laetrile' be charged for?

"C. If you do take 'laetrile' do not stop taking the possibly effective remedies. Cancer is a tough enemy and requires strong measures for control — in many instances a drug will affect normal tissues as it passed by them in order to reach the tumor cells. This results in some damage to normal cells, and side-effects which may be unpleasant.

"These side effects, while unpleasant, are surely worth the potential benefit of tumor destruction. The 'laetrile' literature states that it is compatible with all foods and drugs, so do not give up what your doctor has prescribed.

"D. Realize that cancer therapy is like all other disease treatments — it requires constant dose adjustment, may not always work, and you may have sensitivity reactions, just as some people get rashes to penicillin.

"E. Be comforted by the fact that cancer is a chronic disease, and that the natural history is not usually painful, nor very rapid. Thus, there is no need to panic.

"F. Be aware that cancer patients in B.C. have treatment available to them at no cost, through the Health Insurance Plan and the Cancer Control Agency, which is equivalent to the best anywhere, and is part of a new world-wide Cancer Discoveries Network that now brings the knowledge of new treatments at every Centre in Canada, the U.S.A. and abroad immediately to bear on your problem."

(The foregoing was distributed to members of the International Association of Cancer Victims and Friends prior to a meeting, but was unsigned. I suggest no significance to this, but merely offer it as a fact.)

CHAPTER 28

ANOTHER VERSION OF LAETRILE OFFERED AT PUBLIC MEETINGS

Author's Note:

No Law of Nature ever was established by Legislative Action, Executive Fiat, or Judicial Decision. Fortunately, the Basic Laws of the Universe are not subject to human control.

The proponents of laetrile say that research was done supporting laetrile, but that checking done was biased in favor of predetermined outcome.

The opponents of laetrile say that such checking was adequate, but negative, but appear to take the stand that no further checking should be done, despite doubts, justified or not; that further checking might somehow benefit a method described as "quack."

Some say that the nature of research funding interferes with further research regarding laetrile, because it must be based upon advance prognostication of what to expect. Such requisite would make impossible any meaningful research into a controversial issue, should it control, as alleged.

Research may produce results which are inconclusive, as may occur, or show that laetrile is effective, or not effective, with concomittant circumstances described. In any case, results should be reported in numbers with adequate measurement to establish predictability, or with reasons why predictability may not be established.

In short, the public should be supplied answers which satisfy those who examine them. Such is the thrust of this book, rather than the expansion of the debate.

"Laetrile — Another Version
Malignant Melanoma Case History of
Robert W. Stickle, born February 1, 1918
2422 Prospect Avenue, Cleveland, Ohio 44115

"*November 15, 1968.* Black mole over right scapula removed — St. John's Hospital, Cleveland, Ohio, Dr. William H. Mast, Surgeon.

"*Pathology:* 'Very Active Nevus Cell.'

"*December 8, 1968.* Re-appearance on scar of small pigmented lesion indicated wider biopsy excision. St. John's Hospital, Cleveland, Ohio, Dr. William H. Mast, Surgeon.

"*Pathology:* Report delayed for consultation of several pathologists. St. John's Hospital, Metropolitan and University Hospital pathologists were unanimous in their report that the pathology was malignant melanoma.

"*January 13, 1969.* 10 cm x 15 cm excision of area and removal of right rhomboideus muscle and skin graft. Right axillary disection. St. John's Hospital, Cleveland, Ohio, Dr. William H. Mast, Surgeon. Prior to surgery, Dr. Elden C. Weckesser consulted.

"*Pathology:* All tissue negative.

"*February 13, 1972.* 1.0 cm tumor removed at right periphery of skin graft. Axillary disection performed. University Hospital, Cleveland, Ohio, Dr. Elden C. Weckesser, Surgeon.

"*Pathology:* Tumor — Malignant Amelinoma — Metastatis. Surrounding tissue and tissue from right axila negative.

"*March 27, 1973.* Tumor removed from right axila. 3 cm dia. Surrounding tissue 12 x 5 cm removed from axila. 29 nodes examined by pathologist. University Hospital, Cleveland, Ohio, Dr. Elden C. Weckesser, Surgeon.

"*Pathology:* Tumor — Malignant amelinoma — metastatis. Surrounding tissue and nodes all negative (i.e., pathology — none).

"*August 15, 1973.* Tumor 1 cm dia. appeared in left axila. Dr. John G. Sholl, Cleveland, Ohio, Dr. Robert Kellermeyer, Cleveland, Ohio, and Dr. Elden C. Weckesser, Cleveland, Ohio, consulted. All recommended surgery. Patient refused further surgery.

"*August 23, 1973.* Patient underwent Laetrile therapy at Dr. Ernesto Contreras' Clinic, Tijuana, Mexico. Attending physician, Dr. Abel Mellado Prince, M.D. Therapy consisted of special diet plus one injection daily of 3 grams Laetrile given intravenously plus 9 tablets per day (3 after meals) of Wobe-Mugo (plant enzyme - animal enzyme tablets) plus 2 cc intramuscularly of A-C Factor (highly refined bone marrow). Treatment as outpatient for 21 days. After treatment, tumor had greatly reduced in size. Arthur's Test (Cytological) showed following: 8-24-73 (before Laetrile therapy):

"Structurally altered Nautrophyles 23% (normal less than 19%).

"Structurally altered Monocytes 50% (normal less than 49%)

"Small competent Lymphocytes 30% (normal over 20%).
9-6-73 (Laetrile therapy in progress).

"Structurally altered Neutrophyles — 19%

"Structurally altered Monocytes — 49%

"Small competent Lymphocytes — 34%

9-23-73 (after intense Laetrile therapy)

"Structurally altered Neutrophyles — 19%

"Structurally altered Monocytes — 49%

"Small competent Lymphocytes — 32%

"At present time, patient is taking 3 tablets of 500 mg Laetrile daily, plus 6 tablets of Wobe-Mugos daily plus 1 cc of A-C Factor intramuscularly 3 times weekly. The patient is observing a modified Laetrile diet which consists essentially of *avoiding* coffee, tea, strong spices, alcohol, nicotine, salt, dairy products, animal fats. Ingestion of large amount of fresh, raw vegetables and fruits and juices, certain nuts as well as restricted amounts of animal protein (lean meat, eggs) and white fish is encouraged.

"*December 1, 1973.* Patient in excellent condition, tumor has disappeared entirely. Minute fibrous material can be palpated. Urine test for chorionic gonadotrophin assay by Dr. Manuel Navarro showed negative indications of cancer activity.

"*December 10, 1973.* Chorionic gonadotrophin assay test by Dr. Manuel Navarro showed faintly positive (less than 200 I.U. gonadotrophin hormone).

"*December 15, 1973.* Arthur's Test showed:

"Structurally altered Neutrophyles — 12.7%

"Structurally altered Monocytes — 30%

"Small competent Lymphocytes — 32%

"*January 11, 1974.* Examined by Dr. Abel Mellado Prince at Dr. Contreras' Clinic, Tijuana, Mexico. Patient in good condition. No clinical evidence of Melanoma. Laetrile-Enzyme-A C Factor maintenance therapy continued. Diet continued. Arthur Test negative.

"*June 18, 1974.* Examined by Dr. Lopez, M.D., at Dr. Contreras' Clinic, Tijuana, Mexico. Patient in excellent condition. No clinical evidence of Melanoma. Weight, blood pressure - same as January. Laetrile, Proteolytic Enzyme, A-C Factor therapy continued with reduction in medication. Diet continued. Arthur Test negative.

"*July 1, 1974.* Examined by Dr. W. E. Mishler, M.D. for F.A.A. — 3rd Class Medical for Pilot's license. All SMA tests, electrocardiograph, etc., excellent — normal. No clinical evidence of Melanoma. Doctor remarked to patient that he had 'the cardiovascular system of a 20-year-old.'

"*December 20, 1974.* Patient in excellent condition. No clinical evidence of malignant melanoma. Will visit Dr. Contreras' Clinic in January, 1975, for routine examination and recommendation for continuing medication. Diet continued.

"*February 24, 1975.* Patient visited Dr. Contreras'

Clinic January 22, 1975, for routine physical examination and recommendation on continuing therapy and medication. Patient examined by Dr. Badillo, M.D., who found no clinical evidence of malignant melanoma. Patient in excellent physical condition. However, Dr. Badillo prescribed 2 - 500 mg tablets of activated Amygdalin and 4 - Wobe-Mugo tablets per day. In addition, 1 cc I.M. injections of A-C Factor once per week were prescribed along with 15 drops of A-Mulsin per day (22,500 I.U. of emulsified Vitamin A). Dr. Badillo suggested another visit to the Clinic in about one year for a check-up.

"Arthur's Test showed:
"Damaged Neutrophyles — 6% (excresences)
"Damaged Manocytes — 12% (Halos)
"Small competent Lymphocytes — 46%
which indicated a further regression of the condition.

"*May 1, 1975.* Patient continues with diet. Medication continues with 3 - 500 mg of Amygdalin (Laetrile) and 3 Wobe-Mugo Enzymes daily. No clinical evidence of Melanoma. Patient in excellent physical condition.

"*July 1, 1975.* Patient continues with diet same as before. Weight and blood pressure stabilized at: Weight - 145 pounds; Blood Pressure - 115/65.

"Arthur's Test is negative.

"Dr. Navarro of Manila, Philippines, gives a negative Human Chorionic Gonadotrophin Assay (H.C.G. Assay) Test.

"No clinical evidence of Melanoma.

"*October 1, 1975.* Same as previous. No change. Patient feels good, is very active and in apparent good health. No clinical evidence of melanoma. Lifelong problem of mild eczema has cleared up. Diet is very rigidly followed. Raw foods and juices of raw vegetables and fruits emphasized.

"University Hospitals of Cleveland
"Surgical Pathology Report

"Surg. Path. No. 373-2705-I-II;
"Name: Robert W. Stickle; Age: 55-M
"Hosp. No. 964-685
"Clinical Diagnosis: I- Malignant melanoma
II - R/O metastatic melanoma (Froz.) Sec. Dx.; II - Chronclymphadenitia - Drs. Thomas Laipply and Branimir L. Horvat
"Specimen: I - Lymph node and axillary contents.
"II - Lymph node, right axilla

Date: 3-37-73

"Gross Examination:

"I - Received in formalin is a skin ellipse with attached fibroadipose tissue. The skin ellipse measures 8.0 cm in length by 2.3 cm in greatest width. The skin surface is wrinkled, dull and pale brown. The dermis measures up to 0.2 cm in thickness and is dull and pale gray. The attached dibroadipose tissue is composed of several large and small labules of smooth, glistening, yellow tissue with a delicate, dull intervening stroma. A few small lymph nodes are identified within the specimen.

"Representative sections are embedded under A.

"II - Received in formalin is a tissue fragment previously used for frozen section. It measures 1.3 x 0.6 x 0.2 cm. It is moderately firm, dull and pale yellowish-brown.

"Embedded in toto under B.

"Also received are three similar, irregular fibroadipose tissue fragments varying from 0.9 x 0.4 x 0.4 cm to 0.7 x 0.2 x 0.1 cm. They are moderately soft, glistening and light yellow.

"Embedded in toto under C.

"Impression: I - Skin and fibroadipose tissue fragment —

diagnosis deferred.

"II – Tissue fragments - diagnosis deferred.

Thomas Panke, M.D. (em)

"Slides examined, description omitted.

"Diagnosis: 03-8146 I – *Metastatic malignant tumor* involving one of 26 lymph nodes, clinically from right axilla, see note.

"08-7200 II – Follicular hyperplasia of lymph node, clinically from right axilla.

"1X-0001. Fibroadipose tissue fragments, no pathologic diagnosis, clinically from right axilla.

"Note: The neoplasm is similar to S72-1704.

Thomas Panke, M.D. (em)

Senior Pathologist: Branimir L. Harvat, M.D.

"(signed)"

CHAPTER 29

ERNEST KREBS ON LAETRILE – THE "EYE" OF THE HURRICANE

The following article appeared in the *Cancer Control Journal,* Vol. 2, No. 6, Los Angeles, California, 1974.

"The Nature of Cancer
by Ernst Krebs, Jr.

"(Presented before Cancer Control Society - CCS - Second Annual Cancer Convention, Ambassador Hotel, Los Angeles, California, 1974.)

"It is certainly a pleasure to be here at the Second Annual Convention of the Cancer Control Society – an outgrowth, as you know, of the International Association of Cancer Victims and Friends.

"As I look back through the years marking the immergence of these two fine Societies, I can recall the number of miraculous victories we have had in those intervening years; that it is as true today as it was eleven years ago that Laetrile, Vitamin B17, is the first and last final hope in the prophylacsis in therapy of cancer in man and animals. The reason for this is that Laetrile is a vitamin. It is the 17th of the B vitamins.

"We hear a great deal about its use in terminal cancer, but the time to start with Vitamin B17 is now before the disease becomes clinical. The time to start is the same with any matter of adequate nutrition and that is right now. You may start now by commencing to eat the seeds of all common fruits that you eat. The apricot and peach seeds contain almost 2 percent of Vitamin B17 by weight. The apple seed, although very small, is equally rich in Vitamin B17. So are the seeds of prunes, plums, cherries and nectarines. The only common fruit on this hemisphere that lacks nitrilosidic seeds, are the citrus fruits. This lack has come about by artificial cultivation by breeding and hybridization, since the seeds of citrus fruits on the African continent still contain Vitamin B17.

"Two more rich sources of Vitamin B17 are the simple cereals millet and buckwheat. Macadamia nuts, although expensive and exotic, are very rich in Vitamin B17 and so are bamboo shoots, mung beans, lima beans, butter beans, and certain strains of garden peas. But for convenience, the simplest source for your Vitamin B17 are the seeds of the common fruits.

"We know something about the prophylactic dose of Vitamin B17. For example, we know the Hunza's represent a population that has been cancer-free for over 900 years of its existence. This population has a natural diet, which supplies on the average, between 50 to 75 milligrams of Vitamin B17 a day.

"Hunzaland is a land that has sometimes been described as the 'place where apricot is king.' The Hunzakuts eat the fresh apricots for the three months they are in season and the remainder of the year they eat dried apricots. They never eat a dried apricot without enclosing the seed between them. This supplies them with better than average of 50 to 75 milligrams of Vitamin B17 daily.

"There are many of us in the Western world who don't ingest this amount of Vitamin B17 in the course of an entire year. As a result we're in the midst of a fulminating deficiency of Vitamin B17 or nitriloside, the anti-neoplastic vitamin. Its absence from our diets accounts for the fact that cancer in our population has reached such a pandemisity as to account for its occurrence in one in every three American families. The occurrence is probably much greater than that because it is very late in its development when the cancer is detected. Many who develop cancer are killed by accident or intercurrent diseases before the malignant process has become sufficiently advanced to cause them to have it diagnosed.

"Cancer is a chronic, metabolic disease . . . that is obvious. It isn't an infectious disease, which is caused by bacteria or viruses. It is a disease that is metabolic in origin. A metabolic disease is a disease that is linked with our utilization of food. Most metabolic diseases have as their basis specific vitamins and minerals.

"Let me give you a categorical or axiomatic truth to take with you. One that is totally uncontradictable, scientifically, historically and in every other way. This is that no chronic or metabolic disease in the history of medicine has ever been prevented or cured, except by factors normal to the diet or normal to the animal economy. There have been many erstwhile fatal devastating diseases that now have become virtually unknown. They have been prevented and cured by ingesting the dietary factors and thereby preventing the deficiencies, which accounted for these diseases.

"The one in which you are probably most familiar is Scurvy. A fatal disease that killed mankind by the thousands. A disease that would sometimes wipe out an entire Polar expedition or accounted for about 50 percent mortality among the Crusaders. A disease that is totally prevented and totally cured by Vitamin C or ascorbic acid, a factor normal to an adequate diet. As you know so well from your school days that Great Britain acquired the dominion of the seas, by empirically discovering that by adding lime or other citrus juice to the provisions of the British mariners, the curse of Scurvy from the British sea power was removed. Therefore, Britain competitively gained the ascendency on the seas. Prior to the incorporation of Vitamin C into their diets it wasn't uncommon for three-fourths of the crew to become seriously ill by the end of the voyage and then those who didn't die would mysteriously recover after hitting shore because they would have access to fresh fruits and vegetables rich in Vitamin C.

"Then we have Pernicious Anemia, which had a mortality rate of 98 or 99 percent. And no medical modality under the sun could touch it. Arsenic and its salts, strichnine, iron and hundreds of other remedies were tried, but all to no avail until the researchers Drs. Murphy, Shipple and Minot commenced their classical studies on the relationship of Pernicious Anemia to dietary deficiency.

"While working at the University of California they discovered a very simple remedy for preventing and curing this disease. They simply said to their patients, 'go down to your butcher shop and get a quarter pound of fresh liver. Grind it up and take a tablespoon every day or take the quarter pound and cook it very lightly and just singe the surface and use this as a ration for three days.' And when the patients followed this advice without exception, those with Pernicious Anemia made complete recoveries. Despite this, these men were censored by the Medical Establishment at the time and were criticized for engaging in what was alleged to be Medical quackery.

"The argument was how can respectable doctors advise people with a disease that has a 99 percent mortality rate to ignore all of the established drugs of medical science and go down to the butcher shop and buy some raw liver and take this and expect this to cure a disease that nothing else has cured. Well, raw liver did cure that disease and raw liver did prevent it.

"As the chemistry of raw liver was studied, it was discovered that the factors responsible were Vitamin B12 and Folic Acid. So Vitamin B12 and Folic Acid are now a part of our normal dietary experience.

"So in 1974 the uninformed, the unimaginative, and some of the illiterate are concerned with what to them is a preposterous idea that by eating the seeds of fruit you can prevent a disease that carries a mortality rate almost as high as that once carried by Pernicious Anemia. But scientific truth isn't dependent upon credibility or lack of it. The scientific reality either is or isn't. And this is the scientific reality that the seeds of all common fruits (except citrus) contain Vitamin B17, an anti-cancer vitamin. If we ingest proper quantities of this vitamin either in the pure form or through ingesting the nitrilosidic foods we will be able to prevent this disease just as surely as we are able to prevent Scurvy by the use of Vitamin C or Pernicious Anemia by the use of Vitamin B12.

"There was another disease that is a metabolic or chronic nature and this is Pellagra. At one time it was so endemic in certain parts of the world, particularly the American southwest, that there were entire hospitals given to the treatment of Pellagrans.

"The great Sir William Osler in his *Principles and Practices of Medicine,* written at the turn of this century, said of Pellagra, 'I was at Lenoir, North Carolina during one winter and this winter I visited the Lenoir Home for the colored insane and there 75 percent of the inmates died from the disease. It ran rampant through this institution and convinced me beyond any doubt that pellagra is a disease produced by a virus that is infectious.'

"And then came the fine works of the United States Public Health Service surgeon, Dr. Goldberger, who showed conclusively that the occurrence of Pellagra was related with a deficiency of fresh green material in the diet. So Dr. Goldberger approached this problem first by the use of Brewer's Yeast, which would completely prevent and cure Pellagra. Further studies then showed that the factor in Brewer's Yeast that was most determinate of this effect was Niacin, Vitamin B3.

"So another fatal chronic metabolic disease found total resolution and cure through factors normal to the normal diet or the animal economy. We know that cancer is no exception to this great generalization and to date has known no exception. That is that every chronic or metabolic disease that will ever be controlled by man must be controlled by means that are a part of the biological experience of the organism. Chronic and metabolic diseases can never be controlled, prevented, or cured by factors foreign to the biological experience of the organism.

"Let's make it clear by what we mean by biological experience to the organism. We refer to the experience the organism has had over the million years of its evolution. The organism was exposed to water, air, carbohydrates, fats, proteins, amino acids, and various salts and these factors became integrated with the evolving organism. And the evolving organism became integrated with these factors. And these factors with the evolving organism were incorporated into the beautiful machinery of 'life.' And the vital mechanism of life runs just like the parts of a fine Swiss watch, only infinitely more complex.

"Dr. Thomas of the Sloan Kettering Institute, in a recent article in *Science,* said, 'I'm thankful that my liver works without my knowledge. I do not have the brains to commence to do one-millionth of what my liver does. These things are automatic. So I swallow the food and this infinitely complex machinery takes care of itself.' We could spend years telling you about this magnificent machinery and we still wouldn't touch the surface of this infinite ocean. We do know that there is nothing that we can do to improve upon it. We do know that in the history of medicine there never has been found anything foreign to the indwelling requirements of this machinery that will do the living organism any good. And we can go further to say there has never in the history of medicine been found anything foreign to the indwelling machinery of this infinitely complex system that will not harm the organism. There isn't such a thing as a factor foreign to the biological experience that is not harmful to the organism.

"There is nothing we can add to our air, water and food to improve it. The most we can do is to look at some of our devitalized food and hopefully attempt to replace that which was capriciously removed from it in the process of food refining, manipulation or cooking. There is absolutely nothing that we can add to that food to improve it. These things are basic.

"There isn't any chemical or drug that medical science could suggest that would make us healthier or better adjusted or wiser or give us hope for a longer life. There isn't a single drug or molecule in nature that can unless that molecule exists in normal food. And this probably explains one of the reasons why there is so much resistance to Laetrile, Vitamin B17.

"The application of this science brings us face to face with a lot of things we do not like to face. We have become over-civilized. We are inclined in our delusory thinking to feel that here and there there must be a magic out. That there must be a simple way, a short cut, that somehow or other medical science or some other man-made forces beyond our comprehension will do for us those things we must do for ourselves. And it is slowly dawning on us, perhaps too slowly that this thinking is fraudulent; that it is unsound.

"It isn't in the field of cancer alone where we see this form of charlatanism or quackery. We see it in the area of the human mind. The futile attempts to spare man from the realities that surround him. Above all to spare him from the fact that he is accountable to himself and to his God and that there is no short cut in this accountability.

"It's real at the physical level. And when we are eating less than adequate food, we know better. And when we continue we are engaged in sin. This is the basis for practically all of our physical and mental and spiritual difficulties. We had better be realistic about it. We have them because we don't do the right things. And when we fail in view of our knowledge now to take Vitamin B17 this is a sin against our physical nature. And when we develop cancer we will receive the results of this transgression in the old fashioned Biblical sense that the 'wages of sin are death.'

"If you are not getting Vitamin B17 in your food the best way to get it is in the pure form. If you have cancer, the most important single consideration is to get the maximum amount of Vitamin B17 into your body in the shortest period of time. This is secondary to the medical skill involved in administering it, which is relatively minimal. Then very often there are many supportive measures that are taken in the management of the cancer patient such as the use of materials to build up the blood, to raise or lower the blood pressure or to relieve the pain.

"Pancreatic enzymes and vegetable enzymes are part of the supportive theory. You have the papaya melons as the source of the enzyme Papain and pineapple as the source of the enzyme Bromelain. The demasking effect of these enzymes against the pericellular layer of the malignant cell is something very concrete in the immunology of cancer. Now, I prefer, rather than advising the use of Bromelain or papaya tablets that the individual seeking these enzymes get them directly from the fresh ripe pineapple and papaya fruit. As much as half a pineapple a day should be ingested.

"This is the way to go. You have nothing to lose by eating fresh pineapple and papaya melons. Nothing to lose by eating millet, the seeds of all the common fruits and whole fresh foods.

"Dietary deficiencies arrive primarily from eating less than whole food. This is why the Federal and State governments have made mandatory the artificial enrichment of white flour. Look at any loaf of white bread or white flour that has been enriched by the addition of crystalline Vitamin

B1, Vitamin B2, niacin, iron, and all the rest. What a commentary on the stupidity of our civilization that we put good food through a process that defects it of its essential nutrients and then enforced by the Government mandate requirements that say that we must restore to this food some of the things that have been processed out. One of the most critical factors is removed and that is wheat germ, which contains the Vitamin E and the polyunsaturated fatty acids. It would not be necessary to take it in supplementation if our foods were not manipulated in a way to remove this.

"Now something about supplementations in addition to the Vitamin B17. We can't think in terms of just one vitamin. We get an adequate diet by eating as wide a variety of whole natural foods as possible and as close to their growing period as we can possibly obtain them.

"There are Laetrile therapists who recommend two or three grams of ascorbic acid or Vitamin C in conjunction with the Laetrile program. This is a very moderate recommendation and we can all take up to seven or eight grams of Vitamin C without any problems. This is about the same amount as the higher primates such as the gorilla on a pound-to-pound basis ingest between five to six grams of Vitamin C a day in their normal habitat. Incidentally, the gorilla in his natural habitat eats about 100 to 125 milligrams of Vitamin B17 a day, too. Like the population of Hunzaland, these gorillas are free of cancer, so are bears in their normal habitat. Out in the wilds they don't develop cancer.

"In the San Diego Zoo there was a cage of about ten bears and out of the ten, seven of them developed cancer. To some this was a sign that some mysterious bear cancer virus was loose. But, it wasn't that at all. In the wild state the bears are omnivorous and they eat a lot of wild nitrilosidic berries. Almost all wild fruits are nitrilosidic.

"Keep in mind how far we have drifted from the dietary requirements of the machinery that we now possess. When we evolved and came to our maturity as organisms about 8,000 or 9,000 years ago, the world witnessed the advent of agriculture and horticulture came a little later. The millions of years prior to that time we ate the cherries, apricots, apples, prunes, and the rest of the fruits. They had Vitamin B17 not only within the seeds, but in the flesh, too. Today only wild fruit contain the Vitamin B17 in the flesh. And similarly with maze or Indian corn. This was originally very rich in Vitamin B17, but in the process of hybridization it has been removed.

"The fruit that we eat today is the product of years of manipulation and cultivation for lushness and abundance and so forth, so the meat of that fruit is free of Vitamin B17. To meet our indwelling needs for Vitamin B17, we must either eat the fruit seeds in reasonable quantity or begin supplementing our diet with Vitamin B17 tablets. We can't, of course, do that at present, but we hope to see, before very long, Vitamin B17 available so that we can prevent cancer in the same way we prevent scurvy.

"Several new books are coming out on Laetrile. Both are written by non-medical men — *World Without Cancer,* by Edward Griffin, and *Vitamin B17: Forbidden Weapon Against Cancer,* by Mike Culbert. We are all laymen in the field of cancer. There are more laymen in the Laetrile movement who know more about cancer than some of our most prestigious experts in our most prestigious institutions. These laymen know enough about it to keep alive and not die from it. So you're a pretty rotten expert if you know so little about it as to succumb from it or have your family succumb from it.

"We have many case histories of people that have been helped by Laetrile. Both Alicia Buttons and Mary Henderson were terminal with oral pharyngeal cancer that has a mortality rate of 98 to 99 percent, even in early diagnosis. Both made remarkable recoveries with Laetrile under the guidance of Dr. Hans Nieper in Germany.

"You know we have been meeting ten or eleven years and you've been hearing this story. Each time after the meeting you had 360 days to go home and read newspapers, American Cancer Society Boiler Plate and so forth. In those ten years they haven't told you anything against Laetrile that makes any sense. You can be pretty sure they don't have anything against Laetrile because these people are very uninhibited and the area in which they are most uninhibited is in the area of simple lying.

"If you have any questions about Laetrile, the more critical the better because we are dealing with solid science. We are dealing with a science that admits that there is no rational alternative in the ten years that have passed since these meetings. Nothing has come about to do anything except to make more obvious the fact that Laetrile, Vitamin B17 is the answer to the cancer problem.

"Question: Will cooking millet destroy the Vitamin B17?

"Answer: No, cooking doesn't destroy the Vitamin B17. Almost every food that we eat is better eaten raw. And when we cook a fruit we destroy the enzymes and whereever we have Vitamin B17, we have the accompanying enzyme B-gludosidase naturally. B-glucosidase is destroyed by heat, but Vitamin B17 is not destroyed by heat.

"Question: Is there any way in which a person may be deficient in the enzyme rhodanese?

"Answer: The enzyme rhodanese is a normally occurring enzyme that converts cyanide to the non-toxic compound neocyanate and we evolved with the rhodanese because the Vitamin B17 containing cyanide originally was so large a part of our diet. So far as we know, there is no development of rhodanese deficiencies.

"We must be very realistic that there is absolutely nothing we can do to alter this infinitely complex machinery of the cell and of life. All that we can do is to supply those components that are missing and then hope for the best. It's like being on the freeway with a Cadillac in which the hood is locked and you run out of gas. Now all your knowledge of mechanics is going to be of no avail – just pour gas into the tank and step on the starter and hope for the best that the gas gets sucked into the motor. When the machinery of the cell begins to falter or fail, you put in those factors normal to the operation of that machinery. Since we have no choice, we allow the universe to take its course. We don't go on the presumption that we can successfully tamper with that infinite machinery.

"Do you believe that we should take the Wobenzym enzymes along with the Laetrile?

"Yes, they are good, except I think they are slightly overpriced and I strongly recommend the American Viokase put out by Viobin in Monticello, Illinois.

"Is Laetrile a prescription item in Mexico or Canada?

"I know that it is legal in Mexico, but I don't know the exact situation in Canada at the moment. You may get it without a prescription in Mexico.

"If you get the benefits from the seeds of fruits for prevention, why is it necessary to take the more concentrated forms?

"Like everything else in science, it is self-answering. It isn't necessary, so eat the seeds and you can get an adequacy of Vitamin B17.

"The fact that cancer is a metabolic disease, what role does pollution have in that process?

"Pollutants harm the liver and the liver is a great detoxifying organ of the body. If the liver is detoxifying an excess of estrogen, for example, and the capacity of the liver is impaired by pollutants, the estrogen level then may reach a concentration sufficient to induce cancer. If we are eating apples that have been sprayed with arsenic and we eat enough of these apples, the arsenic may produce a hepatic chirrosis that again will impair the capacity of the liver to detoxify certain carcinogens and thereby contribute to the development of cancer. If we are receiving a very high concentration of Vitamin B17, this will offset the possibility of developing cancer, but these pollutants still can kill us through producing chirrosis of the liver and destroying other vital cells.

"Can the body handle inorganic Vitamin C?

"The Vitamin C on the market is organic and contrary to what is sometimes believed, is not synthetic. The Vitamin C that is produced in this country is produced by fermentation involving the growth of the mold Streptomycetes. So it is a biosynthetic process. This is the cheapest and most efficient way to do it, although this is not a 'complex.'

"How many seeds should we eat?

"I would say that 15 seeds every other day would provide an adequacy and give quite a margin.

"If we are supposed to eat seeds, why aren't we supplied with teeth for breaking through the pits?

"There are societies that have not become too corrupted by the sophistication of modern technology. These people are capable of biting through the pit. We have even seen small dogs break the pit and eat the seeds. Squirrels, chipmunks, bears, higher primates such as monkeys, ordinarily do it.

"Curators of zoos tell us when monkeys and apes are thrown fresh apricots, peaches and plums, in time, if they are thrown enough of them, they cease eating the sweet sugary fruit and they begin hoarding the pits. They manage to break those pits. Primates will take them in hand and hammer them against a piece of concrete. Eating these seeds is universal among the nomads and among the higher animals.

"How do you keep the seeds once they are out of the pit?

"You may keep the seeds indefinitely if you keep them thermatically sealed under refrigeration. If you don't keep them under refrigeration, the Vitamin B17 won't deteriorate, but the unsaturated fatty acids will turn rancid and become carcinogenic.

"Does Vitamin B17 help Sickle Cell Anemia?

"A lot of fine work is being done on this. Robert Houston has done some very brilliant studies along these lines and he has published several top-rate papers. Sickle Cell Anemia crisis is the result of a fulminating deficiency of Vitamin B17 and it occurs in Americans of African origin, who, upon leaving the African continent, become removed from a dietary source of Vitamin B17. Sickle Cell crisis is a Vitamin B17 deficiency disease in the same way that Pernicious Anemia is a Vitamin B12, Folic Acid deficiency disease.

"Do almonds contain cyanide?

"The Romans found that here and there almond trees appeared which had almonds that were completely sweet and no longer had any trace of bitterness. That bitterness is due to the presence of Vitamin B17. So they proceeded to destroy all of the almond trees that had any trace of bitterness and propogated those almond trees that just yielded the sweet kernels. So those almonds that have come to us in the Western world are very rich in the enzyme B-glucosidase, but deficient in Vitamin B17. On the other hand, the Eastern part of the world, such as the Ukraine, Soviet Union, and Red China, have predominately the original bitter almond, very rich in Vitamin B17.

"Is it okay to eat all the legumes raw?

"No, it isn't. It is good to cook most beans. The cooking doesn't destroy the Vitamin B17 content. Although beans eaten raw in small quantities are quite acceptable as food.

"Is it best to take all apricot kernels at once?

"Yes, I should add that it is a good idea to grind them up in a nut grinder. One teaspoon of the material is equivalent to seven or eight seeds. Take two teaspoonfuls and lace a fruit salad or oatmeal or whatever you are eating. You can incorporate it into muffins or use it a hundred different ways. You can take it straight or you can eat it and then follow it with a little honey because of the persisting bitterness.

"Are the broad beans or visa fava high in cyanide?

"Yes, they are splendid. It was one of the staples in the diet of the Roman legions. The legionnaires not only ate broad beans, but they fed them to their horses. This made for a very vigorous infantry in cavalry. Visa fava are also known as Italian beans or flat beans.

"Is Vitamin B17 helpful against devastating effects of excessive quantities of environmental or medical radiation?

"No, and the reason for it is a very common sense one. In all of the exogencies of our evolution and natural selection, the presence of radiation in such horrible concentrations was never anticipated. The organism may be beset with such onslaught and there are no mechanisms including Vitamin B17 to medicate the deadly effects of such excess radiation. This is one of the most horrible assaults on living tissues. The most horrible assault that living tissue can sustain, because it destroys not only the individual of one generation, but it may cripple, if not extinguish, the immortal germ plasm, on which the continuity of the species itself relies."

About Mr. Krebs, Jr.

Ernst T. Krebs, Jr., is a prominent biochemist from San Francisco. He is widely recognized as the co-discoverer with his father of Vitamin B17 or nitriloside, commonly known as Laetrile, for the control of cancer. Also, with his father, he discovered another of the B vitamins – B15 or pangamic acid. In the 1930's and 1940's he studied and expanded the use and knowledge of pancreatic enzymes, particularly chymotrypsin, in the treatment of cancer as originated by Dr. John Beard at the University of Edinburgh, nearly seventy years ago. In 1945 he was instrumental in founding the John Beard

Memorial Foundation to develop and apply the Beardian thesis of cancer on which his work with both the pancreatic enzymes and Laetrile has been based.

In 1950, he perceived that the cyanide that was safely bound in the molecules of Laetrile should be released by enzymes present at the site of malignant cells; the free cyanide should then destroy the cancer. Now he could understand why his father, Ernst T. Krebs, Sr., M.D., had had some good results on cancer with an apricot kernel extract more than 20 years earlier, because he knew that apricot kernels contained Laetrile.

Ernest Krebs, Jr., was born in Carson City, Nevada. From 1938 to 1941, he was a student of the Hahnemann Medical College in Philadelphia, Pa. He received his A.B. degree from the University of Illinois in 1942. He was a graduate student at the University of California in Berkeley from 1943 to 1945 and did research work in pharmacy from 1942 to 1945.

Among the works he has authored are the *Unitarian or Trophoblastic Thesis of Cancer* and *The Nitrilosides (Vitamin B17) – Their Nature, Occurrence and Metabolic Significance (Antineoplastic Vitamin B17).*

CHAPTER 30

IS THERE ANY RELATIONSHIP BETWEEN HUNZA (CANCER-FREE) AND WHAT DR. GERSON SAYS?

Vol. 2, No. 6, *Cancer Control Journal,* contains an article reprinted from *Prevention,* May 1974, entitled, "Death Rides a Slow Bus in Hunza."

Abridged, the article describes the Hunzas as people rugged enough to break the ice to go swimming in the middle of winter, in their tiny country in Northwest Pakistan, 20,000 feet up in the Himalayas.

According to this article, the Hunzas are virtually free of heart disease, high cholesterol, and cancer: "degenerative" diseases, in short.

Many live to be 100 years old, and some men of 90 father children. Old men with 20-20 vision live there.

These people live on raw foods; apricots, fresh and dried, and apricot pits, with meat only on feast days, which come seldom.

The following appears in the *Cancer Control Journal,* Vol. 3, No. 1 and 2, 1975:

"The Gerson Therapy

by Charlotte Gerson Straus, Daughter and Clinical Associate of Max Gerson, M.D.

About Charlotte Straus: She is Dr. Max Gerson's daughter and clinical associate. She was born in Germany and had her early schooling there and left in 1933. She lived and attended many schools in Europe before arriving in New York in 1936 with her family. She finished high school in New York and attended Smith College. She was always interested in her father's work and helped as a practical nurse in his nursing homes in New York. She occasionally made rounds with him, attended his lectures and was raised on his strict ideas of nutrition.

(The following was presented before the Cancer Control Society Second Annual Cancer Convention, Ambassador Hotel, Los Angeles, California, 1974.)

"I welcome you and thank you for being here. I feel that on this platform I always enjoy talking more than anywhere else because usually the speakers that precede me do about half of my work. For instance, Dr. Livingston went into her very interesting work, which I will be able to tie into my father's therapy. Also, Betty Lee Morale's lecture gave a very basic orientation in this direction. I always get an inspiration from these speakers. This includes all the speakers who are so devoted and so enthusiastic and have accomplished such a wonderful job all of these years.

"I will not go back to the development of the Gerson Treatment.

"My father had a genetic background of severe migraines. When he was a young doctor, just out of medical school, he was very ill with migraines, which he usually had three days a week. He had such terrible eye sensitivity and nausea that he had to lie in a dark room and was absolutely unable to function. This was so severe that he was actually despairing of living. He consulted professors and teachers, who had been the authorities to try to get relief. They all told him, 'Well, you know from the books that there is nothing that we can do against migraines. When you are 45 or 55 you'll feel better.'

"So at this point he felt that he would have to help himself. He started to study and read on nutrition, but there was relatively little available. He thought that the first thing babies get and the first thing they can all digest is milk, and then he thought if he were to take nothing but milk, this might help him because surely the body was able to digest milk. He tried that for a little while and he was just as sick as ever and milk didn't do anything for him. Then he thought about that again and he realized in nature there aren't any adult animals that live on milk. Milk is a food designed for babies, which have a fast growth and a completely different type of metabolism. In nature our immediate ancestors, the monkeys in the jungles, do not live on milk. They live on fruits and nuts, greens and vegetables, but mainly fruits and nuts. So he thought this would be a good thing to start with and he put himself on apples. He found that within a very short time he was free of migraines.

"He then used apples as a basis for adding other foods. He lived on apples in all forms and then on other fruit. The minute he added something to this basic apple diet that disturbed his system he would have severe migraines again. He lived on this same diet all his life.

"He soon started practice as a doctor. His shingle read Dr. Max Gerson, Internal and Nerve Diseases.' He had been a student under Professor Ottfried Foerster, the top neurosurgeon in Germany at the time. This was his specialty.

"One day a man came to him complaining of migraines and Dr. Gerson told him very simply, 'The books say there is nothing one can do.' But he did tell the man what he did. 'These foods I eat, these foods I don't eat. Why don't you try it?' The man did and reported shortly that when he stuck to this type of diet he was fine. If he ate the forbidden foods he did not do well and the migraines recurred.

"One day a patient came in for migraines and my father gave him the same migraine treatment that he was using himself. The patient reported a few weeks later and he said, 'You know what, doctor, my migraines cleared up, but on top of that, I cleared up my Lupus.' Now Lupus is skin tuberculosis. So my father said, 'No, that's impossible, Lupus is incurable and it must have been something else.'

" 'No,' said the patient. 'It's not. I have these various lab reports and slides to prove this was Lupus.'

"Father said, 'Let me see.'

"And he observed that these were incontestable lab reports and the man had Lupus and he said, 'Well, let me see the lesions.' No one had ever seen Lupus healing and he looked at a Lupus lesion healing. He was flabbergasted. The next thought he had was, well, perhaps there was a connection between this migraine and the Lupus. He thought the man might have responded because of an allergy which was cleared up.

"Then he asked him, 'Do you know other people who have Lupus? It is a relatively rare disease. I would like to see it on people who have no migraines to see whether this diet really works.'

"You see my father still thought like a specialist. A specific treatment for a specific disease.

"The patient replied, 'Oh, yes, in the hospital where I spent many months with Lupus there were a lot of patients on my floor with Lupus. I will send you some.'

"My father said, 'I will treat them free. I would like to experiment and see what happens.'

"To make a long story short, the other patients without migraines also recovered from Lupus.

"Now, what do you think happened next?

"Father was sued by the medical community for his license. His shingle said internal and nerve diseases and this was a skin disease. He had no right to treat Lupus. This was in Germany, but the judge was not quite the same as some of the judges and courts we are running into here in this day and age.

"The judge asked the doctors, 'Well, do you cure Lupus?'

"And the doctors answered, 'Well, no, it's incurable!'

"And the judge retorted, 'Well, then, why don't you let

this doctor do it?' and then he dismissed the case.

"From Lupus Dr. Gerson figured the body is obviously developing the ability with the right nutrition to kill off the very specific tuberculosis germ and to restore itself to health. Then he went on to other forms of tuberculosis and lo and behold, they also responded.

"In 1928, the wife of Albert Schweitzer, who had contracted lung tuberculosis and was in very serious condition, came to my father. She recovered completely on his migraine diet.

"Now, at this point, my father had no longer called it a migraine diet. He also removed his shingle and became a general practitioner.

"It did not take very long before he realized that patients who were recovering from all forms of tuberculosis, meningitis, etc., often had other complications including arteriosclerosis, arthritis or other diseases. These all cleared up with the same treatment, too.

"He realized that in this approach the basis of the treatment was to see the body as a total organism. When you restore its ability to heal, it will heal itself. And it will not heal selectively. It will not heal skin tuberculosis without healing migraines. It will not heal arteriosclerosis without healing heart trouble. When you have the body healing, it will heal whatever is ailing it.

"You cannot heal cancer selectively without also healing whatever else is wrong with the person. There are many cases in Dr. Gerson's book, *A Cancer Therapy – Results of Fifty Cases,* with the complication of heart trouble and arthritis that were also cleared up when the cancer was controlled.

"What is chronic disease? The beginning of all chronic disease in the body is loss of potassium from the cells. Potassium is lost because of our nutrition. Our poorly grown, artificially fertilized, sprayed foods are low in potassium. The sodium content usually goes up in plants that are artificially fertilized. This fact was published in 1927 in an agriculture publication in Germany: potatoes from fields artificially fertilized had lost their normal potassium content. The sodium content went up with the water content. The potatoes grew nice and big, but this was an edematous potato. Like your body, when your body loses potassium, sodium penetrates the cells and holds the water and your body gets edematous. The water in the cells ties the sodium. If the sodium isn't tied it's toxic.

"Now, in order to reverse this situation, it's become quite clear to you from the talk such as Betty Lee Morales presented that the organic, natural and unprocessed foods are the ones that produce health. But why? Remember what foods go through during processing. First of all they are usually grown on a large corporate farm. They are artificially fertilized and sprayed. They are beautiful, but empty of potassium. They add lots of sugar so that it tastes good and salt so that the flavor is there. The result is a denatured food that is processed, sodium is added, potassium is lowered, and enzymes are killed by processing.

"Now on this do you expect to keep your bodies healthy? You are punishing yourselves. You are punishing your system. Just like you can't put sugar water in your car motor and expect it to produce energy. You know that if you don't give your machines the right fuel they won't work. But your bodies, you don't hesitate for a minute to give denatured, damaged, and changed fuel.

"Now let's go back once more to what we heard. Dr. Livingston showed you the organism, which she feels causes cancer and that it is very closely allied to tuberculosis. I have just told you that with the right nutrition to restore the body's healing ability you can get the body to kill the tuberculosis germ. And you don't have to think very much further to realize that the body can also kill cancer.

"Now I am not going to get into the basic causes of

cancer – whether it is caused by germs, viruses, genetic changes, burns or by various other chemicals. It really doesn't make any difference whatsoever. My father has shown that by taking the cancer patient, he could heal by reversing his body chemistry, which is severely disturbed; by getting the body rid of the excess sodium; by putting a lot of potassium-rich foods plus potassium supplements into the system; by reactivating the digestive system and the body's ability to generate enzymes; and to detoxify itself by establishing the healing mechanism that exists in all our systems, which we suppress. The body heals itself!

"The body will first of all remove the layer of encapsulation or the seal by which the tumor protects itself. If you heard Dr. Nieper you understand that there is a layer around the tumor masses, which protects itself against the body's defenses. Dr. Gerson believed this to be largely a layer of sodium edematous cells. If you attack the sodium excess and remove the edema, you can easily destroy the tumor by forcing in potassium and Lugol Solution (iodine), which he gave.

"However, before you can do anything at all with these severely toxic patients you have to detoxify them. This is the beginning, the middle and the end of the story. You can't do anything until you remove the accumulated toxicity in the body. For instance, I have seen where autogenous vaccine injections had no reaction in the very severely damaged cancer patient. In the advanced cancer patient, which had no more immune reaction this is the big problem. They are so ill the body will no longer react. That's why the immunologists say, 'Well in some people it works and in some people it doesn't work.' The severely ill toxic cases do not react.

"I have seen a case like this who had been inoculated with vaccine, but was so severely toxic that nothing happened. After approximately four weeks of thorough detoxification with juices and enemas, which my father used for this purpose, suddenly there was a reaction to the vaccine and the body was working again. The immune reactions now took place.

"When you know that the immune reactions take place you know that the body is now also attacking the tumor as shown by research work done by immunologists. Dr. Good, an immunologist and head of research at Sloan Kettering, has shown that in order to attack any tumor in the body, a normal healthy system is needed to mobilize certain lymphocytes to attack a sick cell; a cell which they recognize as not normal. Now, all of us might have these sick cells floating around. If we are in reasonably good health, we have these defense mechanisms. We have an immune response in our body and we send the lymphocytes right out to kill and eliminate the foreign and diseased tissue.

"However, we cannot do this if our bodies are so toxic and damaged because the immune system no longer works. Also the enzyme system no longer works because for the enzymes to work they need a high potassium level. When there is too much sodium in the body, large numbers of enzymes are inhibited. I have an excerpt here from a book called *Enzymes* by Dixon and Webb. It shows the various enzymes the body needs to produce. In almost all cases the activating ion needed is potassium. The inhibiting ion? I will give you a guess. It is sodium. So if you have too much sodium in your body you inhibit the enzymes. You inhibit the body's ability to fight. In other words, your first line of defense is a high level of potassium. You obtain potassium in your natural foods, which are unprocessed, unsalted, unfrozen, unbottled, unsmoked, unpickled, etc. You must have natural foods, which support life and are not antagonistic to your body's requirements.

"On this kind of detoxification diet it soon became clear to my father that he could handle severe kidney degenerations. One time he had a patient who was going blind. Her retina was detaching and she had doctored around from one eye doctor to another. Naturally, they were all specialists. The eye doctors tried all kinds of treatments and nothing helped so they were going to operate. She was continually worsening and she was going blind. When she came to my father, he examined her whole body. He found her kidneys severely damaged and infected. He restored her kidneys and the retina grew back and her eyesight became quite normal!

"I am telling you, in other words, that severely damaged kidneys can be restored. We could empty the waiting lists on the kidney machines. There is no need for doctors to go through agonizing decisions. This patient goes on and this one we just don't have room for. He is going to have to die. He does not have to die! Kidneys that are degenerated can be restored. Transplanted kidneys would be unnecessary.

"Now transplanting organs is another great big nonsense. It does not take into consideration the body as a whole. When you transplant an organ you are putting it into the very environment that produced a sick person and made that organ degenerate in the first place. Now you can go on and give these transplant patients immune suppressive agents so that they will not reject a transplant. You further increase the damage to the liver and the whole body. People with transplants are in poor health and usually do not survive. Why not just restore the body and get the damaged organ working again? It can be done and it is not too difficult.

"We can restore sick hearts also. My father had a patient who had six heart attacks in eight days thirty-five years ago and he is alive and well today. He is 78 and fine. He did not need a new heart. He needed his heart restored.

"When it comes to multiple sclerosis, some of the studies in this area point to the possibility that M.S. is caused by lead, viral or some other damage. As far as we have seen it doesn't matter because you can rid the body of the damage caused by the toxicity. You can rebuild the body's ability to heal itself and you can rebuild the damaged nerve sheath and you can get rid of M.S. or whatever other chronic disease you want to name.

"I have seen a severe case of Rheumatoid Arthritis in a girl 24 years old clear up. She had this disease for about three years and she was just about paralyzed in all her limbs. They were all swollen and painful. After three days on a modified Gerson Diet you could see the structures in her skin and in her bones again. About three weeks later, all the deformities in her joints all over her body disappeared. After four weeks she went back to work. There was no more evidence of arthritis after four weeks.

"I hope that I have left you with a very clear understanding that by healing the body you can heal cancer and almost any other chronic disease and it doesn't matter what the cause. I am not going to argue whether it's caused by a virus, trophoblast, gene, radiation burns, or chemicals. It doesn't really matter.

"Remove the toxicity from your body and rebuild the body with the fresh juices from the raw organic foods as my father outlined in his book. When the tumors or toxic masses are removed with this constant detoxification then one can rebuild the organs. The liver is an organ that regenerates itself and after about 16 to 24 months the liver is renewed and most of the time can maintain health even with so-called 'normal' foods.

"Those of you who have read the book called *Death Be Not Proud,* about Johnny Gunther, will remember Mrs. Sealy mentioned in it. Mrs. Sealy was running the clinic for my father. She had a severe case of pancreas tumor, which is deadly. She was completely restored by the Gerson Diet. I accidentally ran across her flying to Florida one day, about 15 years after she had recovered. She had a cigarette in one hand and a cocktail in the other, and she was fine and didn't seem to care. Well, this can happen, the body's organs, if they are really restorable, and not too severely damaged by radiation, chemotherapy or the cancer, can often be restored fully and completely so that the body then will handle its own detoxification and will handle its own health even if you hurt it by going back to bad nutrition. In many cases, of course, this is not possible.

"Some of these cases were so far advanced that they are brought in just days from death and the liver is not fully restorable. The patients could live a normal life within a certain set of limitations. They could not eat junk foods, but they could eat organic meat and other organic foods, and were not nearly as limited as the book showed at the beginning for the early treatment and rebuilding of the body.

"We can handle a complete restoration of the body through the power of the healing mechanism, which must function at all times. Detoxification has to be complete at all times, which means either the body has to be able to handle its own or you have to help it. Detoxification includes the full digestion of foods. The very basic mechanism of health in the body is the digestive system. It must not only provide you with everything your cells need, but it must be able to reduce everything to its end product and eliminate the waste products. If your system is not able to do that, then it needs help or you have to avoid certain foods that your system is not able to break down, utilize and eliminate fully. Either one. If you do not do it, toxicity will start to build up.

"You can think of it in the way a sink stops up. If your sink doesn't drain well and you have a lot of water in there and you keep pouring water in, your level will keep going up and up, instead of draining down slowly, and finally it will overflow. This overflow is the chronic disease. The toxicity in the body is caused by improperly eliminated toxic material that you can build up yourself.

"Our American diet, unfortunately, is extremely high in proteins. If your pancreas is not able to digest the proteins that you feed it and cannot break them down to the end products, utilize what is usable and eliminate what is toxic or should be eliminated, then you are in trouble.

"Albert Schweitzer had severe diabetes when he came to my father. A diabetic is usually told that he can eat nothing but proteins. Dr. Schweitzer had been to the top specialists on diabetes and he was eating proteins and he felt terrible. A sick pancreas, which is producing diabetes, when it is overloaded with proteins, absolutely cannot handle this situation. As you know, very often this leads right on into cancer. Diabetes can be a precondition to cancer, because the pancreas is sick, and then you further proceed to overload it with proteins. It doesn't work. Now would you believe, however, that on this treatment you can give carrot and apple juice with all the sugar it contains? You can even give a baked potato a day to a diabetic. My father gave lots of juices such as the green juices and others, vegetables and salads, and within 10 days he could reduce the insulin dosage to half of what he had been using and within four weeks, no more insulin was needed. Even with all the fruit sugars he was eating, as you very well know, Dr. Schweitzer lived until he was 92. He not only lived, but he was active and working.

"When he came to my father at the age of 75, he said, 'The way I am going, I have no more energy. I am weary and I am tired of living and I don't want to do anything more.'

"But with the pancreas restored, he was able to live an active life again.

"I want to leave you with this thought and that is that chronic diseases are curable. Cancer is only one chronic disease. It is not a specific disease. All chronic diseases are deficiency diseases and they can be healed by the proper approach. And if I get any questions now, such as 'well, is this therapy good for such and such type of cancer, leukemia, or for melanoma, or is it good for Lupus Erythematosus or for any other chronic condition,' I haven't made myself clear."

CHAPTER 31

STARVATION TREATMENT FOR TUMORS

The *Nebraska State Medical Journal*, December, 1965, includes a report by Dr. Albert B. Lorincz and Robert E. Kuttner, Ph.D., describing an effort to starve tumors.

According to the report, malignant tumors demand 1.3 to 11 times the protein level necessary for normal cells.

Patients ordinarily described as terminal cancer patients were used.

Selectively, the amino acids (of which protein is composed) were restricted.

According to the report, some of the patients were even able to resume normal activities.

Such a method would require the attention of a physician intensively trained in nutrition, and probably specializing in it.

Therefore, the details of this highly technical procedure shall not be included here.

CHAPTER 32

MORE ON YOGURT— AND CANCER

The following article appeared in the *Cancer Control Journal,* Vol. 1, No. 4, December, 1973:

"Once Again, Yogurt Stops the Growth of Unhealthy Cells

"Now, at last, the word has gotten to the National Cancer Institute and they have published it in their Journal. The word is that something in yogurt inhibits the growth of cancer cells. One kind of cancer at any rate. Three scientists at the University of Nebraska used laboratory mice for their investigation. They gave two groups of mice regular laboratory chow to eat. One group got plain drinking water. The other was given a bit of yogurt in their drinking water. Then both groups were infected with cancer cells.

"After eight days, an average of 28 percent inhibition of cell proliferation was evident in the mice given yogurt. That is, 28 percent of the tumor cells did not grow, while in the mice which did not get the yogurt the tumor cells continued to grow as expected.

"Say the scientists, 'The above findings suggest that lactobacillic cultures synthesize components which have an anti-tumor effect.' They do not know what these components are and they plan further experiments to find out, if possible. Under no circumstances, of course, would they just recommend to the general public that they eat yogurt daily, since it may contain substances valuable in the prevention of cancer. Such a suggestion would be classified as 'faddist' by these people, we are sure, and by the National Cancer Institute as well.

So, instead, they will proceed, with ever more costly

and lengthy experiments trying to isolate the substance in yogurt which possesses this marvelous ability. Then they will probably try to cure cancer in mice with this isolated substance. And many years from now, perhaps some poor cancer victim may or may not benefit from this experiment.

"Meanwhile, as these Nebraska authors point out, there is evidence from scientists in European countries that extracts from yogurt effectively inhibit growth of two kinds of cancer. This is in addition to the abundant evidence from many sources showing that taking yogurt every day creates healthful conditions in the digestive tract, so that harmful bacteria are discouraged, and helpful ones are encouraged to grow. Considering that digestive disorders plague almost everyone in our population these days, one would think that health officials should be recommending yogurt with every meal.

"Several years ago we reported on using yogurt as a topical treatment for cancer. In the *Journal of the American Medical Association* for December 8, 1969, a physician from Missouri asked about the possibility of applying 'dried yogurt' as hospital treatment for breast cancer. A representative of the American Cancer Society replied:

" 'I suspect the paucity of information about this technique is because it is usually performed by nurses, both to help heal ulcerations and to dispel odors. According to our nursing consultant . . . the rationale for the use of yogurt is to fight bacterial fermentation and growth, and bacteria flourish in an alkaline medium; yogurt produces an acid medium which prevents the growth of odor-forming bacteria.

" 'Yogurt and buttermilk may be used almost interchangeably except that yogurt flakes are more expensive and so are usually restricted to small or virtually inaccessible areas. For example, the flakes would be appropriate for head and neck ulcerations, while buttermilk might be used for a large decubitus ulcer. Buttermilk is effective in irrigations, such as vaginal douches or colostomy irrigations. Yogurt and buttermilk are in daily use at Calvary Hospital in the Bronx, New York, a facility for the care of patients with advanced cancer.'

"We commented at that time that this statement seems to illustrate the tendency of the medical profession to allow just about anything, orthodox or unorthodox, when it comes to *treating* a serious or fatal disorder, but to scoff at the idea of *preventing* ailments with the same treatment. How many human ailments are related to bacteria of the harmful kind? The list is almost endless. How many of these ailments get their start from harmful bacteria that inhabit the human intestine? There must be many.

"When the health seeker manages to control these harmful intestinal bacteria with yogurt or buttermilk, which encourages the friendly or helpful bacteria at the same time, the medical profession declares with one voice that this is imaginery nonsense. A myth. A come-on. A fraud.

"But when the terminal cancer patient is afflicted with a wound so terrible that the odor from the bacteria inhabiting it is unendurable, what is used to overcome these bacteria and establish the healthful acid surroundings that are needed? Yogurt and buttermilk, *applied directly to the wound.*

"If you are a confirmed yogurt-eater, the above information should encourage you never to give up this habit. If you do not regularly buy or make yogurt, now is the time to start. We suggest that you avoid yogurts which have been flavored and sugared. Make your own flavoring by adding fruits, berries, nuts, seeds, or eat your yogurt as part of a salad, with scallions, chives, or cucumbers.

"Your health food store sells yogurt and sells utensils for making it at home, which come with full instructions. It's easy. It's fun. It's healthful!

Here are recipes for two fine salad dressings in which yogurt is a principal ingredient.

"Tangy Yogurt - Garlic Salad Dressing

2 tsp salt sub
2 chopped, crushed garlic cloves
1/3 cup plain yogurt
2 tbsp tabasco sauce
2 egg yolks
juice of 1 lemon
2 tbsp wine vinegar
1/4 cup tomato sauce
2 cups olive oil
1 tsp hot mustard

"Combine salt sub, garlic, tabasco sauce, lemon juice, mustard, egg yolks, vinegar and oil at low beater speed. Add the tomato sauce and yogurt and beat well. Keep refrigerated in covered container.

"Yogurt – Blue Cheese Salad Dressing

4 ounces blue cheese
3/4 cup salad oil
1 cup plain whole milk yogurt
1/4 cup cider vinegar
1 tsp salt sub
1/8 tsp pepper
1 tsp honey
1 tsp garlic powder
1 tsp onion powder

"Mash blue cheese with a fork. With an electric beater at low speed slowly add oil and beat until smooth. Add all other ingredients and beat well. Keep refrigerated in a covered container.

CHAPTER 33

DR. KELLEY'S THEORIES ABOUT PROTEIN AND CANCER

The following articles appeared in the *Cancer Control Journal,* Vol. 1, No. 2, July/August, 1973:

Dr. William Kelley's Three Interviews

"Note: It has been the policy of C.C.S. (Cancer Control Society) to present the views of spokesmen for a variety of non-toxic therapies, even though the therapies may not be equally substantiated or of equal value. It is also to be noted that C.C.S., our Editorial Committee, or other contributors do not necessarily endorse the statements or opinions of anyone quoted in the *Cancer Control Journal.* All information presented in the CCJ is offered solely as an educational service to our readers without recommendation or endorsement.

"The greatest gift that a hopeless cancer patient might receive from any person is information leading to a healthy, enjoyable life. Many previously hopeless patients are convinced that information given by our members has been such a gift.

"This gift of life may now be available to nearly all cancer patients if future results with a new therapy continue to verify the reports received so far by the Journal. This therapy was developed by a Texas dentist. If the early indications are fulfilled, more than 90% of all cancer patients now dying can recover if they start the therapy as little as three months before they would otherwise die (unless damage caused by radiation, chemicals, or surgery has been too severe).

"This therapy was planned so that for most cancer patients:

"1. All necessary materials would be available locally, eliminating any necessity for travel.

"2. The materials would be already approved by the Food and Drug Administration (FDA) for sale in the United States.

"3. Most of the materials would be obtained from animal and vegetable sources in order to generally be safe and non-toxic.

"4. The therapy would be quite inexpensive when compared to the presently used orthodox treatment.

"5. A doctor's assistance would not be essential. However, the assistance of a cooperating physician is desirable if one can be found (many doctors will dare not risk any cooperation). Unless the patient is too weak, he could give himself most of the therapy. A family member or friend could be of considerable assistance.

"6. The essential information would be presented in an inexpensive book written in easily understood language.

"The dentist who developed this new therapy is Dr. William Donald Kelley. The title of his book is *One Answer to Cancer.*

"Dr. Kelley has stated that the techniques of the therapy are very simple but many people are unwilling to change their habits and ways of living to accept these techniques.

"Several people have sent letters reporting good results. We have met others who also report good results.

"*Cancer Victims and Friends* has presented information on several different therapies in the past. We usually state that we consider that the best chances of recovery occur if the patient combined several non-toxic therapies which approach the cancer in several vulnerable directions.

"Therefore, we were quite interested when one therapy combining at least three approaches to cancer was reported to have such good results. Dr. Kelley's therapy includes parts of the scientific thinking attributed to Dr. John Beard, Dr. Ernst Krebs, Jr., Dr. Max Gerson, and others in addition to certain observations of his own.

"We arranged interviews with Dr. Kelley. These interviews provided the material for much of this article.

"Before presenting the interviews, we shall give some background and review of some of the other cancer therapies. This will clarify some of the approaches to cancer and provide a better basis for understanding and evaluating Dr. Kelley's therapy.

"Since its beginning in 1963, Cancer Victims and Friends has worked toward the goal of humane effective treatment for all cancer patients, particularly hopeless ones. We have seen enough extensive evidence to convince us beyond any doubt that several non-toxic therapies produce percentages of recoveries greatly in excess of the percentages achieved by the orthodox treatments of surgery, radiation and toxic or poisonous chemicals.

"There are at least 80 non-toxic therapies. The objective of each of these therapies is to overcome at least one vulnerable aspect of cancer. Some of the therapies approach more than one vulnerable aspect. These various therapies give evidence of varying results with cancer. Even those indicating the lowest percentages of recovery still appear much better than the less than 1 in 10,000 indicated for the orthodox treatment of internal metastasized cancer.

"Dr. Gerson, in his book, *A Cancer Therapy – Fifty Case Histories,* reported 40 to 50% recoveries for internal, metastasized cancer. Although the percentages of recovery can be expected to decrease as the cancer progresses, Dr. Gerson reported on one recovery who came to him unconscious on a stretcher in the last stages of cancer. Dr. Gerson used a practical approach to trying many different things. Those that succeeded, he incorporated in his treatment; those that failed, he rejected. Oversimplifying perhaps, his therapy consisted of two primary approaches to cancer.

"One was to provide an intensive nutritional program to provide the maximum practical amount of the most desirable nutrients needed by all the organs and functions of the body and to provide them in the forms easiest for the body to utilize. Raw fruit and vegetable juices were an important part of this approach. His other approach was an intensive detoxification program to help the body eliminate toxic materials (poisons) which typically accumulate in the blood, liver, intestinal tract, and other tissue and organs in the body and interfere with proper body functions.

"Several other therapies have emphasized either or both of the detoxification and intensive nutritional approaches to cancer.

"About 70 years ago, Dr. John Beard at the University of Edinburgh discovered that the body's primary mechanism for destroying cancer apparently was contained in pancreatin, a secretion from the pancreas that included enzymes for digesting protein (among other things, enzymes digest or liquify foods for absorption by the body; some meat tenderizers use an enzyme from papayas to partially digest or soften meat). Dr. Beard left pictures in his books and papers to show recoveries using pancreatin.

"This was another approach: a direct attack on the malignancy with a substance which did not have toxic side effects on other functions in the body.

"Dr. Howard Beard (no relation) of Fort Worth, Texas, has contributed considerably to the understanding and use of pancreatic enzymes in the treatment of cancer. He and other researchers have indicated that trypsin and particularly chymotrypsin are the most important enzymes in pancreatin as far as cancer is concerned. Dr. Beard also recommended a nutritional program and other things, as stated in his book, *A New Approach to Cancer, Rheumatic, and Heart Diseases.*

"Dr. Ernst Krebs, Jr., of San Francisco, through brilliant

logic and insight, was able to show how amygdalin, a substance contained in many foods, could assist the pancreatic enzymes in destroying cancer. He stated that the amygdalin took advantage of the natural chemistry of the malignant cells in such a way as to destroy them without damaging other body tissue. Amygdalin is one of many nitrilosides occurring in more than 1200 plants. The trade name of these substances as purified for treating cancer is Laetrile.

"Cancer Victims and Friends was formed by Mrs. Cecile Hoffman. She was inspired to do so by her response to Laetrile therapy.

"Even though a person has internal, metastasized cancer, about 70 to 80% appear to recover on Laetrile if they have a life expectancy of one year. The percentage of recovery appears to reduce, as would be expected, as life expectancy grows shorter. However, a few people brought in on stretchers with a few days' life expectancy also appear to have recovered.

"An additional advantage of Laetrile therapy is the reported elimination or great reduction of pain in most cancer patients. Dr. Krebs, Dr. Dean Burk of the National Cancer Institute, and others report that this is due to the natural action of Laetrile in the body.

"Another approach has to do with rehabilitating or supplementing the functions of oxygen in the body. Dr. Otto Warburg stated that cancer did not develop unless the oxygen level available to the cells was too low. Dr. William Koch developed several catalysts for assisting oxygen in removing poisons and toxins from the blood and tissue. Reports on recoveries have varied from 80% to 20%. Dr. Robert Olney, as reported in our last *Cancer News Journal,* has used ultra violet blood irradiation to increase oxygen levels in the blood sometimes by a factor of 4 or 5, for a considerable time after the treatment. There are other oxygenation approaches as well. For instance, eliminating any of the many causes of anemia will raise the blood's oxygen level. At least, it seems entirely reasonable that a patient's strength, sense of well being, will to live, stamina and health are very likely to improve if his oxygen is brought up to normal levels.

"Treatments with herbs have produced many reported successes. The desert creosote bush used as *chaparral tea* or in capsules has apparently produced many recoveries. It has been much in the news recently. Most herbal approaches use a variety of herbs. *The Hoxsey treatment is primarily herbal.* Thousands of successful case histories have been reported with it. The different herbs seem to work in a variety of ways. Some ways are understood and some are not.

"Many other individual materials appear to have been used successfully. Among these are a *mistletoe preparation, raw beet juice,* and *lactobacillus bifidus* — a friendly bacteria cultured from other's milk.

"Let's return to consideration of the Kelley therapy and give a concise description of it.

"*Cancer Control Journal does not consider it wise for a patient to discontinue any non-toxic therapy in order to try Dr. Kelley's relatively new treatment. We believe that a wiser approach is to combine this therapy with other non-toxic methods in order to approach the cancer in as many ways as possible.*

"Dr. Kelley's therapy described in *One Answer to Cancer,* is planned to include at least three of the principal approaches to cancer treatment:

"1. A way of destroying malignant cancer cells directly.

"2. An intensive therapeutic nutritional program.

"3. An intensive detoxification program.

"Dr. Kelley agrees with several other researchers who have said that pancreatic enzymes are one of the body's natural mechanisms for preventing and destroying cancer. Some of these researchers have been Dr. John Beard of Scotland in 1902, Ernst Krebs, Jr. (see *Laetrile: Control for Cancer* by Kittler), and Dr. Howard Beard. Dr. Beard says he has controlled his cancer of the colon for 25 years by using pancreatic enzymes.

"Dr. Kelley says that cancer is an inability of the body to metabolize (digest and utilize) protein, similar to the way that diabetes can be defined as inability of the body to metabolize sugars and other carbohydrates. He contends that malignant tumors are symptoms of the cancer which can grow when the pancreatic enzyme function is inadequate. In a similar sense, the spilling of sugar into the urine is a symptom of diabetes, not the diabetes itself. Dr. Kelley draws other analogies between cancer and diabetes.

"Dr. Kelley considered there may be several different problems with the pancreative enzyme functions. Several of these he gives are:

"1. Inadequate output of enzymes from the pancreas.

"2. Excessive intake of proteins, particularly animal proteins, that use all of the enzymes and create a deficiency of the enzymes that could otherwise digest the malignant cells.

"3. Inadequate minerals and other co-factors required for the pancreatic enzymes to function, even when the enzyme output is adequate.

"4. Poor blood circulation with resultant inability to carry enzymes to the tumor.

"5. Excessive production of anti-enzymes, normally used by the body for keeping the enzymes in check.

"Therefore, Dr. Kelley in his therapy has planned to conserve the body's supply of pancreatic enzymes for the purpose of digesting the malignant cells. The proteins are restricted in type and quantity and are consumed only between breakfast and 1:00 p.m. Digestive supplements including pancreatic enzymes are recommended by Dr. Kelley with each meal to reduce the utilization of the body's own pancreatic enzymes. These are readily available without prescription.

"At 2:30 p.m. and 3:30 a.m. the therapy requires that 5 to 8 pancreatic enzyme tablets are taken orally. Dr. Kelley says that at these times, there is no protein in the intestinal tract to digest so the enzymes enter the blood stream where they digest the malignant cells in the tumors. He states that in a week or two, so much waste material from the destroyed malignant cell is dumped into the blood stream that most peoples' bodies cannot eliminate all of it rapidly enough to keep from feeling sick. If this occurs, he says the enzymes should be discontinued until the elimination processes catch up. Then, he says to adjust the pancreatic enzymes intake so that the patient feels a little bit sick, but not too sick, until the malignant cells are completely destroyed, usually no more than a few months. He says the time depends on the tumor size, and the availability of blood with enzymes at the site of the malignancy. He states that no one should have leukemia for more than a few weeks.

"Dr. Kelley's book outlines an intensive nutritional program including foods, raw vegetable juices (based on Dr. Max Gerson's *A Cancer Therapy – Fifty Case Histories*) and a number of food supplements. These materials are generally readily available. Additional information is provided in the interview.

"The intensive detoxification program is intended to help the body eliminate waste materials which collect in the blood, organs, and intestinal tract. Some of the detoxification program is based on Dr. Gerson's book.

"Dr. Kelley has also developed what appears to be a highly accurate blood test for detecting cancer and monitoring the progress of the therapy. However, he does not consider it an essential part of his therapy, particularly if the patient already knows he has cancer. He considers several urine tests such as the Beard Anthrone Test and the Navarro Immunological Test to be good. He says that the patient should understand, however, that the urine tests will indicate an increasingly positive value in the first weeks of treatment because more of the hormone detected is given off when malignant cells are being digested by the enzymes.

"Dr. John Beard, professor at the University of Edinburgh, Scotland, shortly after 1900, speaking about his trophoblastic thesis and his finding that the pancreatic enzymes are nature's way of destroying cancer: 'God help us if I am wrong.'

CHAPTER 34

VITAMIN C AND LEUKEMIA – IS EVOLUTION TO BLAME?

The following article appeared in the *Cancer Control Journal,* No. 1, Vol. 2, January/February, 1974:

"Megascorbic Therapy of the Disease called 'Leukemia'
The Use of Massive Doses of Ascorbate in the
Control of Leukemic Mortality

Talk presented at the first annual Cancer Convention of
the Cancer Control Society, July 13, 1973
Ambassador Hotel, Los Angeles

Irwin Stone

"In 1912, Casimir Funk, after summarizing the clinical nutrition research of the late 19th century and early 20th century, proposed a new theory of disease causation. He postulated that certain diseases could be caused by the lack of some unknown missing essential constituents in foodstuffs. These unknown missing elements he called vitamins and he recognized three groups to which he assigned the letters A, B and C. Vitamin A was an unknown fat soluble compound, which when missing from the diet of rats, caused a serious eye disease. Vitamin B was later found to be a whole group of water soluble 'vitamins,' which, when absent from the diet, caused a severe nerve disease, a paralytic polyneuritis. Vitamin C, of unknown composition and properties was postulated as causing the deadly disease scurvy when absent from the diet.

"Later work confirmed the correctness of this theory when applied to the vitamins of the A and B groups, but it has been shown to be a gross oversimplification when the vitamin theory is applied to vitamin C and scurvy.

"Our discussion from this point will be confined solely to Vitamin C. For the past sixty years, medicine has unqualifiedly accepted the tenets of the vitamin C theory and it has been the blind acceptance of this inadequate theory which has obstructed clinical research and erected barriers to clear thinking regarding its vast therapeutic potential.

"Twenty years after the theory was proposed, ascorbic acid was isolated, identified as vitamin C and synthesized. This work was so highly regarded that two Nobel Prizes were awarded in 1937, one to Albert Szent Gyorgyi and the other to Walter Haworth. The chemical synthesis has been so improved that ascorbic acid can be obtained in wholesale quantities at about four dollars a kilogram in potentially unlimited quantities, which amounts to about 2500 milligrams for a penny.

"In 1965-67, I demonstrated that frank clinical scurvy was not the simple dietary disturbance, the avitaminosis C, as it had long been regarded, but was the final, pre-mortal symptom of impending death from a genetic, liver-enzyme disease. This disease I named 'Hypoascorbemia' which is caused by humans carrying a defective gene for the production of the liver enzyme, L-gulonolactone oxidase. I have been able to trace the origin of this defective gene to a mutation occurring in a primate ancestor of man about 55 million years ago.

"The lack of this enzyme in the human liver produces an inborn error of carbohydrate metabolism which prevents us from synthesizing our own ascorbic acid (vitamin C) in our livers. This synthesis is common and normal to most mammals and they produce large amounts each day. It is a stress-responsive process and under stress, the mammals produce even greater daily amounts of ascorbic acid. The main function of this large ascorbic acid production during the evolution of the mammals was to maintain homeostatis during biochemical stress. Because of this defective human gene, man, throughout his entire history, has been deprived of this important mammalian protective mechanism.

"Since all living things require ascorbic acid for survival, this defective gene is the reason we humans need an outside source of ascorbic acid or vitamin C. Because of its many functions in the living process, ascorbic acid is required in much larger daily quantities to fully correct the genetic disease, hypoascorbemia, than is the amount of avitaminosis C. It has only been in the last 40 years that we have the technology to fully correct this inborn error of metabolism, which has been afflicting man and his primate ancestors for the past 55 million years. Ascorbic acid and vitamin C have been, up to this point, synonymously used, but since it is not a true mammalian vitamin, but rather a liver metabolite, it will, hereafter, be referred to only as 'ascorbic acid.'

"This defective gene is common to all mankind, therefore, chronic hypoascorbemia is now our most prevalent disease and the basis for our most pressing medical problems. It can be simply corrected with large daily intakes of ascorbic acid, many grams per day.

"Now how does all this fit in for the use of ascorbic acid in the treatment of leukemia? In the first place, these new genetic concepts establish the rationale for the use of large daily doses of ascorbic acid. The genetic disease, hypoascorbemia, cannot be fully corrected solely by consuming fresh foods. The quantities of ascorbic acid existing in foods are so low that it is physically impossible to consume the weight of fresh foodstuffs necessary to give the required gram quantities of ascorbic acid a day. Our digestive systems are just not geared for it. We have to supplement our intake whether we consider ourselves to be in fair health or are suffering from disease.

"The normal mammalian biochemical reaction to stress

is for the liver to increase its production of ascorbic acid in an attempt to overcome the bad effects of the stress and maintain biochemical homeostasis. Because of the defective gene, man is unable to manufacture *any* ascorbic acid in the liver, so any stress just further depletes the usually low body stores of this vital substance. Any stress, without ascorbic acid repletion, only makes the patient's chronic hypoascorbemia more serious. This condition is what was formerly called chronic, subclinical scurvy and has been found in cancer, heart disease and many other diseases. When a patient dies of cancer, heart disease and other fatal conditions, it is the severe chronic hypoascorbemia or subclinical scurvy existing in the patient at the time of death which has prevented his survival.

"Man has existed on subsistence levels of ascorbic acid for so long that medicine has come to regard these low levels as 'normal,' unless frank clinical scurvy results. It is possible that the chronic subclinical scurvy existing in the victim since infancy and even in the womb, with a history of the parents, grandparents, great-grandparents, etc., suffering from the same disease, this may be a factor in initiating the leukemia. These chronic low levels of ascorbic acid may start the wild proliferation of the white blood cells, bringing on the leukemic process.

"While this may be speculation, there is no speculation, but hard clinical facts that leukemics have pathologically low levels of ascorbic acid in their blood plasma. It is not only the biochemical stresses of the leukemic disease which lowers the plasma ascorbic acid levels, but also the abnormally large volumes of white blood cells which scavenge and remove the remaining ascorbic acid from the blood serum. The white blood cells, which selectively absorb up to 40 times more ascorbic acid from the blood serum than the red blood cells, do a fine job of removing the final traces of ascorbic acid from the blood serum and trap it within their cells and make it unavailable to the tissues.

"The fact that there is no ascorbic acid left in the blood plasma deprives the tissues of the body of this most important and essential metabolite. The synthesis of collagen, in the tissues, for maintaining the strength of the tissues, the blood vessels and capillaries is dependent on an adequate supply of ascorbic acid in the blood plasma. If the blood plasma is deficient in ascorbic acid, collagen production will stop and the mechanical strength of tissues, blood vessels and capillaries will weaken and hemorrhage will result.

"Our first line of defense against infection, phagocytosis, is also an ascorbic acid dependent process. Phagocytosis is the gobbling up and digestion of invading bacteria in the blood stream and tissues by white blood cells. Under normal conditions, with a good supply of ascorbic acid in the blood serum, any injury or bacteria getting into the tissues attracts hordes of white blood cells to the area and they immediately get to work swallowing and digesting the bacteria and foreign material. In the process of phagocytosis, the number of bacteria ingested and digested is directly related to the blood serum levels of ascorbic acid. When the ascorbic acid levels are low, or absent, phagocytosis stops and the bacteria grow and reproduce in the tissues and a full blown infection develops.

"It is no wonder that what kills most leukemics is not the neoplastic disease itself, but hemorrhage and infection. This is a statistical fact. Both lack of resistance to infections and hemorrhaging are pathognomonic symptoms of scurvy. They are suffering from uncorrected hypoascorbemia or severe chronic subclinical scurvy in addition to the leukemia. Leukemics require high levels of ascorbic acid amounting to many grams per day to conquer their severe hypoascorbemia. If we can prevent them from dying of the manifestations of scurvy, it may be found that leukemia itself may not be such a serious fatal disease, after all.

"There have been many attempts to treat leukemia with ascorbic acid, as recorded in the medical literature of the past 40 years. All of this work, except one, shows the strong influence of the vitamin C theory in misorienting the clinicians doing this work. Except for one case history, all the clinical investigators used low vitamin-like doses of ascorbic acid of from 100 milligrams or 200 milligrams a day to 900 milligrams a day. On these low dosages, variable and uncertain clinical results were obtained. In the one recorded case where complete remission was achieved and maintained in myelogenous leukemia, the patient took 24,500 to 42,000 milligrams of ascorbic acid a day.

"Let me give you some details from this case history reported in 1954. The patient was a 71-year-old oil executive who was first seen for alcoholic hepatic cirrhosis and polycythemia. Previously he had developed symptoms of chronic rheumatic and arteriosclerotic myocarditis. He was hospitalized and passed a large uric acid bladder stone and a few months later a diagnosis of chronic myelogenous leukemia was established. He also had intractable pyorrhea and his remaining 17 teeth were extracted at one operation. The history so far was indicative of severe chronic subclinical scurvy, but it appears no one thought of scurvy or bothered to look into the ascorbic acid status of the patient. Apparently, on his own initiative, he started taking ascorbic acid at the rate of 24,500 milligrams to 42,000 milligrams a day, because as the case history states 'he reported that he felt much better when he took these large doses.' The reporting physician continues, 'the patient has repeatedly remarked about his feeling of well-being and has continued his vocation as an executive of an oil company. On two occasions, on my insistence, the (ascorbic acid) was discontinued as an experiment. Both times his spleen enlarged to the brim of the pelvis, became soft and very tender, temperature rose to 101 degrees and he complained of general malaise and fatigue. His liver enlarged one finger's breadth, became soft and tender. When the (ascorbic acid) was again started his signs and symptoms were greatly improved, the temperature becoming normal within six hours. The patient continued on this ascorbic acid regimen for over a year and a half and he died at age 73 of acute cardiac decompensation, preceded by a severe attack of epidemic diarrhea' (probably from food poisoning). It was noted that, 'At the time of death the spleen was firm, non-tender and at the level of the umbilicus. It had not enlarged (in the year and a half). The polycythemia, leukemia, cirrhosis, and myocarditis had shown no progression (in the year and a half).' The report concluded with this statement, 'The intake of the huge dose of ascorbic acid appeared to be essential for the welfare of the patient.'

"It seems inconceivable that such exciting results could have been ignored for the past 20 years and has lain dormant in the medical literature. No one picked it up or bothered to try this simple, harmless chemotherapy in some of the thousands of cases of leukemia which appear each year. Fantastic as it seems, this is the case; a search of medical literature failed to reveal any further work in this area.

"What is wrong with our government cancer institutes and the public supported foundations for cancer and leukemia, that they should ignore such provocative results? The medical fraternity is also remiss because this treatment is so simple and uses such a common, inexpensive commodity as ascorbic acid, which any individual doctor could try because it involves no expensive equipment or laboratories or exotic chemicals or biostatisticians to see the results. It is available right now to any doctor — we do not have to wait for years for double blind controlled testing.

"The need for a simple, successful and harmless therapy of this disease is so critical that no suggestion should be left untried, even if the doctor's mental barriers erected by years of misinformation tell him that it cannot work.

"I shall briefly summarize the rationale of the proposed Megascorbic Therapy of Leukemia:

"Leukemia is not a single disease but a combination of a neoplastic blood disease and severe biochemical scurvy. The scurvy can be relieved by massive daily dosing with ascorbic acid or sodium ascorbate. The secret is to empty 25 to 100 grams of ascorbate or more a day, orally or intravenously or a combination of both. Relief of this scorbutic burden will give the patient a fighting chance for his body to battle with the neoplastic process. It may be found that without the severe biochemical scurvy, leukemia may be a relatively benign, nonfatal condition.

"Further, ascorbate, in these large doses, is the only non-toxic, non-specific virucide known. If leukemia is a virus infection, as recent work indicates, then the ascorbate would function, not only to clear up the scurvy, but also to attack the actual causative agent of the disease.

"Because of the brief time available for presenting this talk, many details and much medical data and references had to be omitted or glossed over. All the facts which I have cited in this talk can be substantiated by references in the medical literature. The detailed data and medical references can be found by referring to my new book, *The Healing Factor, 'Vitamin C' Against Disease,* published by Grosset and Dunlap, Inc., in 1972, New York City. It is sold by the Cancer Book House.

"This sort of concludes the scientific part of my talk, but I would like to add a few comments. This talk is based on a scientific paper, of similar title, which I wrote in 1966. It was a paper giving this rationale for the Megascorbic Therapy of Leukemia in an attempt to have the therapy clinically tested. During 1967, I sent the paper consecutively to three cancer journals and three blood journals in an attempt to have it published. It was refused by all the journals. Two of the journals refused publication without even reading the paper. It was returned so fast that they could not have possibly read and understood it. The word 'Ascorbic' in the title prejudiced the editors and reviewers — they just 'knew' it could not work.

"For the past six years, it has been in my files and I cannot help wondering how many thousands of lives could have been saved and how much suffering could have been avoided during this time, had the editors and reviewers just read the paper with an unbiased mind and permitted its publication.

"Thank you."

Questions and Answers

"Q. Did you say 2500 mgs. daily for leukemia?

"A. No, in the case that was reported it was 24,500 to 42,000 mg. a day. This was in a paper that was published in the *Medical Times* in 1954.

"Q. The gentleman asked is there any danger in using too much ascorbic acid.

"A. Ascorbic acid is one of the least toxic substances of similar physiological activity that I know of. Any excess is taken up by the kidneys and excreted in the urine, so there is usually not much of a danger for any serious side effects. Some people, when they take large doses of ascorbic acid are affected with a little diarrhea, but that is only a case of choosing the danger of leukemia or the discomfort of diarrhea, and I think the treatment of leukemia would be preferred.

"Q. What is required for normal maintenance?

"A. Well, in my book I refer to three or four different investigators, Linus Pauling, Dr. Klenner, myself, and a few others. We all agree that the need is for amounts from about two grs. to possibly ten grs. a day under unstressed conditions. Under stress you might have to go up to 100 grams a day, even intravenous use of it. Of course, a doctor would have to give you that. Now, stress includes an awful lot of conditions, such as exposure to heat and cold, pollution, radiation, mental stresses and various diseases that you may get heart disease, cancer, viral infections and bacterial infections.

"Q. That means taking some hourly?

"A. Well, you don't have to take it hourly – you can space it into four or five doses a day.

"Q. Regarding the size of doses of ascorbic acid.

"A. Sometimes taking the large doses of ascorbic acid causes a little gastric distress, due to the high acidity, in those cases, you can use sodium ascorbate, which is the sodium salt and is neutral and tasteless. Ascorbic acid is highly acidic and quite sour in taste. Now, if you can't get the sodium ascorbate, a simple expedient would be to take the ascorbic acid powder and mix it with about one-eighth the amount of sodium bicarbonate. It will fizz and you will form the sodium ascorbate that way. It will be much less acidic. The best way to take ascorbic acid is with food and you usually don't have any irritating effects then.

"Q. Have you done any work with magnesium ascorbate and is there any chance it will be available in this country?

"A. Well it is unlikely that magnesium ascorbate will be available, there's not enough of a market for the drug companies to put it out but you can get the same effect if you take ascorbic acid and magnesium oxide at the same time.

"Q. Is ascorbic acid the natural vitamin C?

"A. Yes, the natural vitamin C is ascorbic acid. That's the material you would be producing in your liver if you didn't have this defective gene. It's the same ascorbic acid that is produced by plants, and it so happens that if you put a plant under stress ascorbic acid will do the same thing for the plant that it will do for the human. It's been used throughout evolution as an anti-stress material.

"Q. Someone who had been giving ascorbic acid to children took the child to the dentist and the dentist, finding some tooth erosion, said the ascorbic acid was taking the calcium out of the teeth.

"A. This is a common condition you will get from imbibing any acidic substance — drink certain carbonated soft drinks, lemon juice, or any acid fruit juice and you will get this condition if you allow the juice to stay in your mouth too long. The best way is to take a glass of water after your drink in order to rinse out the acidity. Long contact with ascorbic acid will tend to decalcify your teeth, but you can get around that by using sodium ascorbate. While talking about children, I'd like to give you the recommended daily intake that Dr. Frederick Klenner uses for his child patients. He gives 1,000 mg. of ascorbate to children for each year of age — a four-year-old would get 4,000 mg. and he increases 1,000 mgs. for each year of age to the age of ten, then gives ten grams thereafter. For instance, children over ten and adults get ten grams per day, 10,000 mgs.

"Q. Since the Herpes viruses are normally present in the body in healthy conditions and apparently cause trouble only when the body's natural defenses break down, is there any nutritional program which will aid in boistering these defenses?

"A. Well, I think there is a program that can be used, and that is to take large daily doses of ascorbic acid. Ascorbate is the only non-toxic, as I mentioned, non-specific virucide that we know of. It can prevent and cure any viral disease, when used properly. We have been working on animals and we can take a dog which is suffering from severe viral encephalitis, which is known as distemper in dogs — the equivalent of sleeping sickness in humans and successfully treat them with ascorbate. We give them a couple of shots of ascorbic acid intravenously — amounting to about twelve (12) grams of sodium ascorbate in each shot, twice a day, and we get rid of the viral encephalitis in two days. I'll give you the details of one case. The owner brought the dog in, to this veterinary hospital, and the dog was practically on its last legs. It could hardly move – it was practically comatose and hadn't eaten for a week. My colleague gave him the injection of sodium ascorbate and put him in a cage. He then went out to the kitchen in the hospital and opened a can of dog food. When he came back the dog was active and jumping around the cage, was voraciously hungry and gobbled the food. In the short time since the injection his temperature had gone down to normal. After a few more shots of sodium ascorbate, the dog was sent home cured, with no signs of brain damage."

CHAPTER 35

BLOOD SUPPLY TO CANCER

Dr. Solomon Garb wrote *Cure for Cancer a National Goal,* Springer Publishing Company, New York, 1968. Dr. Garb is recognized as a research genius, as indicated by an unusual project.

Under his direction, in 1959, Albany Medical College students transplanted some cancer to the hamster cheek pouch.

A blood supply to the tumor developed described by the author as "impressive." Small blood vessels to the cancer developed and, within six days, a small artery. The small artery led to a larger artery in the host animal.

The small artery developed to the size of the internal cartoid artery, one of the largest in the body, as I understand the material.

The arteries thus produced to feed the cancer were not from within the cancer nor manufactured by it, but were produced by the host.

To me, as a layman, this would appear to indicate that cancer must be intended by Nature to serve some survival purpose, whereby cancer cells are protected.

I will not try further to justify this hypothesis here.

CHAPTER 36

IS LACK OF COMMUNICATION A MAJOR CAUSE OF CANCER?

Research represents the public interest only when it is communicated to those who benefit by it. Otherwise, the small rewards given those who conduct the research represent the outside limits of benefaction.

If lack of communication be limiting efforts toward the prevention of cancer to the extent that prevention may be possible, then weakness in communication must represent one of the principal causes of cancer.

Throughout the world are many approaches to cancer. Running down all such information is impossible, and even a sizeable sampling must represent many hours of work, beyond what the average person might be expected to undertake.

Reporting scientific experiments, one by one, may hardly substitute for reporting the direction of cancer research and observation throughout the world.

Observation may represent a viewpoint as important as controlled experiment, inasmuch as some areas of the world are almost entirely, if not entirely, without cancer.

Controlled experiments may or may not offer the reasons why. Observation may represent the most significant criterion, if not the only one, in some instances.

Cases of cancer arrest should certainly be examined irrespective of whether or not produced under conditions of controlled experiment. Even within the history of science, the hypothesis usually precedes whatever results may be demonstrated. Cases of cancer arrest should represent bases for hypothesis, to determine if repetition be possible.

Cases of cancer arrest should not be simply ignored, because a controlled experiment had not been established in advance.

Most of the research done on cancer and in many other fields has depended upon tax money or public contribution for subsidy. Does this establish the "right" of those carrying out the wishes of the public to establish private domains of information, for personal use or the use of the institution conducting the research? Anyone who pays taxes or has contributed to such work as described can understand the validity of the question.

True, the use of information may be abused. But suppose it is not abused. Suppose information is presented in a straightforward manner without distortion or proselyting of opinion.

Is such reporting afforded the same protection given the press, for the same reason, protection of the public?

Within the field of cancer communication exists an internecine struggle to obstruct viewpoints which don't coincide. Outside of pure research, which is usually too technical for the layman and necessarily restricted in area, most books on cancer represent a patently biased effort, not only to "sell" the viewpoint offered, but also to preclude the reader's looking at any other viewpoint as anything but dishonest and venally motivated.

I say that this kind of reporting is inescapably dishonest, even when undertaken by honest people. In short, the system is wrong.

It seems unlikely that a book on cancer may be published without opposition, unless slanted.

Efforts thus far to consult with people have produced only recommended revision of the book to make it a propoganda book, or to meet requirements which probably are not possible to meet, with, happily, some exceptions.

Many requirements have nothing to do with public need, so far as this document is concerned.

No personalities are involved in this dissertation. With

one out of four Americans suffering from cancer, and with much cancer throughout the world, the issue raised here simply reaches far beyond personalities or private interest of any kind.

Do I have any rights in behalf of the public to quote material, to raise questions, rather than allegedly resolve them according to some preconceived pattern?

This question I've raised with my lawyers. If I find I don't have such rights, to the best of my ability, I will make this a public issue.

CHAPTER 37

CANCER CONFLICT AND A POSSIBLE NEED FOR CONSTITUTIONAL AMENDMENT

The American Cancer Society is reputed to be responsible for the study of one million human subjects to determine whether or not cigarettes might be a factor in lung cancer.

Such approach is far different from that taken with Laetrile. Perhaps the benefits of the Laetrile treatment, if any, may stem entirely from diet. But a study of people should be made, to determine (do benefits occur?) and (if they do, why?).

Worse than nothing is research with predetermined answers. The allegation has been made that such "research" has been done in connection with Laetrile.

With such reports as that of Mr. Stickle, further investigation of the matter should not be stopped by the kind of diatribe quoted earlier in this work. Any document getting into personalities cannot be classified as a scientific document, by its very nature.

Much more study needs to be done in relation to human populations, and the proportion of cancer found in them. Mice don't smoke cigarettes. Mice might have been studied from now until doom's day with little substantial knowledge as to the effect of cigarette smoking. Mice may hardly demonstrate to us how much damage may result from robbing food of nutrients, from partially restoring soil through fertilizers without full restoration, from preservatives, and from pollutants within the environment. But conditions in other parts of the world make such comparisons possible.

The shortcomings of animal research should be clarified. For instance, the digestive tract of the human being stretches quite a few miles longer than that of the mouse, and the possible effects of this minor difference, however slight, should be at least mentioned in connection with human diet. Breast-fed babies, for example, get Lactobacillus Bifidus from the mother's milk, not Lactobacillus Bulgaricus.

On the other hand, the significance of some animal research should be clarified. It is alleged that a calf will die within a short time if fed pasteurized milk. If so, why? If so, does this have any relevancy to human beings? Such research is simply ignored entirely.

Might raw milk be produced safely? It might be. Raw milk might both cost and save a lot of money. Would it save lives? The question is certainly relevant. Presently the sale of raw milk is illegal for human consumption, and the case is closed. But the rate of cancer is increasing.

Cancer, Diagnosis, Treatment and Prognosis, by Lauren V. Ackerman, M.D., and Juan A. del Regato, M.D., Third Edition, The C. V. Mosby Company, St. Louis, 1962, under *Biopsy,* page 58, contains the statement:

"It is imperative that pathologic verification of malignant tumors be present before any therapy for them is instituted."

The book is a classic. What is now known must be better used.

The Parade Magazine, for March 28, 1976, by Donald Robinson, discusses "Does Your Doctor Know How to Treat Cancer?"

The author quotes the director of a cancer center as saying that many doctors neither know how to treat cancer, nor do they send patients to a qualified specialist.

The article declares that 85% of all cancer patients go to community hospitals lacking both the equipment and technical skill needed to treat cancer.

It warns that a second opinion should be sought in connection with a diagnosis of cancer. Also, it warns not to let your family physician pick your consultant because he is likely to pick a friend, rather than the most skilled man available.

The article suggests checking with a medical school or call the American Cancer Society.

There is no actual proof that the human mind is capable of understanding the cell well enough ever to explain cancer fully, any more than there is proof that some may be able to describe life after death, although some claim to be able to do this. Maybe some can do it, but proof is something else.

Even if human competence may reach an answer to cancer, the realization of such a hope appears to be far down the road. For example, body rhythm should be considered in connection with drugs, not presently a requisition according to *Body Time*.

I have been told by scientists as competent as any in the field, whom I will not quote by name, to avoid embarrassing them to no purpose, that final answers may be far away in terms of cellular mechanics.

If what is to be observed is to be so restricted, the human race may become extinct before answers may be found, because causes of cancer may out-distance answers, even if they are the right answers.

In addition to trying to destroy cancer, some attention should be given the benevolent forces of Nature, on the assumption that Satan may not rule the Universe, after all. As mentioned, there are places on this planet where cancer is rare if not absent entirely. In such places, cancer-absence should be studied in the manner of studying economics, with microscopes left in the closet. Microscopes are used to look at damage already done, not damage prevented.

For reasons hard to explain, many so-called experts begin consideration of cancer only with the biopsy. The "crackpots," the "faddists," the "lunatic fringe" may be so described for trying to look at cancer beginning with birth, and before.

Whatever the reasons behind this absurdity, they are

not in the public interest.

Unquestionably, the "lunatic fringe" might be helped by highly competent and often dedicated men with eyes presently glued to microscopes.

Even with present knowledge, cancer might well be wiped out in ten years, *if the crackpots be right in some of their contentions about dietary prevention.*

What should a cancer patient do? The cancer patient obviously doesn't care a damn about medical politics, or whatever meddling I may do.

For example, one patient I knew had six pounds of tumor tissue removed. I would not suggest to him that he try to remove six pounds of cancer by fasting.

In short, use the medical profession just as fully as possible.

I would modify diet to make it as adequate as possible. I would satisfy enzymatic, vitamin, and mineral need in a manner to avoid food conflicts.

I would get my intestinal flora in as good a shape as possible. This makes sense at any time for anybody.

Like Mr. Stickle, in the event other things failed, I would certainly resort to treatments ignored in this country. I would certainly not "die with dignity" as a casualty in an ideological controversy.

I would put faith in God, above any human agency, because spiritual serenity must be vital with such an illness as cancer. In most cases of faith healing I have read, the prayers of interested people accompany the healing process, even involving fasting.

To protect the right of cancer victims to life, liberty and the pursuit of happiness, a Constitutional Amendment may be helpful, as indicated:

No cancer patient of sound mind may be denied any treatment whatsoever of his choosing. (Admittedly, the foregoing leaves room for improvement.)

APPENDICES

LIST OF APPENDICES

APPENDIX 1

THE BULGARIAN-RUSSIAN WORK ON BACTERIA AS AN ANTI-CANCER ANTIBIOTIC

"First Report. The Anti-Cancer Action of Antibioticum Bulgaricum on Crocker's Sarcoma [1]

"(Summary)"

by I. Bogdanov and P Pophriotov

"The present report contains the preliminary results obtained from the experimental test of the anti-cancer principle produced by bactericum bulgaricum and called after its name – Antibioticum bulgaricum. This report gives only the results of the application of native filtrates from cultures of bacterium bulgaricum. The experiments for the chemical purification and the results from the test of the chemically cleansed anti-cancer principle are the subject of coming reports.

"The ability to form an anti-cancer antibiotic is also inherent to the 10 strains of bacterium bulgaricum which were tested in our laboratories. According to data obtained until now this property is best pronounced in the production strain L-B-51 which in the course of 9 years was being cultured in our laboratory on the soy bean culture medium described below.

"The production strain does not differ in its morphological and cultural properties from the remaining strains of bacterium bulgaricum.

"The soy bean culture medium is prepared in the following way: 10 percent of well washed soy-beans are being extracted with 90 percent of water at 130 C for 30 minutes. The soy bean extract is filtered and is being sterilized during 30 minutes at 1,5 atmosphere in an autoclave. The culture material is 1-5 to a maximum of 10 percent of the volume of the culture medium. The cultivation is being made in anaerobic conditions at 37°C during 18-24 hours. After a 24-hour cultivation a precipitate takes place which also encloses the bacterial bodies.

"The anti-cancer principle is proved in the precipitate which is readily separated at centrifugation and filtration as well as in the filtrate free from bacterial bodies.

"The experimental specimen for the testing of the anti-cancer action of the filtrates from cultures of bacterium bulgaricum, as well as of the fractions produced through a chemical purification containing the active principle, was Crocker's sarcoma 180. Bits of the size of 1 mm^3, preliminarily treated with a solution of antibacterial antibiotics, were implanted.

"Tumors developed in 98 percent of the implanted animals, the death rate in the control non-treated animals being 100 percent.

"In order to account for the therapeutic action of antibioticum bulgaricum, its application began hardly after the tumors had developed and reached the size of 10-12 mm in diameter. As a rule, this occurred after the 8th day from the implantation.

"The introduction of the filtrates was made intraperitoneally in doses from 0,5 to 1 ml daily, at intervals of 1, 2, 3 to 8 days. In various groups we administered 1, 2, 3, 4 to 15 such doses depending on the therapeutic effect achieved and the general condition of the animals.

"The experiments were carried out on 574 white mice implanted with Crocker's sarcoma 180 – distributed into 119 control and 455 experimental animals.

"Soya broth with an addition of lactic acid in amounts contained in the cultures of bacterium bulgaricum were tested for an anti-cancer action in 40 animals from the control group. The remaining 79 animals were left without any treatment.

"All control animals revealed a normal development of Crocker's sarcoma leading to the animals' death between the

35th and 45th day from the implantation.

"The experimental animals were distributed into groups according to the day on which the treatment was started.

"For a quantitative assessment of the anti-cancer effect following an application of Antibioticum bulgaricum, we introduced the so-called 'necrotic unity.' This is the smallest amount of antibiotic which, being injected intraperitoneally into mice, provokes 18-24 hours later a deep necrosis of more than a half of the tumor mass in Crocker's sarcoma with a diameter of 10-12 mm.

"*Results:* The intraperitoneal application of filtrates from cultures containing at least one necrotic unit (0.5-1 ml), produces during the very first 24 hours alterations in the tumors of the innoculated animals. The dimensions of the tumors decrease, the dense-elastic consistency becomes pasty. The necrotic change leads also to alterations of the color of the tumors — from pink they become almost black.

"On sectioning the tumors reveal macroscopically deep changes reaching a caseoselike necrosis. During the following days the necrotic changes become still more intensified. The tumors continue to decrease in size due to a dehydration of the necrotic tissue. About one week later the necrotic mass falls off and a rapidly closing erosion remains in its place.

"In tumors which cannot be eliminated through a fall off (e.g. metastases in the regional lymphatic nodes), the necrotized tumors are subjected to an organization by the connective tissue growing in them.

"For a complete recovery of the animals one application of Antibioticum bulgaricum is usually not enough in the majority of cases.

"On the 8th, 9th, 10th, 11th and 15th day after the implantation, each animal is innoculated intraperitoneally with 1 ml of filtrate. Then the treatment is discontinued but the involution of the tumors continues — the necrotized tumors fall off and they are replaced by erosions which rapidly cicatrize and become pileous.

"Parallel with the photos of the treated animals there are also photos of one of the control animals illustrating the habitual development of Crocker's sarcoma.

"The histological investigation of the tumor tissue at the various phases of its necrotization shows all the transitions from degenerative changes of the protoplasma and neucleus (pyknosis, caryorrhexis, caryolysis) to a complete caseoselike necrosis in which no cellular elements are discernible.

"All 119 animals displayed a habitual development of sarcoma 180 and perished between the 35th and 45th day from the implantation.

"In 162 animals (36 percent), of the experimental group no recovery was achieved. In 157 animals (34 percent) a complete necrotization of the tumors occurred, but the animals could not survive after the intoxication from the rapid disintegration of the tumor tissue.

"In 136 of the 455 animals (30 percent) a complete recovery was achieved. In the various subgroups (depending on the day on which the treatment was initiated), this percentage varied and in some groups, it exceeded 50 percent.

"The maximal term till which the cured animals were followed up was 220 days. The observed animals did not display any recurrences of metastases. In cases in which the single or repeated applications of the antibiotic did not lead to the complete recovery, recurrences were observed. These recurrences, however, were susceptible to the action of the antibiotic, and creation of resistance was not observed.

"On the other hand, the unchanged activity of the antibiotic, when injected at intervals of 8 days, speaks against the possibility for it to provoke antibodies which would block its action as this is observed in substances of an antigenic character.

"70 of the treated animals underwent second implantations, 27 animals got two successive reimplantations and of

7 animals were subjected to three reimplantations.

"The reimplantations were made at various intervals of time after the clinical recovery of the animals, beginning from the 1st day and going up to the 167th day as shown in Table 3.

"None of the reimplantations were ensued by a development of a tumor whereas in the controls, implanted with the same tumor material, new tumors developed.

"The achieved complete recovery of 30 percent of the animals implanted with sarcoma 180, with a 100-percent-death rate in the control ones, points out the presence of an active cancerolytic principle in the cultures of bacterium bulgaricum."

[1]Brief reports on the results from the test of anti-cancer action of Antibioticum bulgaricum on Crocker's sarcoma were presented at the International Symposium of Anti-Cancer Antibiotics in October, 1958 in Moscow and at the Congress of Antibiotics in May, 1959 in Prague, and in these reports the antibiotic was called after its provisory name Antibiotic L-B—51 (Lactobacterium bulgaricum-51).

APPENDIX 2

BULGARIAN-RUSSIAN EXPERIMENTS ON HUMANS

"Second Report.
"Preliminary Results Obtained From the Therapeutic Action of Antibioticum Bulgaricum in Cultaneous Cancer

"The investigations on the action of Antibioticum bulgaricum (A.b.) in many were initiated in October, 1958, following the observations in Crocker's sarcoma 180 already presented.

"The preliminary observations on animals had convinced us that native filtrates from culture containing A.b. were tolerated by animals without any side effects when innoculated introtumorously and intraperitioneally. Before proceeding with the administration of the preparation in patients with cancer of the skin, we tested on ourselves the tolerance of filtrates from cultures and of purified concentrations of filtrates conventionally called A.b. without any general or local side effects except a pain of short duration in the site of the injection.

"The selection of the cancer of the skin as a first object in man, in order to study the anti-cancer properties of A.b., was not made accidentally. In addition to the advantages which this form of cancer offers for a sure diagnosis and an objective study of the therapeutic results, we took into consideration especially the circumstances that the accessibility of the cancer of the skin makes it possible to experiment in humans without endangering the health and the life of the patient.

"The observations were carried out in polyclinical and clinical conditions in the Scientific-Research Institute of Dermatology and Venerology in Sofia, allowing at any moment to pass without any risks, to classical methods of treatment.

"The total number of patients treated by us with A.b. until now exceeds 40. The present work includes an analysis of the first 18 cases in the order of their admission and treatment. No special selection of the patients involved in our observations was made. The basic requirements included patients with a proved diagnosis and with a localization accessible to manipulation. According to the kind of disease they are distributed as follows:

"Carcinoma basocellulare	6 patients
"Carcinoma spinocellulare	3 patients
"Cutaneous metastases following operated cancer of the breast	2 patients
"Morbus Hodgkin	1 patient
"Mycocis fungoides	1 patient
"Keratoacantoma	2 patients
"Verrucae vulgares	3 patients

"The patients involved in the present work were treated with A.b. only locally in the form of injection into the tumor itself. In addition to this, in individual cases and seances only was the antibiotic also injected into the base of the tumor or circularly around the tumor.

"In our first cases, the single and total dose of A.b. applied to individual patients, as well as the intervals between the separate injections, greatly varied:

"A single dose of 0.1 to 1.0 - 1.5 ml

"Intervals between the separate injections — 2 days to 1-2-3 weeks and longer

"Total number of injections — 2 to 6-8

"Thus the dose applied to humans were appreciably smaller than those administered to experimental animals. In the first patients and in individual cases also later, at the first injection were infiltrated only one part of the tumor mass in order to be able to make a comparative follow-up of the occurring clinical and histomorphological changes in the infiltrated area.

"At about the 4-5th observation we established a constant method which consisted in infiltrating the whole tumorous mass with the antibiotic at the very first seance. The dose necessary for the purpose usually ranged from 0.5 to 1.5 ml but we injected, without inconveniences, over 2 ml at one seance. We applied a second injection, when needed, immediately after the disappearance of eventually occurring phenomena of irritation following the first infiltration.

"Having in mind that we were at a stage of experimentation aiming at ascertaining most generally whether or not an anti-cancer action of the tested A.b. in the carcinoma of the skin in man exists, we deemed it appropriate to form the observed cases into groups according to the kinds of affections. The collection of more observations will allow us later to account for the results in groups: cured, improved, uncured.

"The results obtained in the patients thus treated and followed up are as follows:

"Carcinoma Basocellulare

"1. Maria P., a 38-year-old employee. Clinical diagnosis: carcinoma basocellulare under the right eyelid of three years' standing. The condition previous to the institution of the treatment is shown in Fig. 1 accompanying the article.

"*Treatment:* In this first case we injected on the 9th, 10th and 11th of October, 1958 respectively 0.10-0.15-0.20 ml of A.b. each time only at the right end of the tumor, into the tumor mass itself. On the following day after each injection, one could observe a moderate cold edema of the skin around the site of the injection.

"On the 13th of October, 1958, a general sticking of the tumor was observed. On the 13th of October, 1958, the internal end of the tumor (towards the nose) was infiltrated with 0.20 ml, and on the 20th of October, 1958, the whole tumor mass was again infiltrated with 0.30 ml. On the 3rd of November, 1958, a small epithelizing erosion was discovered, around which the former contours of the tumor, considerably narrowed, were discernible as a shadow (Fig. 2).

"On the 6th day of November, 1958 (Fig. 3) the erosion was epithelized with a scar; along the periphery of the scar one could see, through a magnifying glass, a pearl in the middle of the upper end of the lesion. On the 21st of November, 1958, the lesion was in the same condition without any tendency towards widening. As this was our first observation and in order to examine the histomorphology, the entire residual alteration was excised on the same date.

"Histomorphologically the picture of the typical basaloma was discernible in the region of the residual alteration. On both sides of the residual lesion, in site of the initial situation of the tumor, one could see, under the microscope, a zone in which the derm was subjected to a strong fibronization and hyalinization. At places there were separate piles of inflammatory cells of the count of white blood cells. Controls made on December 22, 1958, on May 10, 1959, and at the end of September, 1960, revealed a smooth postoperative scar.

"2. Zlatko H.T., a 55-year-old retired schoolteacher. Clinical diagnosis: carcinoma basocellulare of the skin behind the right ear conch, of many years' standing, slowly increasing. Beside the basaloma one could see a focus of folliculitis.

"*Treatment:* On October 10, 1958, 0.15 ml of A.b. were injected into the upper and lower poles of the tumor, not more than 0.05 ml remaining within the tumor. On October 11, 1958, the tumor was bluish color, slightly contracted, flattened, softened. On the same date, a second infiltration with 0.30 ml was made.

"On October 13, 1958, the tumor continued to contract, to decrease and to flatten and it lost its distension and the brightness of its color. On the same date, 0.20 ml were again infiltrated into the residual edges. From October 20 till November 30, 1958, two more infiltrations of the residual areas were made with 0.30 ml and 0.20 ml.

"On November 4, 1958, a partial biopsy of the outer half of the tumor was made with a borer, with a view to include a part of the already disintegrated and epithelized upper area and a part of the still not fully disintegrated lower external area. On November 6 and November 10, 1958, two more infiltrations with 0.50 ml on each date were made.

"On November 13, 1958, the whole tumor mass was melted thus exposing a small ulcer. On November 27, 1958, complete epithelization was observed. On December 12, 1958, the lesion had definitely passed, leaving a small smooth scar.

"On January 12, 1959, a granular formation of the size of a grain of wheat appeared on the lower pole of the scar. We considered it to be a recurrence. This growth was infiltrated twice with ½ ml of A.b. each time. Immediately after that, the patient received 3500 r roentgen therapy. Till now [September, 196?] the patient is completely healthy.

"3. Ivan G.R., a 55-year-old peasant-farmer. Clinical and histological diagnosis: carcinoma basocellulare of the skin of the left suborbital region of the face, of one year's standing.

"*Treatment:* At the very first seance on March 12, 1959, the entire tumor of this patient was infiltrated with 0.40 ml of A.b. By the evening of the same day, an evidently visible edema at about 5 c in diameter from the tumor evolved without any general phenomena.

"On the following day, the edema began to decrease spontaneously and slowly, but on March 16, 1959, there still appeared an edema of the skin under and around the tumor. On the same day, a second infiltration was made with 0.20 ml of A.b. On March 20, 1959, the tumor was no longer discernible. In its place one could see a dark small crust.

"On March 23, 1959, a new infiltration with 0.30 ml was made into the entire zone under the crust. On April 16, 1959, at the lower end of the former tumor, next to the remaining part of the crust, one could see a pearly formation. This area was infiltrated again.

"On May 15, 1959, June 15, 1959, and on July 15, 1959, the control examinations showed a soft cicatrix, slightly concave in the middle, non-adherent to the base in the site of the former epithelioma. There was no trace of basalioma.

"On June 4, 1960, i.e., more than one year after the institution of the treatment and one year following its termination, the patient was summoned for a new control examination. In the place of the completely passed basaloma there was a smooth, hardly discernible superficial scar. An excision of the scar was made for a histological investigation. The latter showed moderate fibrosis and hyalinization in the site of the past tumor. No residues from basaloma were found.

"4. Mariika M.H., a 69-year-old housewife. Clinical and histological diagnosis: carcinoma basocellulare of the skin of the right zygomatic region of two years' standing. The lesion was infiltrated thrice (on March 23, 27, and on April 3, 1959, with 0.30 ml of A.b. each time).

"Right after the first infiltration the tumor began to disintegrate and an ulcerative surface was uncovered. On July 15, 1959, the lesion had already completely passed, presenting a smooth, slightly hyperpigmented scar.

"On April 25, 1960, one year after the completion of the treatment, the patient was summoned for a new control examination. In the site of the completely passed lesion, one could discern an extremely superficial, smooth, slightly pigmented scar.

"The scar was excised for a histological investigation. The latter revealed moderate fibrosis and hyalinization of the derm, in the place of the past basaloma.

"5. Milka S.P., a 57-year-old housewife. The observation was made from March 18, 1959, till May 11, 1959. Three infiltrations were made (on March 20 and 23, and on April 3, 1959).

"Owing to the impossibility of continuing the observation of the patient in Sofia, roentgen therapy was applied and the patient was eliminated from our observation.

6. Maria D.K., a 62-year-old housewife. The disease had started at the end of 1968. In 1959, the lesion had been excised but soon after that, recurrence had taken place and it was discernible in the left posterior aural region. The clinical and histological diagnosis was carcinoma basocellulare.

"The lesion was infiltrated five times with A.b. in the course of 45 days.

"The systematic follow-up of the histologic changes before, during, and after the treatment are of particular interest:

"Histological diagnosis— epithelioma basocellulare. The stroma reaction is moderately pronounced. It is chiefly made up of lymphocytes, histiocytes, fibroblasts, and single leukocytes. In the histological preparations made in the course of the treatment, the picture is dominated by a strongly marked perivascular lymphocytic infiltration. This gives the lesion a cicatricial aspect.

"Amidst this stroma are seen scarce epitheliomatous nests made up of a small number of cells. These cells have a preserved aspect only in one place.

"In other places the cells are torn, the nuclei are markedly basophilic and homogenized. In one area is seen a nucleus in a condition of karyorrhexis. A characteristic element of the stroma reaction is the great amount of giant cells of the foreign body type. Usually they are found right next to the destroyed epitheliomic foci and at places — closely sticking to them. The blood capillaries are hyperplasic and most of them are filled with blood.

"Carcinoma Spinocellulare — 3 Patients

"1. Hordan I.M., a 54-year-old gardener. For about four years he had Keratomata-senilia over the skin of the face and the dorsal side of both hands. For six months on one of the keratomas on the left hand developed a gradually increasing and lately ulcerating neoformation.

"Histopathogic diagnosis (December 8, 1959), before the institution of the treatment — carcinoma spinocellulare. The nacroscopic aspect of the lesion following biopsy and previous to treatment is shown. The epitrochlear and axillar lymph nodes were intact.

"*Treatment:* On December 11, 1958, the entire tumor was infiltrated with 1 ml of A.b. On December 13, 1958, the whole central part of the tumor was necrotized and fell off on the dressing, thus uncovering an ulcerative surface occupying the larger part of the lesion. Here and there around the periphery there were still some slightly more elevated edges.

"On the same date and later on December 15, 1958, both edges and the base of the whole lesion were infiltrated with 1 ml of the liquid each. On December 22, 1958, the whole tumor mass disappeared; the edges were not discernible. In their place one could see a superficial ulcer rapidly contracting and epithelizing covered with small crusts.

"On December 26, 1958, the lesion almost disappeared. The central zone was not yet fully epithelized, but there were no infiltrations whatsoever.

"The control ciopsy which was made on December 21, 1958, from the most suspected area of the residual lesion presented the picture of a well differentiated carcinoma spinocellulare.

"Before receiving the results from the biopsy, the patient went, on his own insistence, to his family, but was told to return for a control examination toward January 15,

1959. In February and March, 1959, he had influenza and on account of this, he could not come for the check-up examination.

"On April 20, 1959, we summoned the patient and he came again to the Institute. He informed us that about January 15, 1959, the lesion was completely cured, leaving a smooth scar, and that is why he had not deemed it necessary to come for an examination.

"At the beginning of April, 1959, a slightly painful swelling appeared around the periphery of the scar. On pressure, a drop of pus could be seen under this swelling.

"After cleansing, the whole residual lesion was excised. The histological investigation of the excised area revealed the picture of an initial recurrence of carcinoma spinocellulare. In September, 1960, we found a calm postoperative scar in the site of a past lesion. The cubital and axillary lymph nodes were not enlarged.

"2. Vuna D.A., a 77-year-old housewife. Condition prior to the institution of the treatment – (initial cornifying carcinoma spinocellulare). The neoformation had started about six months previously. The lymph nodes – epitrochlearly and axillarily – were not enlarged.

"*Treatment:* The patient was treated with 3 infiltrations (on May 3, June 8 and June 11, 1959), with ½ ml of A.b. each time. Due to the severe spontaneous pain, the cultural liquid was mixed with a 0.5 percent-novacain solution in a proportion of half of its volume.

"At the second infiltration, half of the liquid was injected circularly around the tumor. As early as June 3, 1959, the larger part of the tumor mass was disintegrated and separated. Following the second and third infiltrations on June 16, 1959, the entire lesion, with the exception of separate points around the periphery, was in a process of disintegration. The spontaneous pain considerably decreased. The wound was dressed only with 5 percent of ung. acidi salicylici. Without any further injection, on June 26, 1959, the wound was clean, contracting and epithelizing at places. No infiltration was found. The pain completely disappeared.

"The treatment was continued with only 5 percent of dermatol-unguent. On June 3, 1959, the wound was completely healed, leaving a smooth scar. In this patient too, after each infiltration, a hard edema as already described, occurred, without any local and general inflammatory phenomena. The control examination in August, 1960, established a smooth scar in the site of the past lesion.

"3. Georgi D.P., a 67-year-old pensioner. For four months he had had histologically proved epithelioma spinocellulare (of the cornu cutaneum type), on the left ear lobe.

"On the 6th day after a single infiltration with 0.30 ml of A.b., the horn fell off and a small crust was seen in the site of the lesion. Three weeks after the single infiltration, the lesion completely passed, leaving a smooth superficial slightly hyperpigmented scar.

"Cutaneous Metastases Following Operated Cancer of the Mammary Gland

"1. Penka I.Z., a 40-year-old housewife. Being placed under our observation, the patient was admitted on January 29, 1959, with the diagnosis: carcinoma mammae utriusque; status post amputationen; metastases cutis.

"The cutaneous metastases were represented by multiple nodular formations of the size from a lentil to a small pea, situated on the skin over the anterior surface of the breasts. Around them and especially higher towards the jugulum, a diffuse erysipeloid redness was seen. In these places, the skin was distended, lustrous, diffusely dense, not allowing the formation of creases (carcinoma erysipelatosum).

"*Treatment:* On January 30, 1959, only two metastatic nodules were infiltrated with several drops of A.b. each.

Three days later, one of the nodules disintegrated and no discernible change was found in the other. An erythematous wreath developed around the disintegrated nodule.

"After a second infiltration, the other nodule was also disintegrated and a bulbous reaction developed around it; the nodule was not seen. On February 23, 1959, both nodules disappeared, leaving superficial scars in their places.

"In the meantime, during the period from February 9 till February 23, 1959, all remaining visible nodules were infiltrated. The daily observation up to February 26, 1959, showed that all infiltrated nodules disappeared – some following disintegration, others dissolved without visible disintegration.

"In the sites of the disintegrated nodules, following the epithelization, hardly visible scars are seen.

"On March 9, 1959, a new granular densification occurred at the inner end of the scar from the already cured first nodule there. An excision was made of the zone of the scar with the new densification and a part of the adjacent erysipeloid reddened skin, for a histological investigation. The latter revealed, in the region of the new densification, in the subcutaneous tissue, solid epithelial new growths whose cells were a pronounced atypism and polymorphism.

"The tumor elements were divided into small nests made up of profusely grown among them connective tissue. The picture was that of a solid carcinoma of mammary gland origin. On the side of this growth, in the zone preliminarily treated with the antibiotic, one could see an area of the derm subjected to a fibrotic and collagenic formation in the midst of which one could discern separate small groups of cells subjected to dystrophic changes. These may be residues of cancer cells, although the strongly marked changes in them make their recognition and classification difficult.

"On March 9, 1959, following the biopsy, 2 ml of A.b., mixed in half with a 1 percent-novacain solution, were injected into the zone of erysipeloid redness between the nodular changes. Following the infiltration there occurred the already known moderate, but clear, edema of the entire erysipeloid plaque and nearby.

"Toward the third day, the edema decreased. The whole plaque was pale in color, considerably softened, slightly wrinkled; the skin then allowed the formation of a crease. The patient herself saw and felt the visible change. Nowhere in the zone thus injected a visible disintegration of the tissue occurred.

"The patient did not allow a second biopsy from the zone thus treated and changed, and was discharged from the In-Patient Department at the Chair of Roentgenology and Radiology.

"2. Ivanka V.I., a 62-year-old housewife. Diagnosis: carcinoma mammae skin; metastases, status post amputationem mammae skin. Already prior to the operation there had been metastases over the head, such a metastatic node, with dimensions 3 x 3 c, could be seen in the right frontotemporal region, and another in the left occipital region. The latter was soft and fluctuating.

"On March 4, 1959, the first node was infiltrated with 2 ml of A.b. Right after that, there occurred a strong edema reaching the upper right eyelid. Towards March 6, 1959, the edema considerably decreased and one observed a melting and softening of the tumor which began to fluctuate.

"Due to the extremely serious general condition of the patient, we discontinued our observation here and placed her under the care of the oncologists-raytherapeutists.

"Keratoacanthoma

"1. Ahten M.M., a 58-year-old housewife. The lesion was of 2½ months' standing. One single infiltration with 0.30 ml of A.b. was made on March 23, 1959. On May 4, 1959, the lesion passed.

"The course of the recovery process essentially differs from the known spontaneous recovery in this self-curing spinalioma.

"2. Krum H.S., a 45-year-old musician. The lesion was of three weeks' standing. On April 6, 1959,, the patient was incorrectly sent for roentgen therapy and our observation was discontinued. Till the moment of the observation, however, the course of the recovery process fully corresponds to that of the former case.

"Verrucae Vulgares

"1. Ludmila A.R., a 21-year-old girl (a university student).

"2. Milcho T.T., a 6-year-old boy.

"The warts were situated on the big toe in the first case and on the dorsal skin of the hands in the second case. In the first case the entire small tumor was subjected to 3 infiltrations from October 10 till October 20, 1958, and in the second case, 2 infiltrations were made into each of the two small tumors on one of the hands.

"The warts remained absolutely unchanged. No necrosis, softening, dissolution was observed.

"3. Hristo L.M., a 44-year-old farmer. He had a vast plaque of multiple cornua cutanea which had developed for one year on ordinary warts over the skin of the ulnar edge of his right wrist.

"The histological investigation confirmed this diagnosis and did not reveal any evidence of carcinoma. One area of the lesion was infiltrated with 1½ ml of A.b. During the following five days, the lesion was not altered, and no local or general reaction was recorded.

"Preliminary General Conclusions

"Incompletely purified concentrations of filtrates from cultural liquids containing A.b. when applied locally within the tissue of the tumor, exert an evidently inhibitory and disintegrative action on the cancer tissue in carcinoma basocellulare and carcinoma spinocellulare, as well as in cutaneous metastases in cancer of the mammary gland, in malignant reticulosis of the skin and in self-curing cutaneous cancer (keratoacanthoma).

"The controls in animals with the ingredients of the medium for the cultivation of the producer show that the results obtained cannot be due to these ingredients, but that they are related to a specific principle resulting from the cultivation of the producer.

"Antibioticum bulgaricum which has been isolated in the meantime by us in the form of powder and the observations made therewith (which are the subject of another report), undisputably confirm the above conclusion.

"In addition to A.b., the filtrates and concentrations of cultural fluid used by us contain also lactic acid in percentages of 5 to 10%. The control experiments with the same concentrations of symthetic lactic acid show that its presence is not indifferent to carcinomas of the skin.

"The extent to which the presence of lactic acid is an important or secondary factor for the results obtained will be shown by further experiments with dry A.b. preparations deprived of lactic acid and applied intravenously, intraperitoneally and locally. The observations made up till now in that respect give us ground to think that the presence and participation of lactic acid in the results obtained by a local application are secondary.

"In a part of the observed by us till now patients with cancer of the skin and treated with Antibioticum bulgaricum, we observed recurrences around the periphery of the treated tumors. The recurrent foci was susceptible to an additional treatment with the same antibiotic.

"The observations which are going on in the meantime also show failures in the treatment of individual cases and a necessity to pass to other therapeutic methods.

"A special further study should be made on the histomorphological and histochemical changes taking place in the cancer tissue and in the tissue which surrounds it, following application of Antibioticum bulgaricum.

"The general tolerance of A.b. used by us so far has been good. The tolerance and the side effects of the already isolated powdered product observed in various forms of application are being thoroughly investigated now.

"The local tolerance of the forms employed till now for the application of A.b. is also good. The product used up to the present in our experiments causes only instantly a slight bearable pain at the moment of the injection. If needed, it can be attenuated or eliminated by adding a novacain solution which does not decrease the efficacy of the antibiotic.

"Special mention should be made of the already described cold edema, lasting 3-4 days, in the base of the tumor and around it, following injection of the more concentrated product. Our impression is that this is a reactive edema and the efficacy of the therapeutic effect is parallel to it.

"The presented observations on the anti-cancer properties of A.b. in man for the time have the value of preliminary experimental data. They, however, give ground to continue the studies by widening the experimentation on animals – in various kinds of experimental, induced and spontaneous tumors – as well as in the clinic in more varied forms of cancer and in more cases.

"These investigations are underway now. It is only after their completion that it will be possible to assess the possibility for the practical use of A.b. in the clinic."

APPENDIX 3

ANTICARCINOGENIC ACTIVITY OF COLOSTRUM FERMENTED WITH LACTOBACILLI

by Dr. Khem Shahani

"Previous studies in our lab have demonstrated the anti-carcenogenic activity of milk cultured with Lactobacilli species. Yogurt, containing a mixed culture of *Lactobacillus bulgaricus* and *Streptococcus thermophilus,* inhibited proliferation of Ascites tumor cell proliferation by up to 28% when fed to male Swiss mice. Further studies were initiated to determine the effect of feeding plain and cultured bovine colostrum upon proliferation of Ascites tumor cells in mice.

"Erhlich Ascites tumor cells were obtained from the National Cancer Institute and maintained in the lab through intraperitoneal transplants in male Swiss mice. Ascites fluid, containing active tumor cells, was withdrawn from donor mice and adjusted to 5 million cells per milliliter in 0.9% saline solution. For experimental work, 0.2 ml of the cell suspension yielding 1 million tumor cells was inoculated into the intraperitoneal cavity of each mouse.

"Cultured product was then mixed with one-third its volume of water and mixed in a blender for 30 seconds at medium speed. The homogenized water-cultured product mixture was then placed in standard water bottles and fed to mice. The control group of mice received only Purina mouse chow and water while the experimental group received mouse chow and cultured product.

"Protocol for inoculation of tumor cells, feeding of cultured product, and enumeration of tumor cells is shown in slide 1. On day 0, 106 cells were inoculated per mouse, day 1 feeding was initiated, and on day 8, tumor cells were enumerated. Tumor cell growth was measured by 1) microscopic count of cells in the Ascites fluid, and 2) Deoxyribonucleic acid (DNA) content of the cell suspension. DNA was estimated by the following procedure: 1) washing the cells in saline, 2) Homogenization of the suspension, 3) purification in cold 10% TCA, 4) extraction of DNA in 2.5% at 90°C, 5) color development with Diphenylamine and 6) measurement of color development at 600 nm in a spectrophotometer.

"A brief review of previous studies in our lab indicates that the bacterial cells are responsible for the anticarcenogenic effect of yogurt. Trials in which the experimental group received plain milk or lactic acid in water showed that neither milk nor lactic acid per se responsible for the anticarcenogenic activity of yogurt. In a similar series of studies in which yogurt was fractionated showed the anticarcenogenic effect associated with the bacterial cells. Further trials in which yogurt cells were homogenized and centrifuged indicate the antitumor activity is closely associated with the bacterial cell wall. The antitumor activity is destroyed by heat processing the cells. Future studies are planned to isolate the antitumor compound(s) by more sophisticated separation techniques.

"Colostrum, the milk secreted the first few days post partum, is thought to provide certain therapeutic value to the newborn due to various immunoglobulins present. Studies were initiated to determine the anticarcenogenic effect of plain and cultured colostrum in male Swiss mice. Frozen colostrum was obtained for the University of Nebraska Dairy Farm at Mead.

"Plain colostrum was fed to a group of mice inoculated with Ehrlich Ascites tumor cells using the protocol given earlier. The experimental group consisting of 6 mice received plain colostrum in a water bottle and mouse chow while the control group of 6 mice received only water and mouse chow. The results of 4 trials clearly indicate that plain colostrum has no anticarcenogenic activity against Erhlich Ascites tumor in male Swiss mice.

"Further studies were initiated in which the anticarcenogenic activity of bovine colostrum cultured with various Lactobacilli species was studied. The first series of trials were conducted with colostrum fermented with a mixed yogurt culture obtained from the Dannon Yogurt Company consisting of *Lactobacillus bulgaricus* and *Streptococcus thermophilus.* The colostrum was incubated with 10% culture at 42°C about 6 hours, until a pH of 4.5 was reached. 150 milliliters of cultured colostrum was blended with 50 milliliters of water, then placed in a water bottle for initiation of feeding. The experimental group received cultured colostrum and mouse chow while the control group received only water and mouse chow. Feeding of colostrum fermented with mixed yogurt culture inhibited tumor cell count by 16 to 35% and the DNA content by 20 to 32%.

"In the next series of trials, colostrum was fermented with *Lactobacillus bulgaricus.* Colostrum was incubated with 5% culture at 42°C for 12 hours. Cultured colostrum was blended with water, placed in a water bottle, and fed to mice according to earlier protocol. The experimental group received mouse chow and fermented colostrum, while the control group received mouse chow and water. Feeding of colostrum fermented with *Lactobacillus bulgaricus* inhibited tumor cell count by 25 to 34% and DNA content by 24 to 34%.

"In the last series of trials, colostrum was fermented with *Lactobacillus acidophilus.* Colostrum was inoculated with 5% culture and incubated at 37°C for 12-18 hours until a pH of 4.5-4.7 was reached. The fermented colostrum was blended with water and fed to a group of mice in the place of water. Colostrum fermented with *Lactobacillus acidophilus* inhibited the tumor cell count by 18 to 38% and the DNA content by 13 to 32%.

"Colostrum cultured with Lactobacilli species inhibited tumor cell count and DNA content of Ascites tumor cell in male Swiss mice by up to 35%. No treatment completely cured the tumor, but inhibited growth. Plain colostrum, in spite of immunoglobulin content, did not inhibit proliferation of tumor growth. The series of studies confirmed earlier studies in our lab in which the feeding of yogurt to mice inhibited tumor cell proliferation. Future studies are planned to understand the anticarcenogenic action of Lactobacilli species in the intestine. Studies are planned to fractionate and isolate the anticarcenogenic compound(s) from the cells."

Slide 1

PROTOCOL FOR INOCULATION OF TUMOR CELLS, FEEDING OR IMPLANTATION OF YOGURT OR YOGURT COMPONENT AND ENUMERATION OF CELLS

Day	Particulars
0	10^6 Cells Inoculated/Mouse
1	Initiation of Feeding or Implantation
2 to 7	Feeding or Implantation Continued
8	Enumeration of Cells

Fig. 1
EFFECT OF IMPLANTING DIFFERENT FRACTIONS OF YOGURT CULTURE UPON TUMOR CELL PROLIFERATION

	TOTAL TUMOR CELLS (Millions/Mouse)			TOTAL TUMOR CELLS (Millions/Mouse)	
Test Group	Control	Experimental Group 1 (Solids)	Inhibition %	Experimental Group 2 (Supernatant)	Inhibition %
1	12.45 ± 1.71	7.58 ± 1.32	39.2	12.33 ± 1.72	0
2	16.46 ± 1.65	10.96 ± 2.3	32.7	16.49 ± 3.16	0
3	18.43 ± 2.5	1.32 ± 2.7	37.9	18.49 ± 1.5	0
4	14.17 ± 1.6	9.98 ± 1.4	30.0	14.07 ± 0.8	0

Fig. 2

EFFECT OF FEEDING DIFFERENT YOGURT FRACTIONS UPON TUMOR CELL PROLIFERATION AS DETERMINED BY DNA CONTENT OF TOTAL CELLS

	DNA CONTENT (μg/ML SUSPENSION)			DNA CONTENT (μg/ML SUSPENSION)	
Series	Control	Experimental Group 1 (Supernatant)	Inhibition %	Experimental Group 2 (Solids)	Inhibition %
1	425 ± 20	430 ± 21	0.0	297 ± 23	30.2
2	442 ± 9	438 ± 29	0.0	330 ± 14	25.6
3	450 ± 20	445 ± 16	0.0	350 ± 18	22.2
4	400 ± 14	410 ± 14	0.0	306 ± 28	23.5

Experimental Group 1 received supernatant fraction.
Experimental Group 2 received solids fraction.

Fig. 3

EFFECT OF FEEDING DIFFERENT YOGURT FRACTIONS (SUPERNATANT AND SOLIDS) UPON THE TUMOR CELL PROLIFERATION

	TOTAL TUMOR CELLS (Millions/Mouse)			TOTAL TUMOR CELLS (Millions/Mouse)	
Series	Control	Experimental Group 1 (Supernatant)	Inhibition %	Experimental Group 2 (Solids)	Inhibition %
1	39.88 ± 2.5	43.68 ± 8.8	0.0	26.14 ± 4.7	34.4
2	40.54 ± 2.6	42.67 ± 9.0	0.0	30.47 ± 2.9	24.8
3	40.46 ± 5.2	43.46 ± 6.7	0.0	31.24 ± 2.9	22.1
4	37.85 ± 2.3	38.98 ± 4.9	0.0	29.59 ± 5.2	21.8

Experimental Group 1 received supernatant fraction.
Experimental Group 2 received solids fraction.

Fig. 4

EFFECT OF FEEDING RAW COLOSTRUM UPON PROLIFERATION OF TUMOR CELLS IN SWISS MICE

Replicate Trial No.	TOTAL TUMOR CELLS (Millions/Mouse)		Inhibition %	DNA CONTENT (ug/ML Suspension)		Inhibition %
	Control	Experimental		Control	Experimental	
1	27.0 ± 2.0	25.4 ± 6.0	5.9[a]	195 ± 48.9	191 ± 34.7	2.1[a]
2	28.6 ± 2.5	28.4 ± 2.4	0.7[a]	227 ± 36.0	235 ± 15.4	0[a]
3	24.0 ± 1.3	24.9 ± 4.3	0[a]	184 ± 38.4	184 ± 19.1	0[a]
4	28.9 ± 2.9	31.2 ± 1.5	0[a]	237 ± 23.1	218 ± 28.4	8.0[a]

[a]Difference not significant at 5% level.

Fig. 5

EFFECT OF FEEDING COLOSTRUM FERMENTED WITH YOGURT CULTURE UPON PROLIFERATION OF TUMOR CELLS IN SWISS MICE

Replicate Trial No.	TOTAL TUMOR CELLS (Millions/Mouse)		Inhibition %	DNA CONTENT (μg/ml Suspension)		Inhibition %
	Control	Experimental		Control	Experimental	
1	35.1 ± 5.5	22.9 ± 7.4	34.8	286 ± 45.3	199 ± 42.2	30.6
2	31.2 ± 4.7	21.9 ± 2.7	29.8	363 ± 21.9	245 ± 19.7	32.4
3	27.8 ± 3.5	25.8 ± 3.0	N.S.	225 ± 19.7	230 ± 21.5	N.S.
4	30.9 ± 1.3	25.9 ± 2.0	16.2	256 ± 17.1	206 ± 24.1	19.5

Significant at 5% level.

N.S.: Not Significant

Fig. 6

EFFECT OF FEEDING COLOSTRUM FERMENTED WITH *L. BULGARICUS* UPON PROLIFERATION OF TUMOR CELLS IN SWISS MICE

Replicate Trial No.	TOTAL TUMOR CELLS (Millions/Mouse)		Inhibition	DNA CONTENT (µg/ML Suspension)		Inhibition
	Control	Experimental		Control	Experimental	
1	27.3 ± 2.1	18.4 ± 1.7	32.6	263 ± 15.1	180 ± 17.1	35.3
2	24.1 ± 1.7	18.0 ± 2.1	25.3	252 ± 20.7	192 ± 17.1	23.9
3	27.8 ± 2.3	18.4 ± 2.1	33.8	291 ± 22.3	193 ± 20.9	33.8

Fig. 7

EFFECT OF FEEDING COLOSTRUM FERMENTED WITH *L. ACIDOPHILUS* UPON PROLIFERATION OF TUMOR CELLS IN SWISS MICE

Replicate Trial No.	TOTAL TUMOR CELLS (Millions/Mouse)		Inhibition %	DNA CONTENT (μg ML Suspension)		Inhibition %
	Control	Experimental		Control	Experimental	
1	22.7 ± 1.2	18.6 ± 1.9	18.1	244 ± 18.2	212 ± 7.9	12.8
2	28.1 ± 2.4	22.5 ± 1.6	19.9	218 ± 5.9	175 ± 11.5	19.5
3	24.9 ± 1.5	15.2 ± 1.1	38.0	204 ± 7.1	139 ± 8.7	31.9

APPENDIX 4

THE ROLE OF LACTOSE IN THE DIET

If the presence of some kinds of bacteria may have a beneficial effect, absence may have a harmful effect. Let's consider this.

The following appeared in the Dairy Council *Digest,* "an Interpretive Review of Recent Nutrition Research Published by National Dairy Council, 111 North Canal Street, Chicago, Illinois 60606," Volume 45, No. 5, September-October 1974, ISSN 0011-5568, "The Role of Lactose in the Diet – Summary." (The National Dairy Council takes no responsibility for other than its own material.)

"Lactose, the main carbohydrate in milk, enhances mineral and protein utilization. Its effect on vitamin synthesis, body composition, brain growth, and intestinal microflora is reviewed. Medical literature in the last few years has revealed an almost international prevalence of adult man's limited ability to digest large amounts of lactose, otherwise known as lactose intolerance. Methods of assessing this ability have been the subject of voluminous investigations. Nutrient utilization in lactose intolerant subjects has not differed significantly from that in normal subjects. More recent studies revealed that lactose intolerance does not denote milk intolerance. It has been demonstrated that individuals with a limited ability to digest lactose can consume nutritionally useful quantities of milk. Based on such evidence as well as the nutritional contribution of milk to the diet, various scientific groups and individuals have endorsed domestic and foreign programs improving milk supplies and milk consumption.

"Lactose, first reported as a constituent of milk in 1633, is the main carbohydrate present in milks of mammals except in certain of the Pinnipedia. Seal, sea lion, and walrus milks contain no lactose (1). The lactose content of other animal milks ranges from about 2.5% in the reindeer to about 6.0% in the mare; human milk with 7.0 to 7.5% is sweeter than cow's milk with 4.5% lactose (2, 3). McCracken (3) and Skala and Lamacova (4) tabulated the lactose content of other animal milks and dairy products.

"A disaccharide composed of the monosaccharides glucose and galactose, lactose is synthesized by the mammary gland late in pregnancy and is hydrolyzed into its component monosaccharides by the enzyme lactase (1, 2). First apparent in the fetal intestines of mammals during the last stage of gestation, lactase reaches maximum activity immediately after birth, and has generally been known to approach low levels in older children and adults of all but those of Western and Northern European ancestry (1, 5-8). The purpose of this *Digest* is to review the nutritional role of lactose as well as to present current knowledge on man's ability to digest lactose.

"Nutritional Significance of Lactose

"Little attention has been given to the role of lactose in the diet. Although its stimulating effect on calcium absorption has been known since the 1930's, no definitive statement on the exact mode of action has been universally accepted. The four main hypotheses presented in the last four decades include: 1) the intestinal acidity theory, 2) the chelation theory, 3) the metabolic theory, and 4) the osteogenic theory(9).

"The effect of lactose on the absorption of other cations like strontium, magnesium, barium, radium, and manganese has also been studied (10, 11, 12, 13), although on a limited scale.

"Since lactose is slowly absorbed in the intestines, it has been reported to promote the proliferation of intestinal bacteria which are capable of synthesizing vitamins like biotin, riboflavin, folic acid, and pyridoxine (12, 14). Particularly in areas where natural vitamin D formation from sunlight is not sufficient to meet the individual's requirements, lactose in milk serves to counteract the development of late rickets and osteomalacia; this suggests that lactose enhances calcium absorption as effectively as does vitamin D (15).

"Sewell and West (16) presented data that lactose plays a physiologically important role in protein absorption and utilization by young pigs and that lactose also improved the digestibility and utilization of protein from plant sources.

"Due to current interest in obesity, it is significant to note that lactose-fed rats showed less fat, more body water, protein and ash (12, 17, 18), a relative increase in the weight of the caecum, liver and kidneys, and an increase in liver protein relative to the total body protein (18).

"Inasmuch as most mammalian milks contain lactose, the major natural source of galactose, it is interesting to speculate that dietary galactose may be useful in the synthesis of brain galactolipids. Varma et al (19) not only reviewed the literature on this subject but also demonstrated that neither the kitten nor the human brain requires preformed galactose for galactolipid synthesis. Further research, however, is needed to elucidate the role of dietary lactose in human brain growth.

"Coello-Ramirez et al (20) studied enteric microflora in relation to carbohydrate tolerance in infants with severe diarrhea. Significant in their findings was that lactose-tolerant patients had the lowest bacterial (klebsiella, escherichia, enterococci, pseudomonas, and proteus species) counts and that bacterial proliferation of these species in the mtestinal fluid interfered with intestinal absorptive mechanisms.

"Lactose Digestion

"If the amount of lactose ingested exceeds the hydrolytic capacity of the available intestinal lactase, a portion of the lactose remains undigested and is transported into the large intestines. Undigested lactose in the large intestines increases the osmolarity of the intestinal fluid and thus draws water from the tissues into the intestines. Undigested lactose may also be fermented by bacteria in the colon, thus generating organic acids, carbon dioxide, and hydrogen. These fermentation products together with the large amount of water drawn into the intestines are largely responsible for symptoms such as bloating, flatulence, cramps, and diarrhea (2, 7, 8, 21-23), all indicative of one's limited ability to utilize lactose. This condition, more commonly referred to as lactose intolerance, was the subject of a previous *Digest* issued in 1971 (24). Since that time, voluminous information on this subject has appeared in the medical literature. An extensive review of dietary lactose and its varied utilization by man has been prepared by Rosensweig (25).

"The Protein Advisory Group (PAG) of the United Nations System felt the need to alleviate confusion with regard to terminology in this subject among the scientific community and the lay public. In a 1972 position statement (26), the PAG recommended, in place of the term lactase deficiency, the word *low lactase activity* defined as 'less than two units of lactase activity per gram wet mucosa.' However, activity of one unit has been regarded by other investigators as low (7, 23). One unit of lactase activity is equal to one mole of lactose hydrolyzed per minute per gram wet mucosa (3, 8). The PAG further defined *lactose malabsorption* as 'reduced absorption of lactose, a consequence of low lactase activity, determined by lactose tolerance test.' *Lactose intolerance* was likewise defined as the appearance of 'clinical signs (abdominal pain, diarrhea, bloating, flatulence, etc.) following ingestion of lactose, mixed in water in standard dose or less, in a person with proven lactose malabsorption.'

"Three forms of low lactase activity have been described

— congenital, primary, and secondary (8, 27, 28). Often regarded as an inborn error of metabolism, the congenital form is an extremely rare occurrence in which lactase is missing from birth throughout life although the histology of the intestinal mucosa is normal. In the primary form — also referred to as isolated or racial — lactase activity is low while the activity levels of the other disaccharidases are normal.

"A secondary form, often a temporary condition, is manifested by a decrease of all disaccharidase activity due to inflammatory or degenerative diseases involving the mucosa. After treatment of the primary disease, disaccharidase activity usually will return to normal values, although on occasion the secondary low lactase activity may become permanent (28).

"The etiology of the primary form of low lactase activity was reviewed in 1971 (24). A great number of researchers favor the interpretation that primary low lactase activity could be a hereditary enzyme defect with late expression occurring with varying frequency in different ethnic groups (3, 29, 30). Other investigators believe that intestinal lactase may be an adaptive or inducible enzyme system whose activity level can be reduced by removal of the substrate and increased by substrate reintroduction (2, 3, 5, 27, 29, 31).

"*Methodology. Biopsy* of the jejunal mucosa has been considered the most accurate and direct approach to measure lactase activity. It is imperative that biopsy specimens be obtained from a uniform location — usually at the ligament of Treitz — since recent findings indicate a gradient of lactase activity along the small intestines from the duodenum to the ileum (5, 8, 32). However, there is a constant ratio between sucrase and lactase activities; thus, this ratio can differentiate subjects with normal and low lactase levels even if specimens are obtained from different areas.

"Indirectly, low lactase activity can be diagnosed by

means of a lactose tolerance test (LTT). 'A "flat" blood sugar curve, i.e., rise of 25 mg% or less following ingestion of standard lactose dose of 50 g/m^2 or 2 g/kg in children' indicates low lactase activity (26, 33). LTT data from various investigators are difficult to compare because of differences in the lactose load administered, blood samples taken, samples time, and methods of blood sugar analysis used. While some investigators find a good correlation among symptoms of lactose intolerance, a low rise in blood glucose following lactose load, and low intestinal lactase levels (34), others do not (35). A more distinct correlation has been reported when blood glucose rise was plotted against the sucrase/lactase ratio (35) and when capillary, not venous, blood samples were analyzed (36). Capillary blood samples are preferable since they tend to eliminate false-positive tests due to delayed gastric emptying; that is, flat tolerance curves of venous blood even in subjects with normal lactase activity and who are asymptomatic from lactose (8, 37).

"A modification of the LTT was suggested by Jussila (38) whereby ethanol is administered prior to the lactose load and blood galactose level is measured. The LTT also has been adapted for field work by the use of Ames Reflectance Meter/Dextrostix method of blood sugar analysis (39).

"The *breath hydrogen test* proposed by Calloway et al (40) is based on the principle that undigested lactose passes into the colon where hydrogen is formed by bacterial fermentation (41, 42). If the mean concentration of hydrogen exceeds 30 ppm in breath samples taken at 30-minute intervals during an 8-hour period after ingestion of lactose, a person may be diagnosed as having lactose malabsorpotion (40). Newcomer et al (43) compared four indirect methods with intestinal lactase values and concluded that breath hydrogen measurement, because it does not require alcohol, istotopes or blood samples, promises to be most suitable for screening large groups.

"Other indirect methods of assessing lactase activity include the oral lactose loading test (44), breath ^{14}C labeled carbon dioxide measurement (45), and radiological test employing barium-lactose meals (8, 46, 47).

"*Incidence.* Less than 15% of Scandinavians and those of Western and Northern European extraction but about 60-80% of Greek Cypriots, American Indians, Arabs, Ashkenazi Jews, Mexican-Americans, American Negroes, and 90% of African Bantus and Orientals have been reported to be lactose intolerant (3, 6, 7, 21, 24, 27, 48-51). The significance of these reports may have been greatly exaggerated because of the testing methods used and the manner of interpreting symptoms. Relatively few studies on incidence in children have been reported. The onset of this condition has been described to be between the ages of 2 and 12 depending on the ethnic group samples as well as on their milk-drinking patterns (5, 6, 29, 51-53).

"*Nutrient Utilization.* Recent studies on the effect of lactose on nutrient utilization have taken into consideration the lactase activity of the subjects. While some researchers report an increase in calcium absorption (54, 55), others do not (56). This conflict prompted a study by Kocian et al (57). Their results indicated that although calcium absorption in lactose-intolerant patients after milk ingestion was poor, calcium utilization and retention were practically the same regardless of the source of calcium and the lactase activity of the subjects. Another study by Calloway and Chenoweth (58) revealed that after adjustments for variations in metabolizable energy intakes, there were no significant differences in nitrogen balance related to level of lactose intake. Unpublished data from the same investigators (58) showed no apparent interference with calcium, phosphorus, and magnesium absorption in lactose-intolerant individuals.

"Luyken (48) reported three investigations that demonstrated 1) the lactose-intolerant children can satisfactorily digest and absorb proteins (amino acids) from milk and 2) the increase in serum albumin in these children on a milk diet was at least as good as those on a lactose-free diet.

"Milk Intolerance

"Milk intolerance due to lactose content has been defined by the PAG (26) as the appearance of 'clinical signs (abdominal pain, diarrhea, bloating, flatulence, etc.) consistently following a few hours after ingestion of milk or milk-containing products in usual amounts in a person with proven lactose malabsorption.' Paige and his co-workers reported that Negro children participating in school lunch programs (59) as well as white and Negro pregnant women of the lowest socio-economic status (33) should not be encouraged to drink milk because of the symptoms experienced after administering the LTT. This suggestion has prompted the scientific community to seek an answer to the question: 'Does intolerance to a 50 or 100 g lactose load indicate clinical milk intolerance?' The PAG (26) objected to equating the symptomatic response to large amounts of lactose to that occurring after ingesting an 8-ounce glass of milk which contains 12 g lactose.

"Leichter (60) reported the intensity of symptoms in lactose-intolerant individuals to be highest with aqueous lactose solution, lower with skim milk, and lowest with whole milk. Tolerance to milk has been reportedly increased by consuming it with a meal, by drinking small amounts several times during the day, or even by taking it as a warm beverage (35, 60, 61).

"The Committee on Nutrition, American Academy of Pediatrics (62) stated that for most children, drinking moderate amounts of milk has no adverse effects and, in fact, is nutritionally beneficial. According to the findings of several investigators (2, 39, 63, 64), the same statement can be made for most lactose-intolerant adults, although one group (65) disagrees. In most foreign nutrition programs, the amount of milk given to a child at one time rarely exceeds 200 ml. Even those children who are lactose intolerant are unlikely to develop symptoms with these amounts of milk supplements (35). A significant finding relative to mass feeding programs for malnourished children was reported by Mason et all (66). They observed that severely malnourished children in Ethiopa responded favorably to feedings of a high-energy milk-based diet. This observation supports the Food and Nutrition Board of the National Academy of Sciences statement (67) that it is inappropriate on the basis of present evidence to discourage programs for improving milk supplies or those that encourage milk consumption in either the U.S. or foreign countries because of the fear of milk intolerance.

ACKNOWLEDGMENTS

The National Dairy Council assumes the responsibility for writing and editing this publication. However, we would like to acknowledge the help and suggestions of the following reviewers in its preparation: W. L. Chenoweth, Ph.D., Assistant Professor of Food Science and Human Nutrition, Michigan State University, East Lansing, Michigan; M. C. Latham, M.D., Professor of International Nutrition, Cornell University, Ithaca, New York; and A. D. Newcomer, M.D., Assistant Professor of Internal Medicine, Mayo Clinic and Mayo Foundation, Rochester, Minnesota.

References

1. Kretchmer, N. Gastroenterology 61:805, 1971.
2. Kretchmer, N. Sci. Am. 227:71, 1972
3. McCracken, R.D. Curr, Anthropol. 12:479, 1971.
4. Skala, I., and V. Lamacova. Nutr. Metabol. 13:200, 1971
5. Bolin, T. D., A. E. Davis, C. S. Seah, K. L. Chua, K. M. Kho, V. Young, C. L. Siak, and E. Jacob. Gastroenterology 59:76, 1970
6. Kretchmer, N., and O. Ransome-Kuti. Proc. Inst. Med. Chic. 28:213, 1970
7. Bayless, T. M. J. Am. Diet. Assoc. 60:478, 1972
8. McGill, D. B., and A. D. Newcomer. Progress in Gastroenterology 2:292, 1970
9. Ali, R., and J. L. Evans. J. Agric. Univ. Puerto Rico 57:149, 1973
10. Featherston, W. R., M. L. Morris, Jr., and P. H. Phillips. J. Nutr. 79:431, 1963
11. Morris, M. L., Jr., W. R. Featherston, P. H. Phillips, and S. H. McNutt. J. Nutr. 79:437, 1963
12. National Dairy Council. *Nutritional Significance of Lactose.* Dairy Council *Digest* 33:1, 1962
13. Lengemann, F. W. J. Nutr. 69:23, 1959
14. National Dairy Council. *Nutritional Significance of Lactose.* Dairy Council *Digest* 20:1, 1949
15. Flatz, G., and H. W. Rotthauwe. *Lancet* 2:76, 1973
16. Sewell, R. F., and J. P. West. J. Anim. Sci. 24:239, 1965
17. Ali, R. A. M., and J. L. Evans. J. Anim. Sci. 33:765, 1971
18. Fervier, C., and A. Rerat. Nutr. Abstr. Rev. 35:1015, 1965
19. Varma, S. N., V. Schwarz, and I. M. Naomi Simpson. Biochem. J. 85:546, 1962
20. Coello-Ramirez, P., F. Lifshiftz, and V. Zuniga. Pediatrics 49:233, 1972
21. Welsh, J. D., Med. World News (special issue on Gastroenterology), 1972, p. 57
22. Rosensweig, N. S. J. Dairy Sci. 52:585, 1970
23. Dill, J. E., M. Levy, R. F. Wells, and E. Weser. Am. J. Clin. Nutr. 25:869, 1972
24. National Dairy Council. *Lactose Intolerance.* Dairy Council *Digest* 42:31, 1971
25. Rosensweig, N. S. *A Review of Dietary Lactose and Its Varied Utilization by Man.* Whey Products Institute, Chicago, Illinois, 1974, In Press.

26. PAG *Ad Hoc* Working Group on Milk Intolerance – Nutritional Implications. PAG Bull. 2:7, 1972
27. Bolin, T. D., and A. E. Davis. Am. J. Dig. Dis. 15:679, 1970
28. Dahlqvist, A., and B. Linquist. Acta Paediatr. Scand. 60:488, 1971
29. Olatunbosun, D. A., and B. K. Adadevoh. Acta Paediatr. Scand. 61:715, 1972
30. Simoons, F. J., Am. J. Dig. Dis. 14:819, 1969
31. Wen, C-P, I. Antonowicz, E. Tovar, R. B. McGandy, and S. N. Gershoff. Am. J. Clin. Nutr. 26:1224, 1973
32. Newcomer, A. D., and D. B. McGill. Gastroenterology 51:481, 1966
33. Paige, D. M., T. M. Bayless, and G. G. Graham. Am. J. Clin. Nutr. 26:238, 1973
34. Welsh, J. D., V. Rohrer, K. B. Knudsen, and F. F. Paustian. Arch. Intern. Med. 120:261, 1967
35. Reddy, V., and J. Pershad. Am. J. Clin. Nutr. 25:114, 1972
36. Bell, R. R., H. H. Draper, and J. G. Bergan. Am. J. Clin. Nutr. 26:1185, 1973
37. McGill, D. B., and A. D. Newcomer. Gastroenterology 53:371, 1967
38. Jussila, J. Scand. J. Gastroenterol. 4:361, 1969
39. Stephenson, L. S., and M. C. Latham. Am. J. Clin. Nutr. 27:296, 1974
40. Calloway, D. H., E. L. Murphy, and D. Bauer. Am. J. Dig. Dis. 14:811, 1969
41. Levitt, M. D., J. Am. Diet Assoc. 60:487, 1972
42. Levitt, M. D., and R. M. Donaldson. J. Lab. Clin. Med. 75:937, 1970
43. Newcomer, A. D., P. J. Thomas, D. B. McGill, and A. F. Hofmann. Gastroenterology 66:754, 1974 (Abstract)
44. Desai, H. G., A. V. Chitrie, and K. N. Jeejeebhoy. Gastroenterologia 108:177, 1967
45. Shanbrom, E. Diagnostic method for determination of lactase deficiency using radioactive lactose. U.S. Patent Office 3, 772, 436, Patented Nov. 13, 1973
46. Walker, J. A., and J. D. Bowdler. Gut 10:78, 1969
47. Thompson, J. R., and I. Sanders. Am. J. Reontgenol. Radium Ther. Nucl. Med. 113:255, 1971
48. Luyken, R. Maandschr, Kindergeneesk, 40:89, 1972
49. Simoons, F. J. Am. J. Dig. Dis. 18:595, 1973
50. Bayless, T. M., D. M. Paige and G. D. Ferry. Gastroenterology 60:605, 1971

51. Bose, D. P., and J. D. Welsh. Am. J. Clin. Nutr. 26:1320, 1973
52. Jones, D. V., and M. C. Latham. Am. J. Clin. Nutr. 27:547, 1974
53. Bayless, T. M. Med. Counterpoint 3:10, 1971
54. Pansu, D., and M. C. Chapuy. Calcif. Tissue Res. 4 (Suppl.):155, 1970
55. Fournier, P., Y. Dupuis, and A. Fournier. Isr. J. Med. Sci. 7:389, 1971
56. Condon, J. R., J. R. Nassim, F. J. C. Millard, A. Hilbe, and E. M. Stainthorpe, *Lancet* 1:1027, 1970
57. Kocian, J., I. Skala, and K. Bakos. Digestion 9:317, 1973
58. Calloway, D. H., and W. L. Chenoweth. Am. J. Clin. Nutr. 26:939, 1973
59. Paige, D. M., T. M. Bayless, and G. G. Graham. Am. J. Public Health 62:1486, 1972
60. Leichter, J. Am. J. Clin. Nutr. 26:393, 1973
61. Cuatrecacas, P., D. H. Lockwood, and J. R. Caldwell. *Lancet* 1:14, 1965
62. American Academy of Pediatrics Committee on Nutrition. Pediatrics 53:576, 1974
63. Nandi, M. A., and E. S. Parham, J. Am. Diet. Assoc. 63:258, 1972
64. Lisker, R., G. Lopez-Habib, M. Daltabuit, I. Rostenberg, and P. Arroyo, Am. J. Clin. Nutr. 27:756, 1974
65. Bayless, T. M., B. Rothfeld, C. Massa, L. M. Wise, and M. S. Bedine. Am. J. Clin. Nutr. 26:465, 1973 (Abstract)
66. Mason, J. B., R. W. Hay, J. Leresche, S. Peel, and S. Darley. *Lancet* 1:332, 1974
67. Food and Nutrition Board, Background Information on lactose and milk intolerance. A Statement of the Food and Nutrition Board. National Research Council. National Academy of Sciences, May 1972.

APPENDIX 5

THE FEDERAL GOVERNMENT SPEAKS

I start with line 19, page 95, of *National Program for the Conquest of Cancer, Report of the National Panel of Consultants on the Conquest of Cancer,* authorized by S. Res. 376 (Agreed to by Senate April 17, 1970), prepared for the Committee on Labor and Public Welfare, United States Senate, April 14, 1971. I finish with line 12, page 101. I make paragraphing consistent with the rest of my book. The quotation is exact:

"How Chemical Carcinogens Induce Cancer

"Research workers have long been aware of the importance of learning what happens when a chemical carcinogen enters a susceptible organism, reaches a target tissue, and acts in some manner to produce cancer.

"Detailed information on the process of cancer formation by chemicals is the soundest basis on which to develop means of protecting the human population against the carcinogenic effects of chemicals in the environment and of inhibiting the processes once started.

"These investigations have been difficult because carcinogenic substances vary widely with regard to many properties such as structure, molecular size, and solubility, as well as in degree and kind of chemical reactivity.

"In spite of the difficulty, investigations in this area have been fruitful, and knowledge of the nature of the carcinogenic processes induced by chemicals has increased greatly in recent years.

"Much of the advance in knowledge has resulted from the development of better model systems. Thus, by the appropriate combinations of chemical carcinogen, of species, and of route of administration, the investigator can now induce tumors in almost any tissue at will.

"Further, cancer can be induced by chemicals in cell culture, and the effects of chemical carcinogens on specific systems can also be studied at the subcellular level. Thus, model systems can be designed in relation to the particular problem under study.

"Metabolism of chemical carcinogen

"Only a very small fraction of a dose of a chemical carcinogen administered to an animal is involved in the induction of a tumor. In most cases the major share of the carcinogen is converted (usually enzymatically) in the body to harmless substances which are eliminated. To the extent that these reactions occur, the deleterious effects of the chemical are reduced. However, another fraction of the administered carcinogen (usually only a small portion) is converted metabolically into the actual carcinogenic form; this chemically reactive derivative, ultimate carcinogen, is directly responsible for the induction of the tumor. In some cases, notably with a class of chemicals called alkylating agents, the carcinogen requires no metabolic activation.

"The cancer-inducing activity of chemical carcinogens varies from species to species, from organ to organ, and probably from person to person. These differences may reflect variations in the cellular enzymes that metabolize carcinogens.

"An enzyme system of this sort which metabolizes polynuclear hydrocarbons has been identified. Its level of activity correlates well with the sensitivity of the cells to the toxic effect of polynuclear carcinogens.

"This system also catalyzes the binding of the ultimate carcinogen to DNA. An inhibitor has been found that blocks its action.

"Measurements of the levels of these activating enzyme

systems may lead to the identification of individuals who may be highly susceptible to certain specific carcinogenic exposures and the enzyme system's inhibition by drugs may lead to a marked decrease in cancer risk.

"**Target molecules**

"Recent studies have shown that the known ultimate carcinogens share a common chemical property in that they are all strong electrophilic reactants (i.e., they contain electron-deficient atoms). As a consequence of their electrophilic character, these ultimate carcinogens, at a class, react chemically with nucleophilic sites (i.e., atoms with excess electrons) in tissues.

"The information-containing macromolecules of the cells (DNA, RNA, with protein) are relatively rich in nucleophilic sites and, in those cases which have been adequately studied, derivatives of chemical carcinogens have been found to be firmly bound to the DNA, RNA, and protein of target tissues.

"Further, in some cases, susceptibility to cancer formation by chemical carcinogens has been correlated with the kinds and amounts of these macromolecule-bound carcinogens.

"Since cancer cells divide to give rise to more cancer cells in the absence of the original transforming agent, the chemical induction of alterations in the information-carrying macromolecules offers one of the most plausible explanations for the induction of tumors by chemicals.

"Complexes of covalently bound carcinogens and DNA, RNA, or proteins have been found in extracts of precancerous and cancerous tissues and in cell-free extracts treated with chemical carcinogens. On the basis of present evidence, such bindings appear to be an essential stage in the carcinogenic process.

"Evidence that ultimate carcinogens bind to a variety of

macromolecules is an important step forward in the understanding of the mechanism of chemical carcinogenesis. Since each kind of macromolecule involved has a variety of important functions, however, it is still not known which of the many interactions is the critical one.

"At this point, it is essential to demonstrate that the carcinogen-bound macromolecules are functionally modified and that such functional changes are consistent with a rational theory of carcinogenesis. This is where research in this area stands today.

"The binding of carcinogens to DNA, the genetic material itself, could be of particular significance. However, the amount of binding of one polycyclic hydrocarbon tested does not correlate with its carcinogenic activity; moreover, transformation induced by certain of these compounds is much too frequent to be caused by mutation, which by definition is a random process. For these reasons, the binding of carcinogens to DNA may not constitute the critical interaction.

"Two possibilities remain: RNA and proteins. Epigenetic mechanisms for tumor induction, akin to those proposed for normal cellular differentiation, are equally attractive. The activities of a cell appear to depend on the selective expression of segments of its DNA.

"Which parts of the DNA are expressed is determined by a complex system of repression and derepression in which other macromolecules, proteins and RNAs, play key roles.

"The altered affinity for critical sites on the DNA of chemically modified repressors or derepressors could greatly modify the responsiveness of a cell and its descendants to homeostatic mechanisms.

"Some studies have suggested that chemicals may trigger the development of cancer through facilitating the expression of latent oncogenic viral genomes in the 'normal' cells.

"Other investigations have emphasized the action of

certain chemical carcinogens — which appear to be generally 'immuno-depressive' — in decreasing the immunological capacity of the host and in thus providing a more suitable environment for the proliferation of abnormal cells.

"The critical question of what is the crucial change involved in chemical carcinogenesis thus remains to be answered. There is no reason at the present time to conclude that the induction of cancer occurs by only one of the above mechanisms. Each mechanism may play a role in the induction of neoplasms in specific cases.

"Cocarcinogensis

"In at least some cases, the induction of tumors is a multistage process, in which each phase is facilitated by specific chemicals that may not be active at other stages.

"This sequence of events has been most clearly demonstrated in the case of mouse skin tumorigenesis. In this model, appropriate doses of certain carcinogens can initiate in an irreversible manner the formation of altered cells with the potential capacity for malignant proliferation.

"However, tumors do not usually develop until another type of chemical called a 'promoter' is applied subsequent to the initiating dose. The promoting agent appears to facilitate the proliferation of the altered cells and in the early stages, its activity appears to be at least partially reversible.

"Knowledge in this area is highly relevant to the testing of new chemicals for their carcinogenicity.

"The Future

"Much further research is needed before complete understanding is obtained of the activation of chemical carcinogens, their cellular targets, the nature of the reactions of the carcinogens with those targets, and the consequences of the carcinogen-cell interactions that are relevant to the induction of malignancy and the proliferation of the altered cells.

"Much of the groundwork for these studies has been laid in the areas of chemical and viral carcinogenesis and in the broader field of molecular biology.

"By providing the information and the tools needed to protect the public from environmental carcinogenic hazards, studies of chemical carcinogenesis can make enormous contributions to public health. Because it is now possible to study the process of cancer formation with new insights, new techniques, and new precision, research in this area is likely to provide new means to prevent, control, or even reverse the cancerous process.

"Areas of Promise in Chemical Carcinogenesis

"In order to achieve the answers to the fundamental and practical problems yet unsolved, it will be necessary to expand our national program in chemical carcinogenesis. Given much increased support, the following studies in chemical carcinogenesis offer great promise:

"1. Development of test systems for identification of chemical carcinogens, with a review of requirements for test systems, and the development of special systems, including use of additional animal species and in vitro systems.

"2. Selection of materials to be tested, these must include those which are highly suspect based on epidemiological and epizoological data, structural features, and mutagenic, teratogenic, and growth-promoting actions as well as those to which man is extensively exposed, including natural hazards, pharmaceuticals, and compounds associated with occupational hazards.

"3. Studies on man, including special population groups, based on geographic pathology, occupational risks, and population 'laboratories.'

"4. Effects of chemical carcinogens on the immunological processes.

"5. Interaction between chemical carcinogens and factors that regulate growth and differentiation.

"6. Role of hormones in chemical carcinogenesis.

"7. Interactions of chemical carcinogens with each other and with other extrinsic factors, such as viruses and radiation, and intrinsic factors.

"8. Identification of target cells in tissues undergoing carcinogenesis.

"9. Distribution, metabolism, and excretion of carcinogens in susceptible and resistant animals.

"10. Nature of interactions between chemical carcinogens and tissue components at the molecular level.

"11. Early events in carcinogenesis, especially in macromolecular synthesis and ultrastructural changes.

"12. Comparison of the biochemical properties of chemically induced tumors with those of the parent normal cells, and the significance of these properties to the carcinogenic process.

"13. Relationship between carcinogenicity, mutagenicity, teratogenicity, and immunosuppressive activities in various species and strains.

"14. Observations on cell population dynamics in relation to chemical carcinogenesis.

"Radiation Carcinogenesis

"Studies in radiation carcinogenesis are directed toward: 1) determining the carcinogenic hazards to humans of both natural and man-made radiation and 2) determining the mechanisms by which radiation produces cancer.

"The realization that ionizing radiation is carcinogenic for man came remarkably soon after the discovery, just before the turn of the century, of x-rays by Roentgen and the purification of radium by the Curies and Henri Becquerel.

"Within a few years, the first skin cancers were beginning to appear on the exposed fingers, hands, and faces of the early workers in the field. By 1908, the injurious effects of ionizing radiation on the bone marrow and peripheral blood were known, and by 1911, the first cases of leukemia began to be reported in individuals previously exposed to significant radiation doses.

"However, the carcinogenic hazards of internally deposited natural and artificial radioactive substances were not appreciated until the now-classic report of Martland in 1931 on the development of sarcomas of the bones in radium watch-dial painters.

"With isolated exceptions, experimental studies of these processes languished until World War II, when the development of the atomic bomb gave a powerful impetus and urgency to such investigations.

"The first systematic studies of the effects of radiation dose and dose rate on longevity and incidence of leukemia in mice were reported in 1947. Since that time, the leukemias and lymphomas have continued to be the most intensively studied of the cancers induced by ionizing radiation in mice and other experimental animals.

"However, a broad spectrum of other types of cancers has also been induced under appropriate conditions, including tumors of the skin, subcutaneous connective tissues, bone, lung, intestine, ovary, thyroid, pituitary, and liver. Moreover, ionizing radiations have proven to be a most useful tool for the elucidation of the fundamental mechanisms of carcinogenesis.

"Mechanisms of action

"Ionizing radiations may induce cancers by at least three different mechanisms: somatic mutation, the activation of latent oncogenic viruses, and the disturbance of growth regulatory mechanisms. The latter two concepts were quite unsuspected 25 years ago, yet today they are well documented.

"On the other hand, somatic mutation, which was the only plausible hypothesis in existence a generation ago, has remained so far unproven. It has long been known that ionizing radiation is powerfully mutagenic, but the frequency of transformations produced by x-rays among cells in culture seems too high to be attributed to randomly occurring mutations.

"The recent successful development of techniques for the induction of radiogenic cell transformations in vitro as well as the new opportunities for the genetic analysis of somatic cells offer great promise for the unequivocal establishment of whether radiation induces cancer through mutations.

"Moreover, since both the dose and dose rate can be calculated with precision and the time of the initial events can be known with certainty, radiation-induced carcinogenesis may well prove to be an important model system for the elucidation of the earliest steps in carcinogenesis, which are inherently more difficult to time with chemical carcinogens or viruses.

"Radiation as an inducer of a mouse leukemia virus

"The leukemias and thymic lymphosarcomas induced in mice by whole-body x-ray exposure were also presumed initially to be the result of somatic mutation. However, in a series of experimental studies, it has been demonstrated conclusively that the results seen in this induction system are not consistent with what would be expected from the induction of mutations.

"For example, although these tumors arose locally in the thymus, local irradiation over the thymic region alone was entirely ineffective in inducing them and shielding of the bone marrow was able to confer a striking degree of protection.

"Finally, and most convincingly incompatible with the

somatic mutation hypothesis, lymphoma development, abolished in irradiated mice by prior thymectomy, could be restored by the later grafting into them of histocompatible thymus glands from unirradiated donors.

"The tumors arose in the thymic grafts and could be shown, by their transplantation behavior and karyotype (chromosome complement), to be derived from the non-irradiated cells of the graft and thus induced by a completely indirect mechanism.

"Were carcinogenesis a result of mutation, it should occur in the irradiated cells themselves.

"Meanwhile, the key to this paradox had been provided by the discovery of Gross that viruses with leukemogenic potentialities could be extracted from the 'spontaneous' leukemias and lymphomas of certain highly susceptible strains of mice.

"Soon thereafter, a similar subcellular, presumably viral, leukemogenic agent was successfully extracted from lymphomas that had been induced by radiation in two low-leukemia strains.

"Since that time, this agent has been purified and proven to be a virus which is closely related to the original Gross mouse leukemia virus with respect to its morphology, its immunogenic characteristics, its vertical transmission from one generation to the next through the embryo, and its ability to act as a 'helper' for the defective murine sarcoma virus.

"However, this agent differs from the Gross virus in its pattern of host strain susceptibility and, most importantly, in its requirement of 'activation' or 'switching on' from a latent, oncogenically inert state, by exposure to ionizing radiation or to a variety of chemical agents. As a consequence, radiation-induced leukemias in mice are now interpreted as being caused by a latent leukemia virus 'induced' in bone marrow cells by radiation. This virus, once released, is capable of producing cancers in thymic cells, whether irradiated or not.

"This phenomenon is of great theoretical interest, since, in many ways, it is remarkably analogous to the extensively studied process of lysogeny and induction of temperate bacterial viruses in their specific bacterial hosts, suggesting that many of the molecular mechanisms of the latter process may have direct applicability at the mammalian level in this 'temperate' leukemia virus system.

"The recent development of quantitative in vitro assays for the mouse leukemia viruses should give great impetus to this field of investigation, which may well have important etiologic implications for the human leukemias as well.

"It has been reported that there is a small but seemingly real increase in leukemia incidence among children born of mothers whose abdomens were exposed in the course of diagnostic radiographic procedures during pregnancy. Those procedures involve very much smaller doses than those which have been estimated to be leukemogenic for adults, which suggests that the human fetus may be much more sensitive.

"Indeed, it may well be that these childhood leukemias are the human counterparts of the latent viral activation mechanism described above.

"Certainly, the extremely low doses of radiation which are known to induce vegetative viral replication in lysogenic bacteria are entirely consistent with such a possibility. These considerations suggest that the specific problem of radiation leukemogenesis warrants much further study.

"Disturbance of growth regulation

"The best, though not the sole, examples of tumors arising by the sustained disturbance of a growth regulatory feedback of equilibrium are those induced by ionizing radiation in the endocrine glands, especially in the ovaries, the thyroids, and the pituitary glands of mice and rats."

From this point forward, the material becomes a mite technical.

I should, however, go back in the book to page 23, to include the following:

"Recently the intriguing discovery has been made of a new kind of antigen, a fetal antigen, associated with human cancer. These antigens, which are released from cells and can be detected in the blood stream, are normally present in embryonic or fetal tissues, disappear in adult life, and only reappear in the cancerous cell. (This reappearance suggests that a gene that is switched on in fetal life and switched off after birth is switched on again during carcinogenesis.)

"One of these fetal antigens, CEA, CEA, is providing the basis for the new immunologic test . . . The second fetal antigen is found in the blood stream of about 75% of patients with cancers arising in the liver. A third fetal antigen is found in association with a variety of other tumors. All of these antigens may be useful in the development of diagnostic tests."

The foregoing information on fetal antigens would seem to suggest consideration of possible relationship between cancer and birth defects, as suggested by previous mention of childhood leukemia. In such case, I shall offer material for the reader to consider, only, no judgments by the writer.

APPENDIX 6

NUTRITION, DIET, AND CANCER – SUMMARY – NATIONAL DAIRY COUNCIL

Courtesy, *Dairy Council Digest,* National Dairy Council. National Dairy Council assumes no responsibility for the contents of this book other than the portions excerpted from the Dairy Council *Digest.*

"Volume 46, No. 5
"September-October 1975

"Nutrition, Diet, and Cancer – Summary

"Cancer is the second leading cause of death in the United States. It is estimated that 80-90% of all human cancer may be related to several environmental factors and, therefore, potentially preventable. Nutrition and diet have been suggested to be among these environmental factors, and nutritional effects in tumor development in experimental animals have been demonstrated. Caloric restrictions, type and amount of dietary fat, deficiencies of certain vitamins and minerals, and dietary content of protein and amino acids all influence induction or growth of tumors in animals. Certain amino acid deficiencies are reported to have tumor-suppressing action. Some vitamin deficiencies enhance tumor development; other deficiencies suppress it. Epidemiologic studies in human populations have implicated high levels of fat or a lack of fiber in the diet in the causation of breast and colon cancer. Differences in the diet may bring about differences in the intestinal microflora which have been associated with variations in the incidence of cancer of the large bowel. More studies are needed to elucidate the mechanism(s) by which nutrition and diet can influence carcinogenesis and to document associations between dietary practices and cancer. While the scientific evidence in experimental animals is suggestive of a relationship between nutrition and cancer, confirmation of these findings in humans is fragmentary. Therefore, other than maintenance of desirable body weight, it is premature to make specific dietary recommendations at present to minimize the risk of cancer.

"A tumor, sometimes called a cancer or a neoplasm, is a new growth of tissue which has lost some, but not all, of the controls which normally keep it in proper balance with the rest of the body (1). Neoplasms may be benign, i.e,. space-filling lesions, or malignant, in which case they invade the surrounding tissues and spread (metastasize) to distant organs via blood or lymphatic vessels. Cancer is synonymous with malignant neoplasm and may occur in all tissues.

"Diseases collectively known as cancer are the second leading cause of death in the United States; in 1974 alone, approximately 355,000 people died from various forms of this disease (2). Of the various types of cancer, death from cancer of the lung, large bowel, and breast (in decreasing order) are the most frequent in this country (2).

"Based on epidemiological studies, it has been estimated that 80-90% of all human cancer may be related to one or more environmental factors (3-6) and, therefore, the majority of human cancer is potentially preventable (7). Barrett (8) presented a comprehensive report of epidemiological and laboratory data suggesting that nutrition and diet may be among the significant environmental factors in the etiology of various forms of cancer including cancer of the esophagus, stomach, liver, colon, breast, bladder, lymph, lung, and skin.

"Nutrition and diet may affect carcinogenesis in either of two ways: 1) food or drink may be contaminated by carcinogens, or 2) the composition of the diet may impose upon the host patterns of enzyme activity and other factors which dictate the yield of naturally occurring or induced tumors (9).

It is in the latter context that this *Digest* will present its discussion of the role of nutrition and diet in carcinogenesis.

"Nutritional Status

"Early reports on the possible relation between nutrition and cancer include a study published in 1909 cited by Tannenbaum (10). Numerous reports on this subject have appeared in the scientific literature since then. Early investigations were based on the concept that tumors develop from living cells and grow by assimilating nutrients from the host. Thus, changes in the nutritional status of the host might be expected to modify (either enhance or depress) both the development of a neoplasm and its subsequent growth (10).

"Because the generic term neoplasm encompasses many different kinds of tumors, it is prudent to avoid generalizations from the response of a single tumor type to a particular nutritional change. Different tumors, benign or malignant, need not be and often are not affected in the same manner by the same nutritional variable. Responses of many types of tumors must be studied before one can draw conclusions about the general affect of a particular dietary component, but a consistent response even of one tumor type is, of course, of great interest.

"*Calories.* Of all the dietary modifications studied, caloric restriction has had the most regular influence on the genesis of neoplasms in experimental animals (10). Chronic caloric restriction inhibits the formation or growth of many types of tumors [with some exceptions (11)], decreases the incidence of neoplasms and delays as well the time at which tumors appear (10, 12-15). However, despite the substantial reduction in tumor risk observed when newly weaned animals were underfed, a regimen of under-feeding during early growth should not be misconstrued as a recommended practice for man (14). The extent of the inhibitory effect of caloric restriction on tumor risk varies with the type of tumor and with the carcinogen used; spontaneous tumors, i.e., tumors arising in animals not intentionally exposed to carcinogens, also are affected (10, 13, 14). In mice, spontaneous neoplasms of the breast and lung are the most affected, followed by induced skin tumors and induced sarcomas (10).

"Body weight is related to tumor risk. Within each group of animals receiving identical diets, the incidence of every tumor type was consistently greater in heavy rats than in lean rats (14). Epidemiological studies have shown that obesity or increased body mass is significantly related to cancers of the endometrium, breast, and gall bladder (16,17). A statistically significant association has been noted between obesity and carcinoma of the large bowel in men but not in women (13). Shils (13) also reported that there is good evidence that cancer of the uterus occurs more frequently in overweight women.

"Tannenbaum (10) and Kraybill (12) summarized several concepts which have been advanced to explain the inhibitory effect of caloric restriction on tumor formation. Mitotic activity of the cells is inhibited by caloric restriction, probably because the amount of carbohydrate and carbohydrate intermediates available for energy production is limited, and this may decrease tumor growth. Caloric restriction may lead to adrenal hyperfunction and a consequent increase in gluconeogenesis and complex endocrine interactions. In the case of mammary cancer in mice, the principal effect of caloric restriction may be one of reducing the production of estrogen (probably a co-carcinogen in spontaneous mammary cancer), diminishing the response of the mammary gland to estrogen, or altering production of other hormones which control growth of mammary tissue.

"*Fat and Cholesterol.* Epidemiological evidence in several countries has shown a direct correlation between fat consumption and mortality rates for breast neoplasms (18, 19). An association between 'Westernization' of the diet and colon cancer has been noted (20, 21). Fat intake is one of the major differences between Western and other diets but fat is by no means the only distinctive component of the Western diet. Multiple cultural and economic differences must be taken into account (21, 22). Furthermore, increasing the level of fat in the diet may well increase body weight because of its high caloric value. Thus, when studying the effects of fats in animals, it is very necessary to take steps to eliminate the excess calories, preferably by reducing the carbohydrate content of the diet (23).

"Increasing the total fat content of the diet from 2 or 5% to 20 or 27% increased incidence of spontaneous mammary carcinomas, induced skin neoplasms, and hepatic tumors and resulted in earlier appearance of these tumors in experimental animals (10, 12, 19, 24-30). However, a further increase in dietary fat from 27 to 61% did not cause a proportional increase in tumors (27). Induction of colon tumors in rats was enhanced by quadrupling but not by doubling dietary fat content (31, 32).

"Although fat-enriched diets augmented the formation of certain tumors, they did not increase the incidence of induced sarcoma, primary lung adenoma, or spontaneous and induced leukemia in mice (10). Also, high-fat diets did not increase the incidence of fibroadenomas and adenomas in general (25).

"In animals, tumor formation and growth seem to be affected not only by the amount of dietary fat but also by the type of fat. In an early study, Miller et al (33) observed a significantly greater carcinogenic potency of paradimethylaminoazobenzene when rats were fed diets containing corn oil instead of hydrogenated coconut oil. Gammal et al (26, 34) reported that a semisynthetic high-corn oil diet enhanced the development of mammary cancer induced by 7,

12-dimethylbenz anthracene in intact female rats.

"This was in comparison to two other groups of similarly treated rats fed a high-coconut and low-fat semisynthetic diet; their average daily caloric intake was similar. Weisburger (32) noted that at low levels of fat intake, colon tumors were more readily induced in rats fed corn oil than in rats fed lard; however, at high levels, no difference was observed. Kaunitz and Johnson (35) noted that the highest incidence of malignant tumors occurred when animals were fed either soybean oil or chicken fat, and the lowest incidence when animals were fed either cotton-seed oil or butter. Increasing the intake of dietary fat and/or the degree of unsaturation of fat has been reported to increase tumor incidence in C3H female mice fed isocalorically (20). Also, mice receiving corn and safflower oil tended to die with gross mammary tumors at earlier ages than those consuming diets containing lower amounts of these fats (30).

"Several explanations regarding the possible mechanism of action of fat-enriched diets in carcinogenesis have been advanced by a number of investigators (10, 36, 37). Rose et al (36) postulated that a high polyunsaturated fatty acid (PUFA) intake could induce the formation of more bile salts, thus increasing the amount of substrate available for the carcinogen-forming bacteria, and hence increase the risk for colon cancer. Mertin (37) reported an inhibitory effect of PUFA on the antigen-induced lymphocyte response. Thus, an increased serum PUFA level might suppress the reaction of the immune system to cancer and favor tumor development and growth.

"Human studies concerning the effect of type of fat on cancer incidence have been based mainly on trials testing the cholesterol-lowering potential of high-PUFA diets. Pearce and Dayton (38) reported a higher incidence of fatal carcinomas in a group of individuals fed four times as much PUFA and half as much cholesterol when compared to a group fed conventional diets. Although the authors noted that many of the cancer deaths in the experimental group occurred among those who did not adhere closely to the diet, they suggested that their results be viewed in the light of animal experiments which suggest that fat intake (especially unsaturated fat intake) affects the incidence of certain types of neoplasm. They cautioned the medical and scientific community that it was premature to make a blanket prescription of a diet high in PUFA for the entire population. On the other hand, data from various investigations (39-42) lend no support to the hypothesis that increased PUFA intake is carcinogenic.

"The possible relationship between blood cholesterol level or cholesterol ingestion and tumor formation has been advanced for several reasons (43-45), among which is the epidemiological association between coronary heart disease and several forms of cancer (18, 36). However, several investigators disagree with this suggested role of cholesterol (7, 36, 46-48). Two studies have demonstrated that serum cholesterol is significantly lower in colon patients than in controls, in contrast to the findings in patients with coronary artery disease, despite the epidemiologic correlations between the two diseases and between them and dietary fat intake (49, 50). Ederer et al (50) compared findings from four separate trials of feeding serum cholesterol-lowering diets conducted in different countries to those of Pearce and Dayton (38). Findings from only one of these studies agreed with Pearce and Dayton's findings of increased cancer incidence and mortality; the remaining three had opposite results. The result of the statistical analysis of the combined data, however, led the investigators (50) to conclude that blood cholesterol-lowering diets do not influence cancer risk.

"*Protein.* Protein, although important in the development of tissues and organs, does not appear to play a significant role in tumor formation and growth (12). Tannenbaum (10) discussed two approaches employed in studies on protein supply in relation to tumor formation. The first utilizes diets in which the amount of protein is varied within proportions that support optimal growth and longevity. The second examines the effect of protein deficiency, in which case the results may be complicated by the effects of altered caloric intake and body weight. This latter approach embraces studies utilizing diets containing inadequate amounts of specific amino acids, particularly sulfur-containing amino acids. For example, induction of leukemia in DBA mice was reported to be inhibited by low dietary cystine (10, 12). Omission of some, but not all, of the essential amino acids from the diets of rats with Walker 256 transplant and of sarcoma-180 bearing mice inhibited tumor growth (13). The tumor-suppressing action of certain amino acid deficiencies may be explained by the different effects on humoral and cellular immunity (51-54). The role of immunity in cancer development is disputed, but cell-mediated immunity may be a means of defense against cancer. Conversely, antibody formation may enhance tumor development by protecting the tumor from cell-mediated immune responses (53). Several studies indicate that deficiencies of certain amino acids or protein restriction can depress antibody production while at the same time, keep cell-mediated immunity intact (51-54). The effects of caloric restriction have been reported to be modified by dietary protein level. In the male rat, both caloric restriction and marginal protein deficiency resulted in an increase in prevalence of other endocrine gland tumors (55). Severe protein deficiency can alter tumor incidence or site, perhaps by altering carcinogen metabolism (55).

"Berg et al (56) cited epidemiological data from 28 countries during 1947-1948 and 1962-1963 that showed significant positive correlations between standardized mortality rates for intestinal cancer and national levels of the intake of animal protein. They also noted a faster rise in mortality from intestinal cancer in 23 countries having the more rapid increases in intake of animal protein over a period of 8-12 years. It is, however, quite difficult to separate the effect of fats since many food items are sources of both animal protein and fat. A significant case-control study implicating various types of meat, particularly beef, involved Japanese migrants to Hawaii. Haenszel et al (57) reported that the increase in beef consumption paralleled the higher risk of large bowel cancer among these Japanese migrants. They added that no example exists of a population with a high beef consumption and a low rate of bowel cancer. From an analysis of international food consumption patterns and from surveys of food consumption in the United States, Howell (21) presented data that supported the findings of the above-mentioned case study. However, Wynder and Reddy (58) feel the need to determine whether the relationship of beef to colon cancer is real, and whether beef contains carcinogenic components as such or increases the incidence of colon cancer by contributing significantly to the overall fat intake of a population.

"*Vitamins.* Vitamins have differing effects on tumor formation and growth; while certain vitamin deficiencies tend to enhance tumor development, other deficiencies suppress it. Vitamin excesses can also influence tumor development in either direction. Again, it is necessary to take into account nonspecific effects of caloric intake and body weight.

"Vitamin A deficiency has been related to the development of odontomas and salivary gland tumors (13), precancerous lesions of the gastric mucosa (12), and colon tumors in rats under some, but not all, conditions (31, 32). High levels of vitamin A sometimes inhibit the development of certain tumors although an enhancing effect has been reported (59). In hamsters, vitamin A excess has been reported both to depress and to enhance growth of respiratory tract tumors (60) and to depress gastric tumor growth (61). The mode of action of vitamin A is not understood; it has been shown that its protective effect against carcinogenesis may be partly due to its inhibition of enzymes that convert certain chemicals to their carcinogenic form (62). Also, vitamin A compounds may stimulate the immune system to be more effective in countering malignancy (62). Vitamin A controls epithelial differentiation in many tissues through unknown mechanisms which may influence carcinogenesis (63).

"Riboflavin deficiency has been shown to retard the growth of certain spontaneous and transplanted tumors (64, 65). The mechanism underlying the anti-tumor effect of riboflavin deficiency is not known. One explanation might be the starvation of the rapidly multiplying tumor of the flavin coenzymes that are vital for metabolism (64).

"Other B-vitamins (folic acid, vitamin B_{12}, and choline) in conjunction with the amino acid methionine, a group of nutrients termed lipotropic agents, influence tumor induction in rats. Deficiency of these nutrients is associated with enhanced induction of tumors in the liver, colon, and esophagus by several different chemicals (66). This deficiency in rats is an experimental model for human alcoholic cirrhosis, a disease associated with increased cancer of the liver and esophagus. Excessive levels of vitamin B_{12} in the diet enhanced markedly the carcinogenic effect of paradimethylaminoazobenzene in rats fed a methionine-deficient diet (67).

"The possible protective effect of ascorbic acid against cancer has been suggested. Clayson (9) has reported that ascorbic acid reduces sodium nitrite to nitrogen oxides. It thus inhibits the nitrosation of secondary and tertiary amines, amides, and ureas to form potentially carcinogenic nitrosamines and nitrosamides. Cameron and Pauling (68) have postulated, but not presented evidence, that high levels of ascorbic acid might prevent cancer by maintaining the hyaluronidase inhibitor, believed by some to control cell proliferation, at an adequate level.

"*Minerals.* Inorganic minerals such as arsenic, beryllium,

chromium, radium, lead, nickel, and cadmium have been implicated in tumor development and increased cancer mortality (10, 12, 69, 70). Fortunately these are not normally consumed in large amounts. There are conflicting reports on the influence of sodium, potassium, calcium, magnesium (10), and selenium (71, 72) on carcinogenesis. Deficiencies of certain minerals have been associated with an increased incidence of tumors (13, 16). For example, a diet low in iodine has been related to increased incidence of thyroid cancer in man (16), and thyroid tumors and pituitary enlargement in rats (13). Magnesium deficiency in rats has been associated with thymus cancer (13).

"*Fiber.* Fiber is another dietary component which in recent years has received wide attention from the scientific community for its role in the etiology of cancer of the large bowel (colon plus rectum). Colonrectal cancer is a major cause of cancer death, second only to lung cancer in the United States (73, 74). The geographical variations in the occurrence of colonrectal cancer have been explained epidemiologically by some investigators through differences in the diet (21, 56). Burkitt (75) noted a lower incidence of colon cancer among Ugandans and concluded that this was a result of their higher consumption of unabsorbable fiber compared to that consumed by Western man. Walker (76) pointed out an epidemiological relationship between fiber intake and the incidence of large bowel cancer. However, to date, definitions and measurement of dietary fiber are still in dispute (77).

"Although the relationship between fiber content and colon cancer is as yet unclear, several mechanisms have been suggested to explain how dietary fiber may reduce the incidence of colon cancer. First, fiber decreases intestinal transit time, thereby reducing the duration of exposure to fecal carcinogens (78-84). Second, fiber influences bile salt metabolism, thereby reducing the formation of potential carcinogens from bile salts (81, 83). Third, fiber may exert a solvent-like effect in that it dilutes potential carcinogens by its bulking effect and ability to bind water, sterols, bile acids, and fat (80, 83, 84). Fourth, fiber may influence the intestinal flora, resulting in decreased bacterial degradation of bile salts (83-86).

"Intestinal Microflora

"It has been postulated that specific intestinal bacteria produce carcinogens from dietary fats or from bile acids. Hill et al (87) reported that fecal flora of individuals consuming a Western diet in high-incidence colon cancer areas (England, Scotland, and United States) contain a higher concentration of anaerobic species such as bacteroides and lower counts of enterococci and other aerobic bacteria than those of individuals in low-incidence colon cancer areas (Uganda, South India, and Japan). The feces of Western people also contained higher concentrations of steroids which were more extensively degraded. The bacterial strains in the feces of Ugandans and Indians had less potential to degrade the bile acid, cholic acid, to deoxycholic acid, which has been suggested as a possible carcinogen or co-carcinogen.

"Similar findings were reported by Reddy and Wynder (88) in their study of the fecal microflora of Americans consuming a mixed Western diet and of American vegetarians, Seventh-Day Adventists, Japanese, and Chinese. They also observed increased levels of microbial beta-glucuronidase activity in the feces of Americans on a Western diet. Glucuronidase activity is a measure of the degree of microbial capacity for the enzymatic hydrolysis of various complex conjugates in the large bowel.

Hill (89) has suggested that bacteria, particularly certain clostridia, metabolize bile acids to produce unsaturated products which act as carcinogens or co-carcinogens. He added that diet determines the fecal bile acid concentration and the intestinal bacterial flora and, consequently, the amount of carcinogen or co-carcinogen produced. In support of this hypothesis, he cited the effects of various dietary regimens including those high and low in fiber, meat, and fat.

"Cultured dairy foods, largely lactobacilli-fermented types, have been known to contain anti-tumor components (91). Reddy et al (90) reported a substantial inhibitory effect of yogurt (milk fermented with *Lactobacillus bulgaricus* and *Streptococcus thermophilus*) on the proliferation of Erlich ascites tumor transplants in mice. More work relative to the nature and mode of action of the active compound in yogurt is needed.

"Thus, alterations in the bacterial composition can be reflected in the metabolic potential of the intestinal microflora. The effects of dietary regulation of bacterial composition and bacterial metabolic activity may have relevance to colon carcinogenesis. Further studies to identify critical enzyme systems in the intestinal flora of human subjects to explain metabolic pathways are warranted (91).

"Much needs to be done in order to elucidate the role of nutrition and diet in carcinogenesis (92). The many areas to be studied include 1) the impact of diet on hormonal balance, on digestive secretions, on hepatic, enteric and other tissue metabolism of carcinogens, and on the composition of and the substrates available to the enteric flora; 2) interaction between diet and carcinogenic stimuli that may affect cellular and genetic stability, differentiation, metabolism, the immune cellular and genetic stability, differentiation, metabolism, the immune status, and undoubtedly many other factors; and 3) nutritional status of population groups which can be related to cancer incidence. Detailed cancer statistics are available for counties and economic divisions of the United States which show marked variations for some cancers and some areas (93). Such epidemiological data, when validated with control studies, may be useful in programs designed to prevent cancer."

ACKNOWLEDGMENTS

The National Dairy Council would like to acknowledge the help and suggestions of the following reviewers in its preparation: D. B. Clayson, Deputy Director, The Eppley Institute for Research in Cancer, University of Nebraska Medical Center, Omaha, Nebraska; S. L. Gorbach, M.D., Infectious Disease Section, Tufts - New England Medical Center, Boston, Massachusetts; J. T. Kalberer, Ph.D., Associate Director for Program Planning, Division of Cancer Research Resources and Centers, National Cancer Institute, Bethesda, Maryland; and A. F. Rogers, M.D., Senior Research Scientist, Department of Nutrition and Food Science, Massachusetts Institute of Technology, Cambridge, Massachusetts.

References

1. Willis, R. A., *Pathology of Tumors,* 3rd edition London: Butterworth Co., 1960
2. Gasner, D. Fam. Health 7:27, 1975
3. Ackerman, L. V. Nutr. Today 7:2 (Jan.-Feb.) 1972
4. Anon. *Lancet* 2:1133, 1973
5. Campbell, H. Proc. R. Soc. Med. 65:641, 1972
6. Drasar, B. S., and M. J. Hill. Am. J. Clin. Nutr. 25:1399, 1972
7. Asvall, J. E., A. V. Chaklin, R. A. Melnikov, and H. P. Rhomberg, Neoplasma 21:131, 1974
8. Barrett, V. K. Dietary Factors in the Etiology of Cancer, National Cancer Institute Report No. 18, March 1975
9. Clayson, D. B. Nutrition and Experimental Carcinogenesis: A Review Paper presented at the Conference on "Nutrition in the Causation of Cancer," Key Biscayne, Florida, May 1975
10. Tannenbaum, A. Nutrition and Cancer, *Physiopathology of Cancer,* 2nd Edition, F. Homburger (Ed.), New York; Hoeber-Harper, 1959, pp. 517-562
11. Comings, D. E. Proc. Natl. Acad. Sci. 70:3324, 1973
12. Kraybill, H. F. Clin. Pharmacol, Therapeutics 4:73, 1963
13. Shils, M. E. Nutrition and Neoplasia. In: *Modern Nutrition in Health and Disease,* R. S. Goodhart and M. R. Shils (Ed.), Philadelphia; Lea & Febiger, 1973
14. Ross, M. H. and G. Bras. J. Natl. Cancer Inst. 47:1095, 1971
15. Goldstein, S. New Engl. J. Med. 285:1120, 1971
16. Wynder, E. L., and K. Mabuchi, Prev. Med. I:300, 1972
17. de Waard, F. Breast Cancer Incidence and Nutritional Status with Particular Reference to Body Weight and Height. Paper presented at the Conference on "Nutrition in the Causation of Cancer," Key Biscayne, Florida, May 1975
18. Lea, A. J. *Lancet* 2:332, 1966
19. Carroll, K. K., E. B. Gammal, and E. R. Plunkett, Can. Med. Assoc. J. 98: 590, 1968
20. Wynder, E. L., T. Kajitani, S. Ishikawa, H. Dodo, and A. Takano, Cancer 23:1210, 1969
21. Howell, M. A. J. Chron. Dis. 28:67, 1975
22. Anon. Br. Med. J. 1:309, 1974
23. Clayson, D. B. Personal communication
24. Carroll, K. K. and H. T. Khor, Cancer Res. 30:2260, 1970
25. Carroll, K. K. and H. T. Khor, Lipids 6:415, 1971

26. Gammal, E. B., K. K. Carroll, and E. R. Plunkett, Cancer Res. 27:1737, 1967
27. Boutwell, R. K., M. K. Brush, and H. P. Rusch, Cancer Res. 9:741, 1949
28. Tannenbaum, A. Cancer Res. 2:468, 1942
29. Harman, D. Int. Cong. Gerontol. 5:259, 1966
30. Harman, D. J. Gerontol, 26:451, 1971
31. Rogers, A. E. and P. M. Newberne, Dietary Effects in Chemical Carcinogenesis in Animal Models for Colon and Liver Tumors. Paper presented at the Conference on "Nutrition in the Causation of Cancer," Key Biscayne, Florida, May 1975
32. Weisburger, J. Dietary Factors and Cancer of the Large Bowel. Paper presented at the Conference on "Nutrition in the Causation of Cancer," Key Biscayne, Florida, May 1975
33. Miller, J. A., B. E. Kline, H. P. Rusch, and C. A. Baumann. Cancer Res. 4:153, 1944
34. Gammal, E. B., K. K. Carroll, and E. R. Plunkett. Cancer Res. 28:384, 1968
35. Kaunitz, H., and R. E. Johnson. J. Japan Oil Chem. Soc. 22:411, 1973
36. Rose, G., H. Blackburn, A. Keys, H. L. Taylor, W. B. Kannel, O. Paul, D. D. Reid, and J. Stamler. *Lancet* 1:181, 1974
37. Mertin, J. Br. Med. J. 4:357, 1973
38. Pearce, M. L., and S. Dayton. *Lancet* 1:464, 1971
39. Singman, H. S., M. Archer, and L. Bergner. Mt. Sinai J. Med. N.Y. 40:677, 1973
40. Miettinen, M., O. Turpeinen, M. J. Karvonen, R. Elusuo, and E. Paavilainen. *Lancet* 2:835, 1972
41. Malmros, H. Bibl. Nutr. Dieta. 19:108, 1973
42. The Committee on Diet and Heart Disease, National Heart Foundation of Australia, Med. J. Aust. 1:663, 1974
43. Bortz, W. M. Metabol. 22:1507, 1973
44. Siperstein, M. D. Trans. Am. Clin. Climatol. Assoc. 83:156, 1972
45. Addleman, W. New Engl. J. Med. 287:1047, 1972
46. Westlund, K., and R. Nicolaysen, Scand. J. Clin. Lab. Invest. 30 Suppl. 127:1, 1972
47. Deutscher, S. J. Natl. Cancer Inst. 46:217, 1971
48. Nydegger, U. E., and R. E. Butler. Cancer Res. 32:1756, 1972
49. Bjelke, E. *Lancet* 1:1116, 1974
50. Ederer, F., P. Leren, O. Turpeinen, and I. D. Frantz. *Lancet* 2:203, 1971

51. Anon. *Lancet* 1:303, 1973
52. Good, R. A. Proc. Natl. Acad. Sci. 69:1026, 1972
53. Worthington, B. S. J. Am. Diet. Assoc. 65:123, 1974
54. Ross, M. H. and G. Bras, J. Nutr. 103:944, 1973
55. McLean, A. E. M., and P. N. Magee. Br. J. Exp. Path. 51:587, 1970
56. Berg, J. W., M. A. Howell, and S. J. Silverman. Health Serv. Rep. 88:915, 1973
57. Haenszel, W., J. W. Berg, M. Sezi, M. Kurihara, and P. B. Sock, J. Natl. Cancer Inst. 51:1765, 1973
58. Wynder, E. L., and B. S. Reddy. J. Natl. Cancer Inst. 54:7, 1975
59. Smith, D. M., A. E. Rogers, B. J. Herndon, and P. M. Newberne. Cancer Res. 35:11, 1975
60. Smith, D. M., A. E. Rogers, and P. M. Newberne. Cancer Res. 35:1485, 1975
61. Chu, E. W., and R. A. Malmgren. Cancer Res. 25:884, 1965
62. Maugh, T. H. Science 186:1198, 1974
63. Cohen, B. F., and I. K. Cohen. J. Immunol. 111:1376, 1973
64. Anon. Nutr. Rev. 32:308, 1974
65. Rivlin, R. S. Cancer Res. 33:1977, 1973
66. Rogers, A. E. Cancer Res. 35:2469, 1975
67. Day, P. L., L. D. Payne, and J. S. Dinning. Proc. Soc. Exp. Biol. Med. 74:854, 1950
68. Cameron, E. and L. Pauling. Oncol. 27:181, 1973
69. Woolrich, P. F. Am. Ind. Hyg. Assoc. J. 34:217, 1973
70. Berg, J. W. and F. Burbank. Ann. N.Y. Acad. Sci. 199:249, 1972
71. Shapiro, J. R. Ann. N.Y. Acad. Sci. 192:215, 1972
72. Anon. Food Cosmet. Toxicol. 10:867, 1972
73. Silverberg, F., and A. Holleb. Cancer 23:2, 1973
74. National Cancer Institute. *National Cancer Institute: Factbook.* DHEW Publ. No. (NIH) 73:512, 1973
75. Walker, A. R. S. Afr. Med. J. 46:1127, 1972
76. Burkitt, D. P. Cancer 28:3, 1971
77. Eastwood, M. A., N. Fisher, C. T. Greenwood, and J. H. Hutchinson. *Lancet* 1:1029, 1974
78. Spiller, G. A., and R. J. Amen. Food Prod. Dev. 8:30, 1974
79. Southgate, D. A. T. Plant Food for Man 6:45, 1973
80. Scala, J. Food Technol. 28:34, 1974
81. Anon. Nutr. Rev. 31:110, 1973
82. Harvey, R. F., E. W. Pomare, and K. W. Heaton. *Lancet* 1:1278, 1973
83. Sherman, W. C. Food Nutr. News 45:3, 1974

84. Anon. Food Process. 36:24, 1975
85. Burkitt, D. P. *Lancet* 2:1229, 1969
86. Burkitt, D. P. J. Natl. Cancer Inst. 47:913, 1971
87. Hill, M. J., B. S. Drasar, V. Aries, J. S. Crowther, G. Hawksworth, and R. E. O. Williams. *Lancet* 1:95, 1971
88. Reddy, B. S., and E. L. Wynder, J. Natl. Cancer Inst. 50:1437, 1973
89. Hill, M. J. Metabolic Epidemiology of Dietary Factors in Large Bowel Cancer. Paper presented at the Conference on "Nutrition in the Causation of Cancer," Key Biscayne, Florida, May, 1975
90. Reddy, G. V., K. M. Shahani, and M. R. Banerjee. J. Natl. Cancer Inst. 50:815, 1973
91. Gorbach, S. L. Personal communication
92. Gori, G. B. The Diet, Nutrition and Cancer Program of the National Cancer Institute – National Cancer Program. Paper presented to the National Cancer Advisory Board, July 16, 1975
93. Mason, T. J., and F. W. McKay. Atlas of Cancer Mortality for U.S. Counties. 1950-1969. DHEW Publ. No. (NIH) 75-780

APPENDIX 7

WHICH ANIMALS HAVE CANCER?

The following appeared in the August, 1973 edition of *Dr. Shelton's Hygienic Review:*

"Over forty years ago, Dr. John Round, D.Sc., in an article on *Flesh Eating and Cancer,* wrote: 'According to Rayer, cancer is common among birds of prey and extremely rare in those that are non-carnivorous. Eagles and vultures in captivity often die of cancer. The common barnyard owl is particularly subject to cancer. One of the most horrifying discoveries made in recent years is the prevalence of cancer among fishes . . . Cancer in fish is most prevalent among those raised in captivity as in the so-called fish hatcheries . . . Cancer has been found in reptiles — the salamander, the frog and the python.

" 'On the other hand, of all domestic animals the horse seems to be the one of the least liable to cancer. Next to the horse, cancer is most infrequent in cattle. Cancer is rare in sheep and very rare in goats. In rabbits it is so rare that we do not know of a single case. *Per contra,* again there is much cancer among such scavengers as rats and mice. It is more common in those that have been fed on animal food. Wild animals kept in captivity sometimes get cancer. Cancer also occurs with alarming frequency in the cat. Of all animals studied, however, with the exception of the mice, the dog is most subject to cancer.

" 'Semner found 8 percent of cancerous dogs in 3,525 animals examined. All the principal types and varieties of cancer found in human beings have been found also in dogs. Now, the dog is a carnivorous animal, and the domestic dog is often given too much meat, in addition to which he is apt to consume a good deal of very inferior meat and scraps, which he loves to find in dirt heaps.

" 'On the immune side again, the monkey appears to be, of all the animals examined, the least liable to cancer. In fact tumors of all sorts are extremely rare among the monkey tribe. Monkeys prefer a diet of nuts, and their almost entire immunity from cancer is a highly important fact.

" 'Turning to ourselves, we find that cancer is common in proportion to the amount of flesh we consume. This may not [always] be true of individuals, but it is certainly true of nations and tribes.'

"Discussing cancers found in plants, he says: 'Cancers, of sorts, are found in some trees. It is most interesting to notice that these vegetable cancers are common in trees that grow in soils that are saturated with sewage, in other words, in trees that are over-nourished with nitrogenous material. Sugar beet that is over-nourished is apt to develop a disease known as "crown-gall," a form of plant cancer. Crown-galls on sugar beets have a horrible resemblance to cancers as seen in animals, not omitting human cancers.' He quotes Professor E. F. Smith, of the Laboratory of Plant Pathology, Washinton, D.C., who says 'Plant cancer is most likely to occur in plants which are over-fed . . . Like human cancer it is almost certain to reappear when removed. Plant cancer, in time, destroys the plant on which it grows.'

"Over-feeding and excess nitrogen, particularly of inappropriate nitrogenous material, are thus seen to be antecedents of cancerous development. My good friends of the 'organic gardening' persuasion should learn a valuable lesson from the foregoing facts about cancers in plants and should realize that over-composting, particularly with rich nitrogenous materials, provides a very poor food for man or animal. Flesh-eaters should see in the greater prevalence of cancer in flesh-eating animals, even in the wild state and its relative absence, even in domestication, from vegetarian and fruitarian animals, an indication of the unfitness of animal proteins for human nutrition.

"Aluminum cooking vessels, tarred roads, aniline dyes, boracic and salicylic acids, radium burns, and other 'causes of cancer' that are so much discussed today, are not primary causes of cancer. Ancient peoples who suffered with cancer did not have tarred roads and aluminum cooking vessels. They did not suffer with x-ray and radium burns. These things are not the causes of cancer in the fish of the sea, nor in the eagle and the owl on the wing. We need a common factor to account for cancer in man, animals and plants, and to account for its frequent failure to develop in the presence of these much talked of 'causes of cancer' to get the headlines. An impaired metabolism consequent upon bad feeding habits, a state of systemic poisoning, growing out of surfeit and improper fare, supply the universal substratum upon which rest the development of tumors and cancers."

APPENDIX 8

CHEMICAL PROTECTION AGAINST AGING

The following are excerpts from *Chemical Protection Against Aging,* by Denham Harman, Professor of Biochemistry and Medicine, University of Nebraska College of Medicine, Omaha, Nebraska 68105:

"Aging, an individually unwanted biological phenomenon — at least to man — would seem to play a useful role and possibly a necessary one, in the evolutionary process by aiding to remove old organisms after they have provided new 'experiments' for evaluation against the environment. Probably because of the importance of the death of individual organisms to evolution, the basic aging process(es) built into each species has been protected from extraneous influences in such a manner as to insure that all will be dead by some age appropriate to the species.

"Degradative changes in an organism leading ultimately to death may be regarded as being due to the basic aging process(es) on which disease states are superimposed and intertwined. From this viewpoint disease serves merely to hasten the death made inevitable by the basic aging process(es). The life span then of any given organism, in the absence of non-age associated accidential death — and collectively, the mean life span — is determined by the combined deleterious effects of the basic aging process(es) and disease states while the maximum life span of the species is the value observed when these effects are minimized.

"Efforts to decrease degradative changes in man, largely through improved medical care, nutrition, and public health facilities, have resulted in significant increases in mean life span but not of maximum life span. Thus, in the United States the life expectancy at birth increased from about 45 years in 1900 to 70 years by the mid-1950's while the maximum life span remained unchanged at around 100 years.

"In terms of mean life expectancy, the most that can be achieved by further disease-oriented biomedical research is about 15 years. For example, the current mean life expectancy in the developed countries – 70 years – would be increased by about 10 years if cardiovascular diseases were eliminated as causes of death while the corresponding figure for cancer would be about 2.5 years (1, 2). The 15 years' difference between the potential mean life span of around 85 years and the maximum life span of about 100 years arises from non-age associated accidental deaths and individual variability in life span in the absence of overt disease.

"Considering that the mean life span in the United States has remained essentially constant at around 70 years since the mid-1950's, the rate of increase in mean life span in the future is likely to be low unless new approaches can be found to inhibit the rate of biological degradation in man. One promising approach to the problem of increasing the useful, healthy life span of man is based on the possibility that degradative changes – both from aging and disease processes – may be due in part to free radical reactions (3, 4), reactions that are ubiquitous in living systems (5). This approach offers the prospect of an increase in the mean life span to beyond 85 years as well as the possibility that a significant number of people will live to well beyond 100 years.

"Free radical reactions gain their name from the transient presence during the course of the reactions of highly reactive intermediates known as free radicals (6, 7); a free radical is an atom or a group with an unpaired electron. Free radical reactions are commonplace: (1) reaction of oxygen with gasoline, as in an automobile engine, (2) smog formation, (3) drying of linseed oil paints, (4) formation of many of our commonly used plastics, (5) development of rancidity in butter. Because of the high chemical reactivity of the intermediates (due to the unpaired electron), free radical reactions give rise — generally — to a variety of products. In addition, free radical reactions are almost invariably irreversible; for example, it is not possible by any simple process to take the CO_2 and water coming from an automobile exhaust and get back the original gasoline and oxygen. . .

"The rate of free radical reactions involving molecular oxygen is enhanced by catalysts such as copper, iron and manganese (6), which increase the rate of formation of new radicals, and inhibited by antioxidants, which increase the rate of removal of free radicals.

"By a properly selected natural diet is meant one that provides essential nutrients but with a minimum intake of substances such as copper and polyunsaturated fats that might be expected to significantly increase more-or-less random-free radical reactions.

"If a search for suitable inhibitors of the basic aging process(es) is successful, assuming that free radical reactions are involved, then an increase in mean life span to beyond 85 years may be achieved along with a significant increase in the maximum life span to well over 100 years.

"Summary

"Aging, an individually unwanted biological phenomenon, is important to evolution. Changes in an organism, such as man, leading ultimately to death, can be looked upon as being due to a basic aging process(es), 'built-in' by evolution to insure death — and largely determining the maximum life span, on which disease states are superimposed and intertwined. These degradative changes — both from aging and disease processes — may be due in part to free radical reactions. Experiments based on the above hypothesis have been encouraging. . .

"It is suggested that the addition of one or more free radical reaction inhibitors to nutritionally adequate and acceptable natural diets, selected to minimize the intake of substances (such as polyunsaturated fats and copper) that might reasonably be expected to significantly increase more-or-less random in vivo free radical reactions, may increase the average age at death of man by five or more years with accompanying increases in the years of useful, healthy life.

"References

"(1) B. Woodhall and S. Jobolon, *Prospects for Further Increases in Average Longevity,* Geriatrics 12, 586-591 (1957).

"(2) R. R. Kohn, *Human Aging and Disease,* J. Chron. Dis. 16, 5-21 (1963)

"(3) D. Harman, *Aging: A Theory Based on Free Radical and Radiation Chemistry,* J. Geront. 11, 298-300 (1956)

"(4) D. Harman, *Role of Free Radicals in Mutation, Cancer, Aging and the Maintenance of Life,* Radiation Res. 16, 753-763 (1962)

"(5) I. Isenberg, *Free Radicals in Tissue,* Physiol. Rev. 44, 487-517 (1964)

"(6) W. A. Pryor, *Free Radicals,* (McGraw-Hill, Inc., New York 1966)

"(7) C. Walling, *Free Radicals in Solution,* (John Wiley & Sons Inc., New York 1957).

APPENDIX 9

DIATHELIC IMMUNIZATION

The Veterans Administration Work Experiment with Development of Cancer Immunity Through Injection of Cancer Cells into Udder of Cows at Roberts Bomb Shelter for Cows at Elkhorn, Nebraska

by Richard E. Ogborn, M.D.

"Current Progress to 2/16/66

"Objective

"We have produced, we believe, active antibodies by diathelic immunization utilizing the cow as the antibody producing animal and the C3HBA mouse tumor as the antigen. The presence of antibodies have been shown in agar immunodiffusion precipitan tests and in neutralization tests. When lactoglobulin from the sensitized cow is used, tumor takes are fewer and delayed. The animals so treated survive longer.

"Methodology

"The neutralization tests used lactoglobulin from the sensitized (immune) cow No. 331, that of the control (non-immune) cow No. 208, no lactoglobulin (incubated controls), and no incubation (direct controls). Comparisons were made of number of tumor takes, time of tumor take, and time of death.

"The oncogenic material used is tumor cell suspension made by homogenizing tumors in Ten Broeck homogenizers with physiological phosphate buffered saline, containing antibiotics. The tumor cell suspensions have been sterile. Some of the lactoglobulin samples have had bacteria. The cows have remained free of detectable bacterial and viral infections as shown by tests of the milk and blood.

"Technic

"I. The tumor cell suspension was prepared and used as planned. The instillation was done for five weeks. The experimental cow became severely debilitated so that instillations were halted for a while and then later resumed. Twenty-four instillations have been done to date (February 15, 1966). Histopathology has not as yet been done.

"II. The milking data point out:

"There is not a significant difference in the greater amount of cream given by the experimental cow No. 331.

"Neither cow has gotten a bacterial or viral infection since the start of the experiment.

"Cow No. 331 comes into heat frequently, but has not been able to conceive by artificial insemination, whereas cow No. 208 has not come into heat lately.

"Although neither of the cows had many white blood cells in their milk prior to instillation, cow No. 331 exhibited clumps of them once instillations started and sympathetically cow No. 208 exhibited considerably more after instillations had begun on cow No. 331.

"The cows are kept in adjacent stalls in the bomb shelter.

"There is no significant difference in the amounts of milk from the two cows. The total amount of milk and percent butter fat is about the same as is expected of similar cows in the outside.

"The lactoglobulin recovery from cow No. 331 milk is generally greater than that from cow No. 208 milk.

"Cytotoxic (Neutralization)

"Neutralization is an *in vitro* testing procedure. The oncogenic material is intermixed with the material to be tested (immune lactoglobulin) and incubated (37°C.) for a given period (4 hours). To test if the oncogenic material has been 'neutralized,' the mixture is injected into mice. The results of these neutralization tests are shown in the graphs where the effects of the immune lactoglobulin is compared with that of non-immune lactoglobulin, no lactoglobulin during incubation and no incubation.

"Neutralization experiments have been the only cylotoxic tests done to date.

"Chemistry

"The crude lactoglobulin has been recovered as planned. The material is not amenable to electrophoresis* (paper, gel, or liquid) as is. By taking the lactoglobulin slurry prior to lyophilizing,** centrifuging and passing it through a millipore filter, it becomes more amenable to gel electrophoresis and more active in agar immunodiffusion plates.

"Disc electrophoresis has shown that there are two major areas of interest in lactoserum (whey). One, the globulin area, comprises about twenty per cent of the proteins found, and this ratio does not vary appreciably from sample to sample. The second area is generally considered to be the albumin area; however, in lactoserum, the beta lactoglobulin fraction appears in this area. This area is consistently about forty (40) per cent of the sample.

"The relative composition ratio does not vary from the control to the experimental animal. However, there is an easily detectable difference in the concentrations. From these data, identification of the next fraction(s) responsible for the production and/or transportation of the antibodies cannot be made. Methods for separating these fractions for testing individually have thus been initiated. Fractions in samples obtained from the experimental animal are approximately thirty-three (33) per cent more concentrated than the corresponding fractions obtained from the control animal.

"**Immunology**

"In addition to diathelic immunization, immune antibodies were produced in rabbits by standard procedures to the C3HBA tumor, the Freund virus and normal tissues in both cases. The antibodies to the C3HBA tumor have been demonstrated by agar immunodiffusion plates. Using Hyland plates specific for antigen A, M, and G gamma globulin, the tumor cell suspension has shown similarities with both A and M gamma globulin. Attempts to show antigen-antibody reaction by other methods such as agglutination or precipitation have been unsuccessful.

"A chromatographic separation of the antigen from the tumor cell suspension has been accomplished."

*Electrical shaking **Freeze-drying

(Author's Note: From the foregoing it would seem that Nature intended milk at least to serve as a potential anticancer agent. Obviously, this calls for further experiment.)

Diathelic Immunization

Project Leader R. E. Ogborn, M.D.

"History and Significance

"The number of scientific papers in the field of tumor virus attests to the possibility of tumor control by regulation or inhibition of viral agents. (1, 2, 3, 4) Lactoserum has been shown to provide other animals with passive protection against such bacteria as Salmonella pullorum (5). Thomas and Leclerc (6, 7, 8) produced diathelic immunity in cows by injecting first a suspension of inactivated foot-and-mouth virus (highly virulent O strain) and then subsequently the live virus.

The lactoserum protected guinea pigs against the fully virulent virus. In the same way, injection of large quantities of unconcentrated lactoserum into heifers protected them against a 10^4 ID 50 (median infective dose).

"Finally, they used the lactoglobulin and by intravenous injection protected fully exposed cattle from the viral disease. In 1960 Sekla and Holeckova (9) immunized ewes by the diathelic method against rat cancer. Rats were implanted with equal number of Walker 256 tumor cells which had been incubated with normal and immune milk. Controls (no incubation of cells) had a 70% take of tumors. Rats implanted with cells incubated in normal milk had an 85% take and rats implanted with cells incubated in 'immune milk' had a 45% take of the transplants. Other tests revealed prevention of significant takes of implanted tumor by using milk serum I.P. They also showed the cytotoxic effect of immune milk serum by cell count pre- and post-incubation of freshly prepared tumor cells in immune milk serum. They surmised that 'any system capable of immune reaction is able to produce antitumor factors passively transmissable, and active in inhibiting tumor growth in susceptible animals.'

"Dr. Edwin E. Osgood has evolved a theory on the concept of cancer growth (10). He portrays an inhibitor from 'n' cells which regulate 'A' or alpha cell division. The quantity of 'n' cells regulates the concentration of the inhibitor factor in a direct proportionality within this system. Xanthine oxidase is an enzyme responsible for the regulation of the final degradations of nucleic acids and is considered a 'rate-limiting step' in nucleic acid degradation, i.e., it controls the catabolism of nucleic acids. (11) Xanthine oxidase is not found in cancer tissue. Cancer resistant mice have a higher level of xanthine oxidase in their mammary tissue.

"A question is raised with the foregoing in mind. Is the inhibitor factor normally present in the healthy (non-malignant bearing) individual an autoimmune (antibody) type of substance produced in a perfect aequilibria state within the host (i.e., plasma cells, etc.). Secondly, can an inhibitor be exogenously supplied by exciting or stimulating the reaction within a secondary producer and the inhibitor be passively used by the initial host to re-establish the equilibrium? Does the excitation increase catabolism regulators such as xanthine oxidase?

"A second and more direct question raised is, 'Can antibodies be produced which will prevent, cure or palliate tumor growths?'

"Objective

"We propose to attempt to produce an antibody (or other substance, i.e., inhibitor factor) by diathelic immunization procedures utilizing the cow as the antibody or inhibitor producing animal and the C3H mammary tumor mouse as the test animal. If a substance is produced which has cytotoxic effect, preventive effect, and/or palliative or curative effect, we propose to apply this technic in humans suffering from incurable malignancy as the experimental subject.

"Methodology

"1. Diathelic immunization will be carried on in Guernsey cows as performed by Sekla and Holeckova in ewes.

"2. Lactoglobulin fractions will be used in

"(a) a cytotoxic experiment with C3H mammary tumor cells.

"(b) a preventive experiment in suckling mice (C3H mammary tumor type)

"(c) a comparative tumor growth experiment will be conducted in C3H mammary tumor mice

"(d) comparison of transplant takes in control animals and those immunized with immune milk products

"(e) comparison of death rate between tumorous animals diathelically immunized and controls "(f) comparison of time of tumor take between animals challenged with oncogenic material treated with lactoglobulin from immunized and non-immunized cows.

"3. If (1) and (2) do not show positive results, try

"(a) absorption, i.e. lactoglobulin from cow instilled with oncogenic material subtracted from lactoglobulin from cow instilled with normal mouse tissue

"(b) instillation with oncogenic material separated by

"(I) gradient centrifugation, open

"(II) electrophoresis

"(III) immuno electrophoresis

" Diathelic Immunization Technic

"I. Sacrifice C3HBA and C3H mammary tumor mice. Isolate tumors with sterile technic. Prepare histopathological slides of a representative section. Prepare cells by sterile homogenization in Ten Broeck. Dilute cells in PBS saline (with antibiotics). Count representative samples in Coulter Counter (VA Annex). Instill 1 x 10^8 into each quarter (Mr. Slatin). Milk every 12 hours. Repeat technic weekly for five weeks.

"II. For two weeks previous to and all milkings following instillation, the following is recorded on all milk samples.

"1. Quantity, volume/milking/day/weight

"2. Butterfat

"3. Bacterial count and culture — (daily-slides; monthly-cultures)

"4. Time of milking 6-7 am - 6-7 PM

"5. Cellular count and differential (polymorphs, mononuc)

"6. Lactoglobulin content possible (salt out and centrifuge)

"7. Milker

"8. Code by number the milking for use in future experiments

"9. Virus culture, etc., on blood sample of cow

"10. Visible difference in cow and milk to milker and recovery chemist

"III. Test with friend virus in Swiss mice."

"Diathelic Immunization*

by Richard E. Ogborn, M.D.

"The production of antibodies against viral and bacterial antigens within the lactating mammary gland of the species has been proved (1). Sekla and Holeckova have suggested and published the results of preliminary experiments which support the theory that antibodies or an 'inhibitor' factor may be produced in a lactating mammary gland of a species using this technic against certain malignant tumors (2).

"For the past sixteen months the VA Hospital research program with major support from Roberts Dairy Company has been pursuing experimental technics in diathelic immunization to try to establish the authenticity of Sekla's et al previous work.

"We have proven that diathelic immunization is practical in a tumor system. We have verified Sekla et al in a different tumor system, i.e., C3H mice, C3HBA tumor and cow.

"In neutralizations, the recovered immune lactoglobulin prevents tumors from appearing in some animals, always delays the appearance of tumors and always allows the animals to live longer.

"In prevention, the recovered lactoglobulin, injected at the time of injection with tumor cell suspension, will at least delay the appearance of tumors and allow the animals to live longer.

"The recovered immune lactoglobulin also exhibits *in*

vitro activity as does serum of immunized rabbits in agar immuno-diffusion plates.

"Continuance of the preventive experiment is underway. Comparative tumor growth and long term preventive experiments await availability of investigators, time, and finances.

"Purification of the 'inhibiting factor' is dependent upon the most modern subtle chemical separatory technics. The scientific manpower is available as is the instrumentation upon suitable financial backing.

"It is known, this technic, i.e., Diathelic Immunization, is a practical source of antibodies against viral and bacterial agents. With the identification of the 'pure' substance in the milk which is the inhibitory or antibody agent, this technic could become an inexpensive, efficient source of infectious disease preventives in animals and humans. This can be developed as an industry within a year following a six-month research period. Either a large pharmaceutical company could be invited to establish a branch in Nebraska and secure the raw material from the Roberts Research Institute or Roberts could supply this to interested sources.

"*Diathelic immunization is the act of inciting antibody production within the mammary gland of a species from the injection of dead or viable antigen material. These antibodies are then transferred to and are collectible in the milk. Antibodies so produced are not effective when given orally to other specie recipients, but efficiently immunize the same or cross species when injected into the organism."

(Author's Note: Dr. Ogborn gave me his material before he died.)

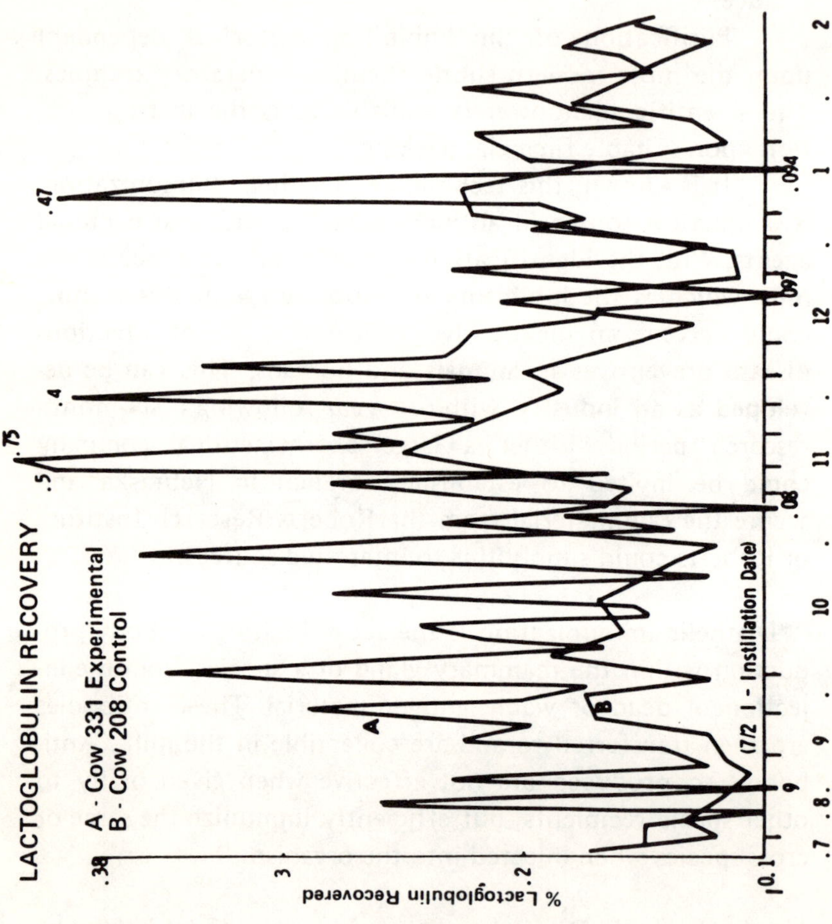
LACTOGLOBULIN RECOVERY
A - Cow 331 Experimental
B - Cow 208 Control
% Lactoglobulin Recovered
(7/2 I - Instillation Date)
.38
3
.2
0.1
.7 .8 9 9 10 11 12 1 2
.47
.4
.75
.5
.08
.097
.094
A
B

NEUTRALIZATION IV

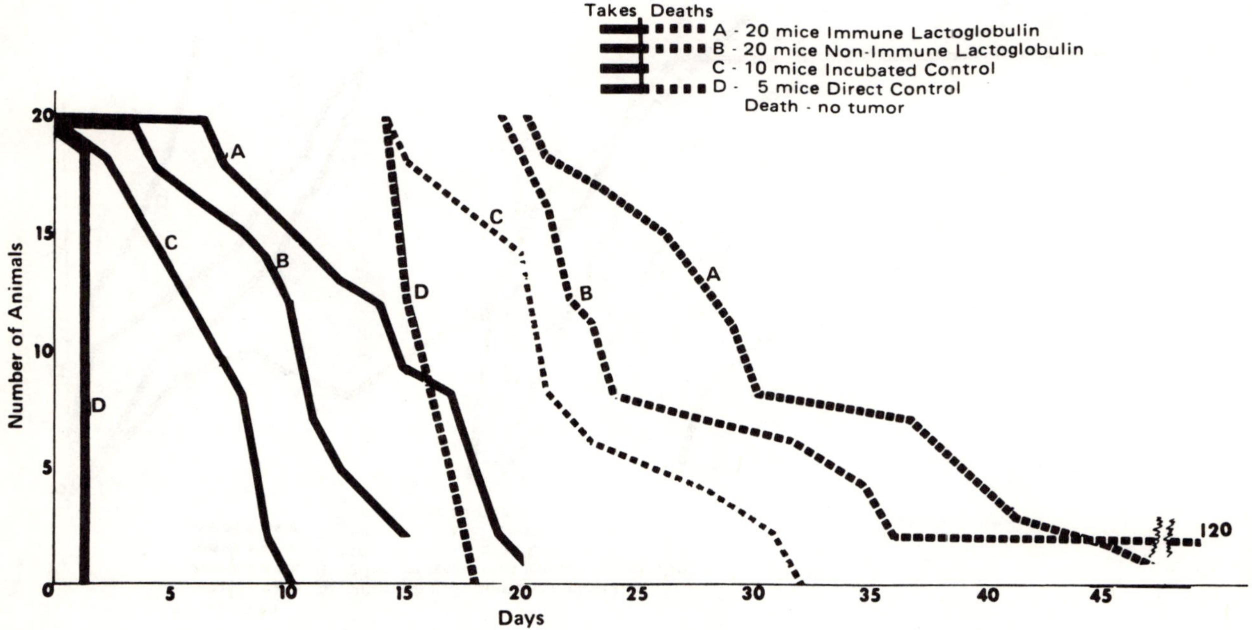

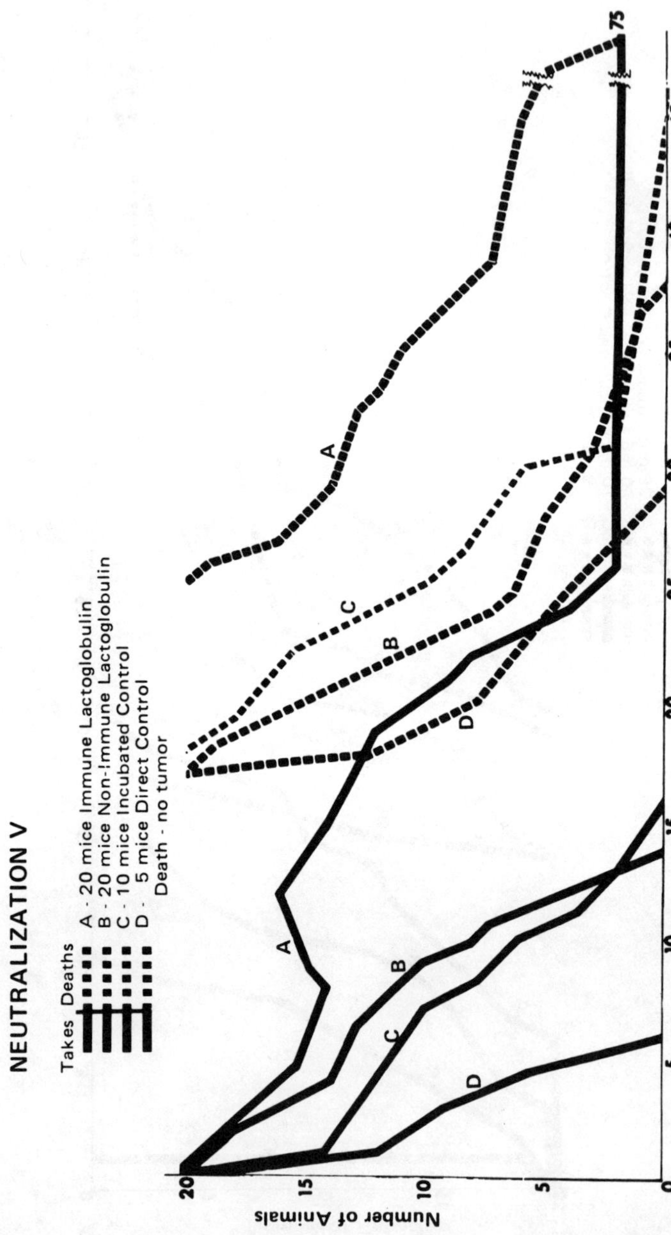
NEUTRALIZATION V
Takes Deaths
A - 20 mice Immune Lactoglobulin
B - 20 mice Non-Immune Lactoglobulin
C - 10 mice Incubated Control
D - 5 mice Direct Control
Death - no tumor
Number of Animals
Days
A
B
C
D
0
5
10
15
20
25
30
35
40
45
75

NEUTRALIZATION VII

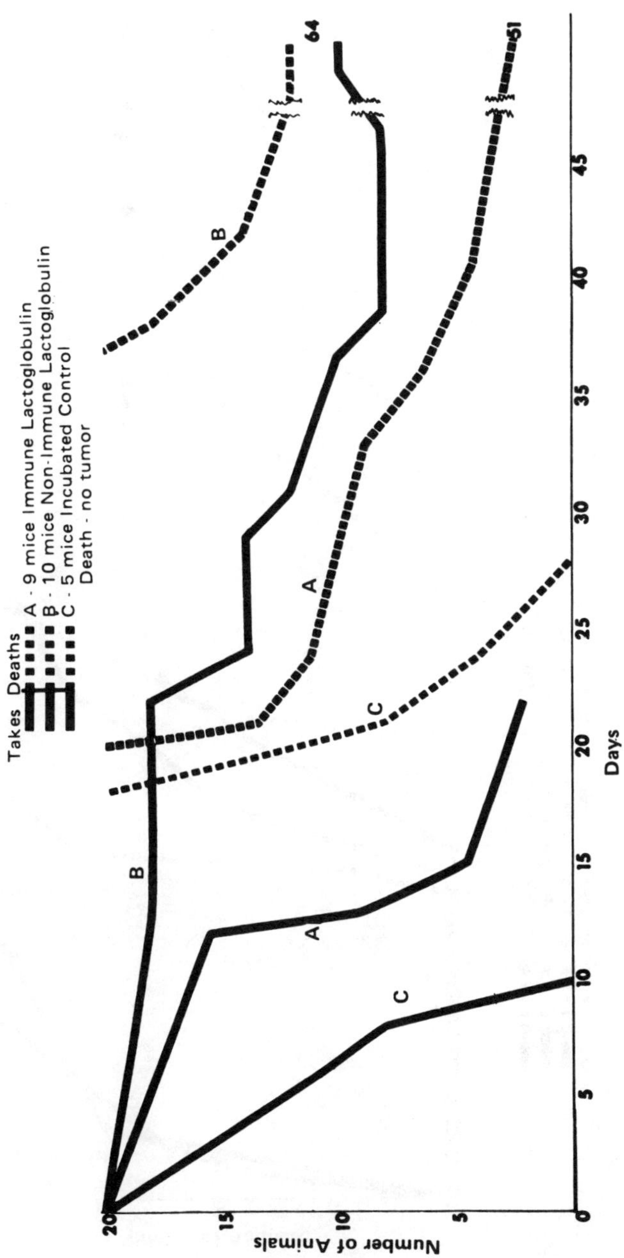

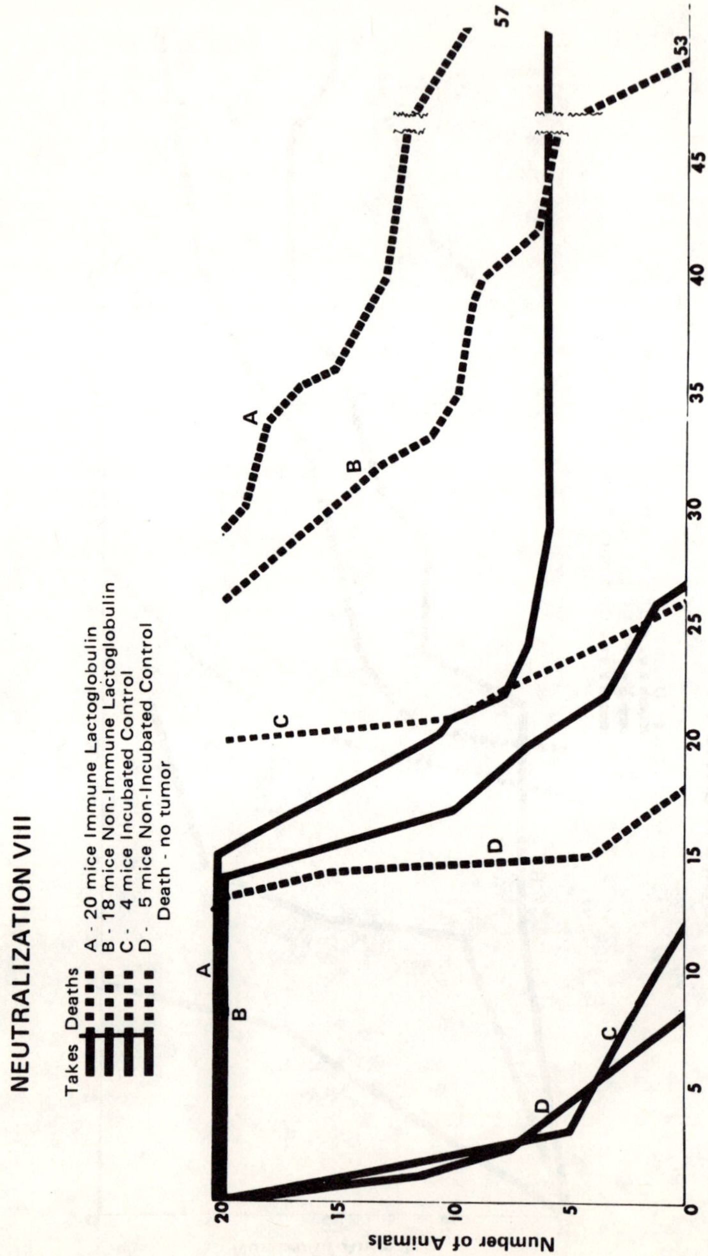
NEUTRALIZATION VIII
Takes Deaths
A - 20 mice Immune Lactoglobulin
B - 18 mice Non-Immune Lactoglobulin
C - 4 mice Incubated Control
D - 5 mice Non-Incubated Control
Death - no tumor
Number of Animals
Days
0
5
10
15
20
25
30
35
40
45
53
57
A
B
C
D

NEUTRALIZATION IX

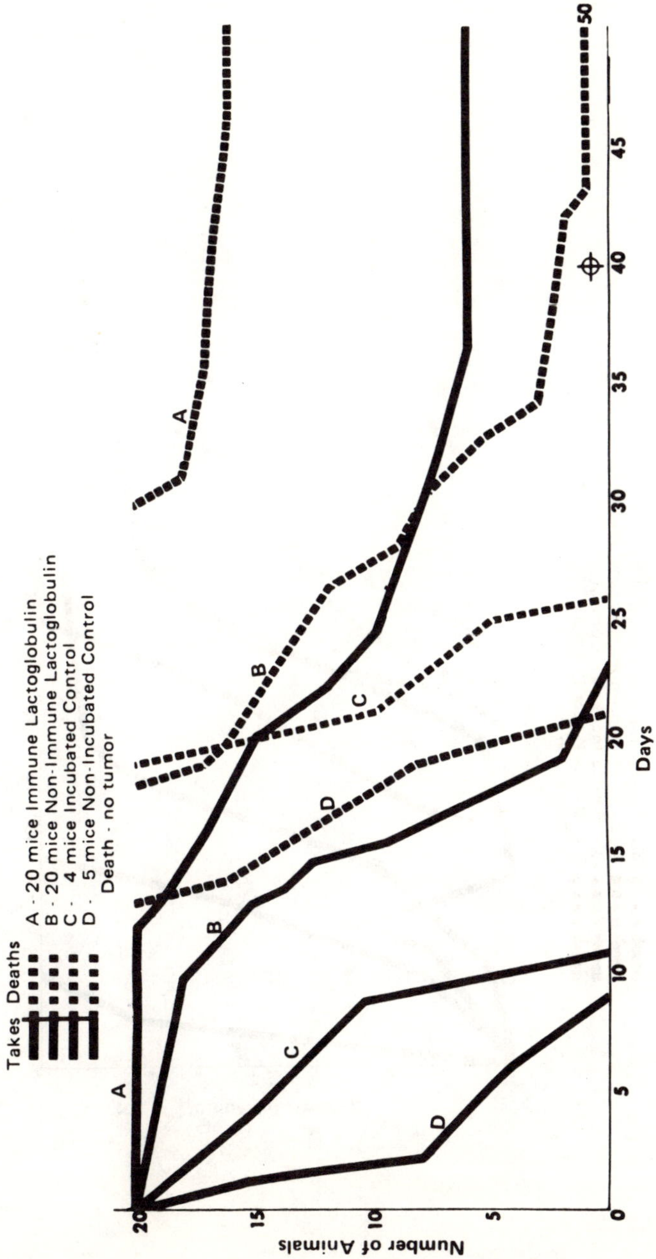

NEUTRALIZATION X

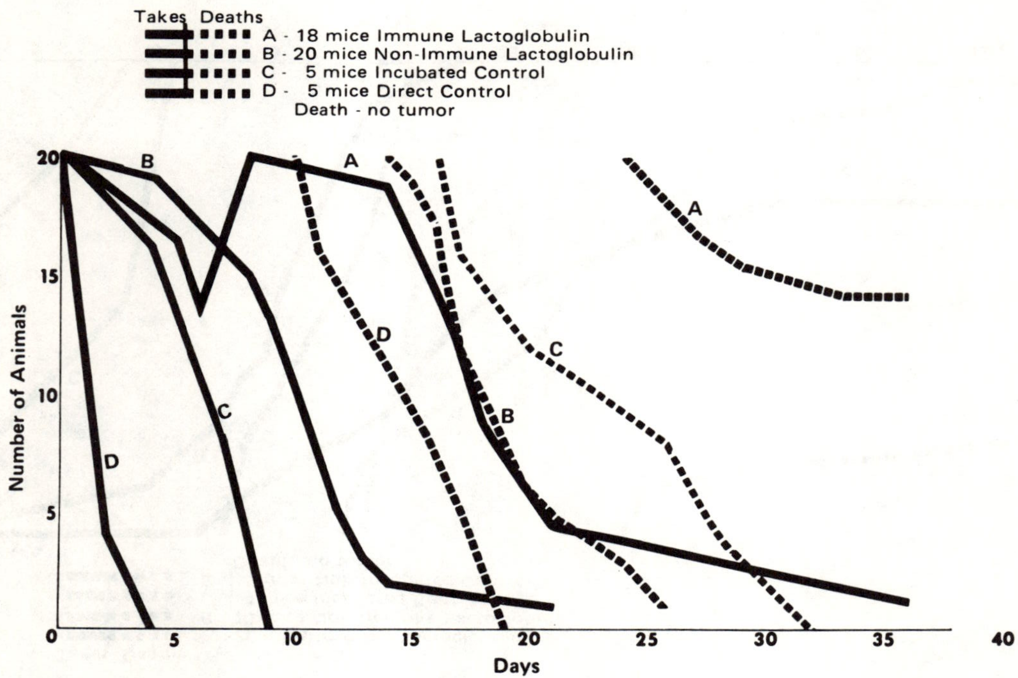

APPENDIX 10

THE NUTRITION BATTLE

The following appeared in the *Cancer Control Journal*, Vol. 3, No. 3, 1975, by James Privitera, M.D.

"The Nutrition Battle

"I am first going to give you a brief resume of how I became interested in nutrition. Even before this interest in nutrition, when I was working at Roswell Park Memorial Cancer Institute, New York, where I am from, we were doing studies with viruses and tissue cultures.

"We always found that there was contamination in the cultures. The interesting thing about this was that no matter how antiseptic the conditions, this contamination always appeared in the cultures of viruses that were supposedly causing cancer. They called these pleural pneumonia-like organisms, PPLO.

"The interesting thing today is that under a dark field microscope Dr. Virginia Livingston of San Diego sees these fungi. It was not visible under a light field microscope, so we couldn't see it.

"I think possibly this Cryptocides fungus is an invader, but Dr. Livingston thinks it is a cause. I think it is an invader because cancer has a difficult time living in a high oxygen level as shown by Dr. Otto Warburg, Dr. Dean Burk and Dr. William Koch.

"In 1965 we were doing some work in my medical school training at Creighton University, Omaha, Nebraska. We found that alcoholic patients were losing magnesium and zinc in their urine. This was very interesting. Then in my internship in Seattle, Washington, there was a lot of talk in the magazines about magnesium and zinc. A lot of diseases were shown to be associated with deficiencies of magnesium and zinc. Zinc caused healing to increase by about 50 percent in surgical entities such as pylonoidal cysts.

"At that time I was taking Spartase for my allergies. It contained potassium, magnesium aspartase, which was sold on prescription. I felt pretty good on this and it was also known to make the French Foreign Legion feel good as it reversed their fatigue from the heat. All of a sudden the government told the company that produced Spartase they had 30 to 60 days to prove efficacy or it was going to be removed from the market. They dropped it from their line of products because it wasn't profitable since it was only a minor product in their line. It wasn't worth the research. That's when I began to get interested. I walked into a health food store and started learning about what's really going on with regard to vitamins and minerals.

"In 1970 I took a fellowship in Allergy and Immunology at Scripps Clinic in San Diego.

"I then set up a practice in Covina. A patient came to my office and begged me to inject her with a vial of Laetrile and so I did. She was terminally ill and had a huge liver. She said, 'Dr. Privitera, I know this helps my pain. I know it's not a cure. I know I am not going to live very long. Would you please give me this so I don't have to go to Mexico?' This relieved her pain and I was quite impressed. When she didn't get it, her pain returned.

"Another patient had cancer of the kidney which had been diagnosed by biopsy. This man took Laetrile and the whole nutritional program including enzymes and diet. A later biopsy at Kaiser Hospital, San Francisco, was then reported to be negative.

"This I thought was quite impressive. These two cases then led me to go to Ernst Krebs, Jr., co-developer of Laetrile, where I met Dr. John Richardson. I listened to Krebs, Jr. and other people talk and became involved in this nutrition controversy.

"This led to my arrest by the California Food and Drug in July, 1974. About 15 agents came into my office and arrested me on the charge of selling Laetrile and other substances in the diagnosis, cure and alleviation of cancer.

"In Citrus Municipal Court, West Covina, on February 3, 1975, Judge Sam Cianchetti declared this statute unconstitutional. This was the first time any judge in all of the United States, especially in California, which is a test state, declared such a statute unconstitutional. I believe he is a very brave man.

"Here is the amazing part. October 4, 1974, I received a phone call from Sergeant Barclay of the Covina Police at one o'clock in the morning and he told me that my office was broken into. I went down to my office at one o'clock Saturday morning and there were two agents from the San Diego District Attorney's office to arrest me on a felony charge — conspiracy. The charge was conspiracy to commit the crime of unlawful sale of drugs, compounds, devices in the alleviation or cure of cancer.

"They handcuffed my hands behind my back and I spent the night in jail as did Carroll Leslie, who was arrested the same morning. What you have here is plain and simple harassment. There was no need to arrest us on a weekend at one o'clock in the morning as we were not going anywhere. I later found out this is standard operating procedure when the government wants to harass anyone.

"I have also read the law, which states that *before you are even arrested, they must give you a hearing and if the hearing goes against you, they must give you a cease and desist order.* This was also quite true for Dr. Richardson and other people harassed throughout California on this same charge. According to Health Code 1707.4, they are supposed to get a hearing and a cease and desist order and none of them have had it.

"Recently in Ohio, a man was brought before the Medical Board for using Laetrile and they gave him a hearing. So California is much harder and more vicious than Ohio. In Ohio they are civil; in California they are not civil. In San Diego we brought this motion up and the judge denied this motion for a cease and desist hearing and he gave no reason.

"In a Superior Court in San Diego, January 2, 1975, a historical victory was won in a Decision and Order Overruling Demurrer The People of the State of California versus William Turner, Winifred Davis, James Privitera, M.D., Carroll Leslie and Phyllis Disney.

"Judge Ben Hamrick said you can use Laetrile and any other nutrient in treatment of the whole person as long as it's articulated to the patient that it is part of the treatment for the whole person. You cannot treat the tumor or cancer per se. He did not nullify the statute, but he did emasculate it, which is a plus, but not a total plus.

"We are having a lot of trouble with the courts and this is a real problem. The trial is now in progress in San Diego and that includes Bill Turner, Wynn Davis, Carroll Leslie, Phyllis Disney and myself.

"Phyllis Disney of Hollywood, who was selling Laetrile and Vitamin B15, has already plead nolo contendere for financial reasons. Just to show you how vicious things are, they are still harassing her with this conspiracy charge.

"Now the other case in West Covina is on appeal. Although the judge in the municipal court declared this particular cancer statute unconstitutional, the State Food and Drug has appealed it. So it's now in the Superior Court of Appeals and will soon be decided.

"So much for that. Now let me give you some of my thoughts on cancer and nutrition.

"Natural vitamins may cost a bit more than synthetic vitamins. It costs a little more to go first class, but it's worth it.

"There are two recent articles in the *Prevention Maga-*

zine about Vitamin A and C deficiencies in animals and humans with cancer. Now we're seeing more articles explaining the dangers and diseases resulting from vitamin deficiencies.

"Recent data shows that cities that have fluoridation have a 20 percent higher cancer incidence.

"You probably noticed in the newspaper recently that Dr. Rosemond, president of the American Cancer Society, said that one out of two people are going to be cured of cancer. When he was asked further about this statement, you know what he said? 'Well, I must admit that we just kind of picked this figure out of the air.' Greenburg of the *Washington Post* then went on to say, 'Well, actually *the American Cancer Society juggles its statistics and there haven't been any improvements in its statistics since 1955.'*

"When Raucscher was asked about this, he said, 'Yes, those figures are correct.' So here we have the American Cancer Society trying to generate optimism about the government's multi-million-dollar program for cancer, admitting in the paper, virtually, that they lie.

"Many of the doctors have been so educated that they have abandoned common sense. They are very intelligent and they know a lot about drugs and radiation. I can tell you stories about so many patients I have seen.

"One of the most heart-rending stories was a woman who came to my office who had had radiation therapy for cancer of the cervix. And guess what? She now has a colostomy and cancer of the cervix. They don't want you to know about this. I suppose the best thing that happens is that she will probably tell 50 people about it. So they are having a lot of trouble trying to sell chemotherapy and radiation these days.

"Recently in the *American Medical Association News,* Dr. Powers, who is the head of the Internal Medicine Department, Wayne State University, stated that we were only eating 50 percent of the fruits and vegetables that we ate 20 years ago. He further went on to state that if doctors don't get interested in nutrition, they will be mortgaging their future . . . because patients are demanding more knowledge about prevention. They are tired of having doctors treat their diseases after they get them. I think this is very encouraging.

"There actually have been a lot of articles in the standard medical journals about nutrition such as articles on bran in the prevention of colon cancer. The Africans rarely get cancer of the colon because of their intake of bran.

"Here's another thought on radiation. You don't give radiation or chemotherapy to a well person, but Western medicine has no compunction in giving these to a sick person, as a first hope rather than a last resort!

"One of the most toxic drugs is 5 FU and 50 percent of the stock is owned by the American Cancer Society. One of the side effects is death. That's written right on the circular. I wonder how many doctors tell their patients about the side effects?

"Goggins, a Democrat from San Bernardino, wants to tie standard therapy to malpractice. In a bill before the California Legislature, this Democrat is proposing that a doctor must do standard therapy. Forty percent of my practice is standard therapy and 60 percent isn't. So they probably would tell me, 'Well, Dr. Privitera, I am really very sorry, but you see you just don't do standard therapy and we just can't give you any malpractice insurance.' My malpractice insurance is supposed to go up to $4,000 by October. Now I have never been sued by a patient. The only people who have sued me are the Government.

"There are many problems involved.

"The problem with a lot of people who have come to my office is that they have been sold a bill of goods. They have had a lot of radiation and chemotherapy. The problem is they are not using nutrition as a first benefit; they are using nutrition as a last rite.

"Doctors should tell their patients that with a lot of radiation and chemotherapy it is more difficult to respond to nutrition because they are less resilient. Their immune system isn't as good as it should be. So we have two problems. We have a person with cancer plus we have an immune system which has been knocked down. These people do not respond as well as the people who are what I call 'clean cases,' who do not, or have had little or no chemotherapy and radiation.

"Unfortunately, what's happened is a lot of people have come to me or Dr. Contreras, Dr. Richardson or Dr. Jones when it was really too late and too much destruction has taken place. When 50 percent of their liver is destroyed by cancer and they are emaciated, it is usually too late.

"We have patients that come in and say, 'What are your statistics?'

"The problem is, it depends on where they are. Have they had chemotherapy? What's their age? What's their previous medical history? What's their nutrition like? What's their immunity like? What is the environment in the home? Are they cooperative? Many factors are important. Statistics are kind of meaningless for this type of patient. You could categorize some 10 different types of patients with regard to age and other factors I just mentioned.

"I have been on frequent T.V. and radio shows and I keep telling these people, 'Listen, stop asking me how my patients are doing. Ask my patients.' Also, if they talk to me and then go back to their other doctors, it's just doctors talking against doctors. It's one doctor saying nutrition is worthless and another doctor saying you must have some radiation and chemotherapy. You know UCLA and USC use it, don't you think we know what we are doing? We couldn't use it if we didn't think it was good. So I just have to give them analogies like Columbus and Galileo and others the establishment said were crazy and who were locked up, ignored and harassed. History proved Columbus and Galileo correct.

"A big problem the Medical Establishment has from a research standpoint is that they cannot see a deficiency disease under the microscope. They could not find the answer to scurvy by taking tissue from a patient with scurvy and looking under the microscope nor tissue from a patient who had pernicious anemia. They wouldn't find it. It's not there. Vitamin C or B12 was not there. These are deficiency diseases and that's the problem. And so it is with cancer and Laetrile (Vitamin B17, amygdalin), abscisic acid and nutrition.

"I have seen patients take abscisic acid after they had done everything else. They had pain and that went away completely after taking 1 to 20 milligrams of abscisic acid a day. It's not a cheap material. It is a fat soluble nutrient found in the apricot oil.

"I think here again nature is right when you eat the whole apricot kernel. You violate nature when you remove the oil from apricots and make Aprikern (defatted apricot kernel powder) because abscisic acid is in the fat portion. For this reason, I put most of my patients on approximately 10 apricot kernels a day plus their Laetrile. This way they will get the full complex in the kernel plus the abscisic acid.

"Hippocrates, the Father of Medicine, said, 'Leave your drugs in the chemist's pot if you can heal the patient with food!' In other words, use nutrition and foods first and drugs last. However, many doctors now are using drugs first and nutrition last. That is why we are in a very sorry state.

"Hippocrates also said in the Hippocratic Oath, 'For the good of the sick, to the utmost of my power.' He didn't say except if there is a state regulation that may hinder what you may want to do or except if your peers in the local community don't do it. He said no, 'for the good of the sick, to the utmost of your power' — not with exceptions. The reason this Cancer Quackery code is so basically absurd is because it goes against the Hippocratic Oath.

"The medical license in California says that you can use any and all remedies, which will help your patient. It doesn't say except.

"Another discriminatory thing about the cancer statutes is that they only refer to cancer. It is discriminatory against the cancer patient and restricts him. No other disease is so restricted by politics.

"I know a lot of medical nutritionists who are afraid to treat a patient with cancer because they know the government doesn't want anybody to interfere with the normal routine standard therapy for cancer.

"It is also discriminatory against the Negro because Laetrile helps sickle cell anemia. This has been validated by Robert Houston, who has done brilliant work.

"It is discriminatory against the poor because the poor can't afford to go to Mexico or Germany like Mrs. Jerry Henderson or Mrs. Red Buttons.

"So here we have a great case for the American Civil Liberties Union. Where is the ACLU?

"People with cancer do not belong in an American hospital because they are not prepared to give them a nutritional program. They don't have fresh juices and they are not trained in detoxification.

"My therapy also consists of oxygenation because it is difficult for disease to live at a high oxygen level. It consists of enzymes. It is a well known fact that the pancreas dumps its enzymes into the small bowel and that cancer is extremely rare, like 1/10 of 10 percent. We use a lot of minerals for activation of enzymes and also to increase oxygenation and therefore increase metabolism. We use a detoxification program. It depends on the individual patient exactly which program we set up.

"Therefore the trouble with the treatment of cancer is just that . . . Western medicine believes in treating the cancer.

I believe we have to go back to Hippocrates' viewpoint of treating the whole patient and hopefully the patient will throw off his cancer.

"I do agree that we have to fight this battle in all the arenas including the press, public meetings, courts and especially the Legislature in the hopes of knocking this discriminatory statute out, which limits the nutrition of patients with cancer."

About James Privitera, M.D.

James Privitera, M.D., graduated in 1962 with a B.S. degree in Biology and Chemistry from Canisius College, Buffalo, New York. Later he took Biochemistry at the University of Buffalo Graduate School. He gained research experience at Roswell Park Memorial Institute, Buffalo, New York, but decided to go into medicine.

In 1967 he graduated with his M.D. degree from Creighton University School of Medicine, Omaha, Nebraska; followed by a one-year Internal Medicine Internship at Providence Hospital, Seattle, Washington. For the next year he took an Internal Medicine Residency at Presbyterian Hospital, San Francisco, California.

From 1969-1970 Dr. Privitera took a Clinical Fellowship in Allergy, Immunology and Reumatology at Scripps Clinic and Research Foundation, La Jolla, California. From 1970 on he entered a private practice of Allergy and Nutrition.

APPENDIX 11

THE LEGAL FIGHT OVER LAETRILE

The following article appeared in the *Cancer Control Journal,* May/June, 1973, Vol. 1, No. 1:

"Department of Health, Education, and Welfare
Public Health Service
National Institutes of Health, Bethesda, Maryland 20014

"Room 4E-16, Building 37
National Cancer Institute,
Bethesda, Maryland 20014
May 30, 1972

"Honorable Lou Frey, Jr.
214 Cannon House Office Building
Washington, D.C. 20515

"Dear Congressman Frey:

"Pursuant to your letter to me of May 4, 1972, I am pleased to submit to you the following comments and attached enclosures regarding the current status of the anti-cancer agent variously known as Amygdalin (the chemical name given to it upon its discovery in 1830); Laetrile (a contraction of its long chemical formulation); B-17 (vitamin B-17); or, more generally, nitriloside.

"**Food and/or Drug.** Amygdalin occurs natively in over one thousand species of plants, many of which are edible, and in this lay sense it is fundamentally and historically a *food* constituent or supplement. It becomes a *drug* in a legal sense when it is purified in a pharmaceutical preparation for specifically indicated medical purposes; of which anticancer activity is the most prominent of several activities reported in the scientific literature on Amygdalin.

"**Chemical Composition and Crystalline Form.** Pure Amygdalin is a chemical compound containing one molecule of benzaldehyde, one molecule of cyanide, and two molecules of glucose (blood sugar), all bound together so tightly that at ordinary temperatures it can be decomposed into its indicated components only by the action of a very special enzyme, glucosidase, found in many plants and in some animal tissues. Like many chemical compounds, Amygdalin may exist in several crystalline forms, depending upon the number of molecules of water of crystallization attached (e.g. 0, 1, or 3 H_2O), all of which forms, however, when dissolved in aqueous media, yield one and the same Amygdalin.

"**New vs. Old Drug.** One particular crystalline form of Amygdalin containing one molecule of water of crystallization, known as Amygdalin-MF, is many times more readily soluble than any of the other known forms, and was first prepared by the McNaughton Foundation about eight years ago, and, with regard to potential anticancer activity, is classed by the U.S. Food and Drug Administration as a *'New Drug'*. Other crystalline forms may perhaps be regarded as *'Old Drugs'* under the so-called Grandfather Clauses (a matter still requiring Court adjudication), since they entered into commerce and medical usage either before passage of the Federal Food, Drug, and Cosmetic Act of 1938 or more particularly before passage of the Kefauver Amendment to this Act, the 'Drug Amendment of 1962' (public Law 87-781, 87th Congress, S.1552, October 10, 1962) – which amendment added the further requirement of demonstration of drug efficacy in addition to drug safety, and an amendment whose constitutionality with respect to safe anticancer drugs remains to be tested (see below).

"Furthermore, prior to passage of the Kefauver Amendment, Judge W. T. Sweigert of the San Francisco Federal District Court ordered limited distribution of supplies of

Amygdalin (laetrile) to the McNaughton Foundation of Canada and to certain American physicians for investigation with, or treatment of patients (cf. Case 38179, Exhibit A, Proviso, May 17, 1962 et seq.) thereby federally recognizing the elements of commerce and pharmaceutical medicine with respect to Laetrile before October 10, 1962.

"**Interstate Commerce.** The various forms of Amygdalin are currently enjoined by the FDA from interstate commerce when they are prepared as pharmaceuticals for *human* medical investigation or use, but not when they enter commerce as chemicals such as now sold by many leading chemical and biochemical firms, with published catalog price listings.

"In this connection, Dr. Earl L. Meyers, Bureau of Drugs, FDA, has written Mr. A. R. L. McNaughton, President of the McNaughton Foundation, on April 7, 1972: 'There is nothing to prevent you from importing Amygdalin-MF for *animal* testing if you choose to do so' (emphasis added.)

"Thus, on such a basis, I have recently received 300 grams pure Amygdalin-MF sent from Mexico, and across state lines, to my laboratory here in Bethesda, for continued conduct of animal experimentation with normal and tumor-bearing mice; as have similarly Drs. Saul Schepartz and John Venditti (Drug Research and Evaluation Branches, NCI) for experimentation with various cancer-bearing mice and rats, and likewise 5,000 grams Amygdalin to Mrs. Helen Nauts, Executive Director, New York Cancer Research Institute, for experimentation with cancer-bearing dogs and cats at the New York Animal Medical Center Laboratories, under the experimental supervision of Drs. William Hardy and Lloyd Old of the Sloan-Kettering Institute for Cancer Research, all in accord with Dr. Meyers' directive.

"Parenthetically, I may add that the patient-care-use of medical drugs, New or Old, is not under the intrastate legal control of the federal FDA, on bases of either IND (Investigational New Drug) excemption or NDA permit therefrom, *if* they are nontoxic as prepared and dispensed under the supervision of a within-the-state M.D. and are no threat to the within-the-state public health. Indeed, there are also exceptional instances where this is also true even interstate (cf. 38 Corpus Juris Secundum, pp. 726, 804; Brennan vs. Titusville, 14 S. Ct. 829, 153 U.S. 289, 38 L Ed 719; 12C Juris, p. 20), as, for instance, when a drug gift for a donee living in another state may be delivered by the donor to a third party who delivers it to the donee for the donee's use.

"Dr. A. C. Ivy, M.D., Research Director, Ivy Cancer Research Foundation, Chicago, has been proceeding on this basis in the State of Illinois for a number of years with respect to the potential anticancer agent, 'carcalon,' without effective challenge or restraint.

"**Current Human Usage of Laetrile.** In spite of the aforementioned FDA prohibition of Laetrile in interstate commerce, there are well over 2,000 cancer-afflicted persons in this country using Laetrile for cancer treatment and amelioration, and a goodly number of non-cancer persons using it merely with prevention of development of cancer in view, and these various persons include M.D. physicians as well as laity.

"I have had considerable personal experience in this regard, for in the past year alone at least 750 persons, including more than 50 physicians, have contacted me for information on the use and availability of Laetrile, and I know of others with approximately the same quantitative extent of similar experience. In over 20 countries of the world, well over 5,000 cancer patients have been treated with Laetrile, with, significantly, no demonstratable noteworthy clinical contraindication of its use either along or in conjunction with virtually any other anticancer agents, chemotherapeutic, radiological, or surgical.

"Laetrile at physician-prescribed dosages is nontoxic by a factor of 100-1000 times when compared to essentially all anticancer drugs now used with FDA approval on an IND or NDA basis. The human use of Laetrile is growing rapidly, in and out of the United States; partly because in the last two or three years, five factories have been developed for its production in Mexico, Monaco, Italy, Germany, Yugoslavia. Court and legislative actions to facilitate American usage are in progress (see below).

"Although the foregoing Laetrile utilization in this country is proceeding, as indicated, in spite of FDA prohibition, it is even more so *because* of unwarranted FDA procedures, and lack of FDA scientific and medical justification for its stand, extending to probable unconstitutionality, concerning which many thousands of cancer-afflicted persons and their relatives and physicians are rapidly becoming aware.

"In this connection, I have hundreds of letters sent to me enclosing FDA information sheets and pronouncements, in which the senders of these letters point out the extensive falsification, duplicity, deviousness, red herrings, and literal lies (the preferred euphemism of the ever-chivalrous Hon. James Symington is 'mendacities') promulgated by the FDA with respect to Laetrile, as well as similarly on the part of a limited number of certain high officials (though scarcely ever rank-and-file members) of the American Medical Association, the American Cancer Society, the U.S. Department of Health, Education and Welfare, and state agencies (most prominently the California Cancer Advisory Council, see below), as I have specified in detail on pp. 706-707 and 714-720 of the herewith enclosed material taken from the Hearings before the Subcommittee on Public Health and Environment of the Committee on Interstate and Foreign Commerce, House of Representatives re H.R. 8343, H.R. 10681, S. 1828, September 15 - October 11, 1971, that led eventually to the passage of the 'National Cancer Act of 1971,' and as I more extensively documented by further submissions requested by the Subcommittee and staff for their files, to the extent of some 400 pages.

"In any event, it is becoming evident that the current generation of cancer sufferers is coming to regard the intransigence and palpable lies of the FDA and the above-indicated related organizations with a marked measure of contempt on the basis of prima facie evidence provided by these organizations themselves as to their integrity and credibility and that something of a Boston Tea Party mode of action is being undertaken by an increasing number of cancer-sufferers in this country, who intend to be hoodwinked no longer; in short, an active backlash is developing even at the grass-roots level and along various lines, some of which follow:

"**Proposed Congressional Action.** The enclosed letter from Jay M. Hutchinson, Chairman, *'Test Laetrile Now Committee,'* reports on the first petition of 1,000 signatures of Americans who ask for the clinical testing of Laetrile on human cancer sufferers who have given their informed consent, which requests: 'We the undersigned citizens petition your committee to recommend to the Congress that special authority be immediately granted for the clinical testing of Amygdalin-MF (Laetrile, an internationally used cancer controlling agent) by recognized medical authorities in accordance with the testing data submitted by the McNaughton Foundation for the Investigational New Drug (IND) No. 6734 of the Food and Drug Administration.'

"Other 1000-signature petitions will follow in large number,* and will be sent to various U.S. Senators and Congressmen, as the first one already has and will proceed from all parts of the country, the first one coming mainly from the San Francisco area.

"I may add that I have been reliably informed by the staff member in charge of handling IND applications in one of the largest cancer research organizations in the country, that the McNaughton Foundation IND applications made by

**Over 20,000 by February 1973*

and granted to said cancer research organization, and this in spite of the report of the 'kangaroo court and jury' of the FDA described in my testimony on pp. 719-720 of the enclosed Hearings by the Rogers Subcommittee on Public Health and Environment (cf. also letter of Jay M. Hutchinson, paragraph 8).

"A Bill, H.R. 12092, has already been introduced (December 7, 1971), herewith enclosed, and along the lines of the aforementioned Petition, that is intended to cover not only Laetrile but a large number of safe and nontoxic drugs, foods, vitamins or other substances for study and use on cancer mitigation in human patients, and that directs the Director of the National Cancer Institute to pursue activities along such lines as part of the expanded, intensified and coordinated cancer research program to which the Institute is now committed by the National Cancer Act of 1971.

"A similar Bill is being proposed for introduction into the Senate, with respect to anticancer agents that are safe and nontoxic at dosages far less toxic than the 'safe' anticancer drugs or substances now approved and allowed by the FDA, and far below any dosages producing even mild or moderate sublethal effects.

"The National Cancer Act of 1971 would appear to raise a question as to conflict of jurisdiction of authority between the National Cancer Institute and the Food and Drug Administration as to which agency shall hereafter set standards of safety and care regarding *cancer* patients being treated with biological materials and other therapeutic substances (cf. Section 407, (b)(5)). The legislative intent as to disposition of IND authority is not clear as yet, apparently.

"**Proposed Court Actions.** An action is scheduled* for initiation in a U.S. District Court by a New York law firm acting on behalf of a Plaintiff Mrs. Joan Andrews and a number of co-plaintiffs who suffer from cancers in various

**For hearing in the Federal 4th Circuit Court ca. April 2, 1973, in Baltimore.*

forms, to enjoin the United States Post Office, the U.S. Customs Office Service, and the Secretaries of the Treasury and the Department of Health, Education and Welfare from preventing entry into the United States and into Interstate Commerce, the material known as Amygdalin (Laetrile) for personal use pursuant to a physician's prescription.

"The scope of the action is a narrow one, i.e., it will not attempt to permit introduction of such material into interstate commerce for commercial purposes, but rather permit freedom of individual use. No claim will be made in this litigation as to the anticancer efficacy of Laetrile, but rather only that it is safe for humans at applied physician-prescribed dosages.

"The position taken is that the efficacy standard of the Kefauver Amendment, as applied to a narrow class of persons who are cancer patients and diagnosed as such is unconstitutional, violating, among others, the Ninth Amendment constitutional right to privacy. The action may well proceed through District and Appellate Courts to the Supreme Court.

"Parenthetically, I may add that I have been reliably informed by a co-writer of the Kefauver Amendment that the original legislative intent was not concerned with agents, nontoxic or toxic, against what were then regarded as essentially noncurable (or noncured) diseases such as cancer, but was directed against diseases essentially curable on a large scale, such as pneumonia or tuberculosis, for which a number of effective agents were then already and otherwise available.

"A Court action with respect to the Grandfather Clause status of Laetrile (hereinbefore referred to) is under consideration, following upon similar Court actions now underway with respect to a number of quite different drugs and substances where it would appear that the FDA has taken inappropriately retroactive measures with respect to the Kefauver Amendment, and such Court action has already reached the Court of Appeals.

"**Constitutional Free Press Court Action.** On March 31, 1971, the Attorney General and Deputy Attorney General of the State of California, as attorneys for the Plaintiff, Louis F. Saylor, M.D., Director of Public Health of the State of California, instituted an action (no. 999731) in the Superior Court of the State of California for the County of Los Angeles to restrain the Defendants: International Association of Cancer Victims and Friends, *Cancer News Journal*, National Health Federation, certain officials of these organizations, and Does I through XX, from making any representations that Laetrile has any value in arresting, alleviating or curing cancer, in violation of section 10400.1(d) of Title 17, California Administrative Code. At the hearing of the case on May 3, 1971, Superior Court Judge Wisot refused to issue the preliminary injunction sought by the state authorities, basing his decision on the finding that the requested prohibition would violate the First Amendment of the U.S. Constitution guaranteeing freedom of the press. Judge Max Z. Wisot said he could not deviate from the principle that individuals have the right to determine their own course of action and to be influenced by or to ignore what they read.

"Judge Wisot further pointed out that the very statute in question had declared that nothing therein contained shall be deemed to abridge the freedom of the press. Freedom of the press has been construed down through history since the enactment of the First Amendment to the Constitution as applying to every means of communication, including books, pamphlets, films and verbal expressions, as well as newspapers and magazines.

"The protection aimed at by the writers of the Bill of Rights was not solely for persons in intellectual pursuits unrelated to action. The First Amendment is a charter for government, not for an institution of learning, and 'Free trade in ideas' means free trade in the opportunity to persuade to action, not merely to describe facts.

"In a closely related, widely cited case, Near vs. Minnesota, the Supreme Court reversed the decision of the trial court that had ordered a certain periodical abated, and had enjoined the defendants from distributing it; the Supreme Court held that the Minnesota authorities' actions were unconstitutional as imposing an unconstitutional *previous restraint* and censorship upon the defendants' right to freedom of the press.

"Mr. Chief Justice Hughes wrote the opinion that 'it is the chief purpose of the guaranty to prevent previous restraints upon publication.' Earlier, Blackstone had written, 'The liberty of the press is indeed essential to the nature of a free state; but this consists in laying no previous restraints upon publications, and not in freedom from censure for criminal matter when published. Every freeman has an undoubted right to lay what sentiments he pleases before the public.'

"In view of the foregoing, rather well-known, elementary considerations, one can but wonder how and why the California officials involved should ever have attempted to institute a suit of prior restraint amounting to total blanket injunction along lines contraindicated since the time of Blackstone.

"The concluding points and authorities cited by the California officials to the effect that a competing consideration should take precedence, namely that of 'The interest of a person who wants her cancer treated with a drug which medical and scientific evidence shows is worthless,' is odd, to say the least, even from a legal point of ivew, but is further demerited by the consideration that in the year 1971 Laetrile is indeed already regarded, medically and scientifically, as far from 'worthless' by many authorities, granted that the matter, like most scientific and medical matters, is controversial.

"For, it is a widely held maxim that 'In science one cannot prove that there is no ghosts.' The California administrative authorities have widely overstepped the bounds of science here, and, similarly, the bounds of medicine also. Their action may be likened to the well-known state legislature that attempted to declare that thereafter in that state the value of π, the numerical ratio between the circumference and the diameter of a circle, would be an even 3, instead of 3.1416 . . . One cannot help but wonder whether the California officials introduced the suit mainly to tighten up their own pseudo-medical loopholes by a legal but scarcely scientific device.

"Judge Wisot denied the requested restraint, but added, 'without prejudice to any application for renewal, in the event there can be or is shown to the Court any greater need or any greater grounds than an invasion of constitutional rights of speech.' Apart from the aforementioned dubious scientific and medical groups, the California officials would be well advised to recall first that state laws and regulations can extend and go further than federal laws and regulations by the legal rule of pre-emption (supersession) an instance of which was very recently confirmed and upheld by a decision of the U.S. Supreme Court dated March 22, 1972 (92 Sup Ct 1029, Supreme Court Reporter).

"In the May 3, 1971 Hearing before Judge Wisot, the constitutional issues were ably presented by the Defendants' lawyers, Kirkpatrick Dilling of Chicago and Charles Pratt of Virginia, both of whom have had legal experience on food and drug matters for over 35 years, and both of whom are frequently called upon to protect small businesses against tyrannical and unwarranted acts of the FDA involving, e.g., illegal search and seizure, electronic snooping and entrapment, scare techniques, 'book burning,' jury softening and intimidation, all extensively described and documented in *The Dictocrats: Our Unelected Rulers* written by Omar Garrison (1970), to which I may invite your careful attention.

"**Red Herring Ploy**: On a more academic level, it is a

very commonly employed ploy on the part of administrative and health officials to attempt to pass hypothesis off as fact, as in the following very recent instance so advanced by Ralph W. Weilerstein, M.D., Executive Secretary, California Cancer Advisory Council (Department of Public Health): 'The use of Laetrile in early cancer cases to the exclusion of conventional treatment might well be dangerous since treatment with acceptable, modern curative methods (surgery or radiation) would thereby be delayed potentially until such time as metastases had occurred and the cancer, therefore, might no longer be curable.' (College of Marin Time, Kentfield, California, April 26, 1972.)

"The line of 'reasoning' can be run across hundreds of times, and was indeed a ploy frequently set forth by the recently removed Director of the National Cancer Institute and his letter-writing assistants, and, it is to be hoped, will be discarded by the newly-appointed Director, Dr. Frank Rauscher.

"Of the 350,000 cancer patients dying of cancer in the United States every year, and of the twice this number suffering currently from cancer, I doubt if proponents of this idea could produce as many as ten instances, even five, perhaps even one; certainly to my knowledge, they never have, and may herewith be presented with the challenge to do so.

"Of the thousands of cancer patients who have contacted me, I have yet to find one who had not been treated with 'conventional' methods before seeking Laetrile, and nearly all of those so seeking were in 'terminal' or near-terminal cancer status. (As earlier stated, I know of non-cancer persons who do take Laetrile, in one form or another, with prevention in view.)

"This is, of course, a growing number of cancer patients who come to take Laetrile along with 'Conventional Treatments,' in view of its widely recognized nontoxicity, and lack of medical contraindication of such a course of action.

"The Editor of the College of Marin Times, which had just earlier printed 'prolaetrile' material, editorialized, 'We are at a loss as to which side (pro-laetrile and anti-laetrile) has the right story. You can be sure that one of the sides is fraudulant.' In the opinion of the undersigned, there is little doubt as to which one is.

"**Conventional Failure:** Let us now examine more closely the implications of 'conventional treatment' so referred to above by Dr. Weilerstein (as well as by countless others). To set an appropriate stage, let us begin with citing Benjamin Rush, M.D., Surgeon General of the Continental Army of the United States, and Signer of the Declaration of Independence, 'To restrict the art of healing to one class of men and deny equal privileges to others will constitute the Bastille of medical science. All such laws are un-American and despotic . . . and have no place in a republic . . . The Constitution of this Republic should make special provision for Medical Freedom as well as Religious Freedom.'

"The 350,000 cancer deaths a year in the United States referred to above represent patients almost exclusively with disseminated, metastatic cancer, their deaths occurring on the average many years before otherwise allotted time.

"They represent the number who failed of the benefit of 'acceptable, modern curative methods' cited by Dr. Weilerstein. Estimates of the percentage of disseminated-cancer patients who survive more than a very few years vary most frequently between 5 and 15%.

"Thus, at a White House Press Conference following immediately upon the swearing in of Dr. Frank Rauscher, Jr., as new Director of the National Cancer Institute, Dr. Rauscher reported a figure of about 7.5% as follows: 'of the 100 cancers that afflict man, about 15 percent of those can be treated extremely well, to the point of at least 50 percent 5-year survivals' (15% x 50% = 7.5%). A considerable part of the 7.5% is in fact made up of leukemias, and only a much smaller fraction by patients with solid tumors (sarcomas and carcinomas). According to Dr. Albert Sabin, '85% of cancers do not respond to any drugs.'

"This is also confirmed approximately by citations listed in the enclosed 'A Very Grim Picture,' which gives direct quotations from a number of prominent physicians reporting in the Sixth National Cancer Conference Proceedings, published July 1970, under the auspices of the National Cancer Institute and American Cancer Society, who selected the reporting physicians.

"At a very recent, heavily attended Chemotherapy Conference held in the main auditorium of the NIH, Dr. Charles Moertal of the Mayo Clinic stated at the end of his lecture on May 18, 1972, after being introduced by Chairman Dr. Stephen Carter (NCI) as 'probably one of the country's foremost, if not the foremost expert in this area (of gastrointestinal cancer)': 'Perhaps some small and hesitant progress has been made, but it is evident that in this year of 1972 there is no remarkably effective specific therapy for any types of gastrointestinal carcinoma that cannot be surgically extirpated. There are none that can be accorded the stature of treatment of preference. Our most effective regimens are fraught with risks and side-effects and practical problems, and after this price is paid by all the patients we have treated, only a small fraction are rewarded with a transient period of usually incomplete tumor regressions.'

"At the beginning of his lecture, in which a large variety of experimental anticancer agents studied by Dr. Moertal were reported in detail, Dr. Moertal said, 'Our accepted and traditional curative efforts therefore yield a failure rate of 85%. These patients with advanced gastrointestinal cancer present us with one of the most frequent major disease problems encountered in medical practice today . . . The patient with gastrointestinal cancer is still getting the same old 5-Fu he got 14 years ago. Some patients with gastrointestinal cancer can have very long survival with no treatment whatsoever.'

"Dr. Moertal was followed by Dr. Bernard Fisher of the University of Pittsburgh on the subject of breast cancer, who spoke inequally frankly pessimistic vein on breast cancer, with respect to current, available therapies.

"The two physicians just referred to, and the some 15 others reporting in 'A Very Grim Picture,' are unquestionably men of highest integrity, sincerity, and effort, and one may well ask Dr. Weilerstein where are all the modern curative methods to which he, the California Cancer Advisory Council, and indeed so many administrators so glibly refer? One must bear in mind here that 'trilingual' English is often met with: (a) M.D.'s speaking frankly among themselves, (b) administrators speaking to Congressional Appropriations Committees, and (c) for patients and their families. No, disseminated cancer, in its various forms and kinds, remains by and large as 'incurable' as at the time of the Kefauver Amendment 10 years ago, or the California Cancer Commission 20 years ago — Dr. Weilerstein or no Dr. Weilerstein, FDA or no FDA, ACS or no ACS, AMA or no AMA, NCI or no NCI.

"Their practicing M.D. spokesmen say so, as I have very briefly indicated, in their plain, unadulterated English, class (a).

"And what about Laetrile, by comparison? Leading Laetrile physicians (M.D.'s) claim about the same kind of 5-15% objective benefit, though they do not do so on particular bureaucratically required forms of e.g., the FDA or the California Cancer Advisory Council. But, with these added benefits: (a) no such bodily harm of the type produced by virtually all toxic drugs now contentionally employed and recommended; (b) much higher percentages of pain relief than the 5-15% objective benefit.

"That the various administrative agencies claim Laetrile is worthless, may be dismissed (as indicated above) as unscientifically based, together with the fact that few or none of such claimants have ever worked personally with Laetrile and patients, nor have they seriously if at all, ever visited hospitals and clinics where Laetrile is used, and their alleged medical basis goes back to the 1953 report of the California Cancer Commission which described no patient ever receiving a *total* dosage of Laetrile as great as is now the current standard *daily* dosage (3 gram/day or more).

"Fewer and fewer people are being hoodwinked by this last consideration, unless it be the indicated agencies repeating it over and over to themselves.

"As for the conventional pain-relievers employed, one of the speakers at the May 18-19, 1972 NCI Chemotherapy Conference said: 'Our primary responsibility is relief of pain . . . after centuries of experience dating back to Paracelsus and beyond, it is astonishing how little we really know about relief of pain with oral medications.

" 'Our prescribing habits are usually guided by such unimpeachable sources as the physicians' desk reference, or the detail man's testimonial or the throw-away literature that accompanies the free ball-point pen.'

"Many cancer patients on Laetrile have reported heretofore usage of conventional pain-relievers has been reduced greatly, even completely. Pain, of course, is a subjective consideration, but by and large, the patient himself is the highest authority, with respect to himself.

"A popular fallacy (rather than intentional ploy) found almost universally among practiced employers of the ploy, is the concept that if an agent cannot harm the body it cannot harm cancer.

"The fatal weakness in this view is that wherever cancers differ from normal body cells (and they in several well-established ways do, e.g. metabolically, catalase content, water content – broadly speaking) then an anticancer agent may have specificity against cancer compared to the normal cell.

"This specificity may be absolute or relative. It may yield anticancer efficacy as distinguished from pharmacologic harm. Even a simple ordinary body compound, such as glucose (blood sugar), has been shown in the very extensive work of Manfred von Ardenne to have remarkable anticancer activity, and the more so when used in multitherapy involving several simultaneously employed anticancer agents, all used, of course, under predetermined optimizing conditions.

"**The Carcinogenicity of Conventional Anticancer Drugs.** A recent report from the Southern Research Institute, dated April 13, 1972, several hundred pages in length (see enclosed Summary first 11 pages), conducted for the National Cancer Institute (Contract PH-43-68-998), shows that a majority of the common clinically used 'Weilersteinein conventional' anticancer drugs are highly carcinogenic in rats and mice, and in a surprising variety of organs thereof.

"The suggested indication is that virtually all such conventional toxic anticancer drugs will yield the same result when the studies are fully completed.

"These are the drugs now approved by the FDA for cancer treatment, on an IND or NDA basis, before or after the enactment of the Kefauver Amendment. As Dr. Saul Schepartz has remarked to me — this is something we will really have to start worrying about when and if some of these drugs get to producing several years — 'cures' — for after that time carcinogenicity will rear its ugly head. Ironically, when it comes to *foods* the FDA is required by the Delaney Amendment to preclude usage of any compounds in foods for which the slightest carcinogenic effect has been reported in animals so fed.

"The gap in thinking here is almost infinite, but currently *sotto voce*. The rationalizing argument made is 'efficacy vs. risk' (as in so much of medicine) or, in plainer language, 'the lesser of two evils.'

"**New Animal Experimentation with Laetrile.** I have referred in column 2 of this letter to Laetrile experimentation with animals about to be taken up anew, in the National Cancer Institute by two separate groups, and by the New York Institute for Cancer Research, with mice, rats, cats and dogs, and may add that currently similar studies with, in addition also rabbits, is underway in the Paris laboratory by Dr. T. Metianu of the Pasteur Institute.

"These can certainly be interesting academic and scientific studies, and where positive might particularly aid in studies with humans, though the same cannot so readily be said where negative, because as with all searches for anti-cancer agents, variability of efficacy, as distinguished from pharmacology, can vary enormously from organ to organ, species to species, cancer type to cancer type, etc., as every-one knows or should know. Pharmacologic results with animals are far, far more readily transferable to humans than are anticancer efficacy studies.

"**New Food Containing Laetrile**. Recently, starting in Europe, efforts are underway to produce food products relatively rich in Laetrile, where (a) it will not be a drug, and (b) can be consumed in sufficiently small food quantities yet provide current daily recommended Laetrile dosages of the order of several grams/per day, at approximately one-tenth the cost per unit of Laetrile now otherwise prevailing.

"Thus flours may be made from bitter almonds (extensively available in Europe), or apricot kernels (extensively available in this country), or other kernels of the Prunus family.

"A variety of foods are under consideration, including bread, pastry products, even milk shakes. The bitter almonds themselves have long been readily available in European grocery stores, just as the apricot nut kernels have been here.

"I have found that adult mice can live indefinitely when their normal chow diet is made up to contain 50% defatted apricot nut flour. This provides them with approximately

125 mg amygdalin per mouse per day, or 4000 mg amygdalin/kg mouse/day, and is in addition excellent food material, rich in protein and minerals.

"Sickle Cell Anemia:

"**Other Laetrile Possibilities.** There are about two million persons in the United States with the sickle cell trait, and some 50,000 with actual sickle cell anemia, which very recently has been found to be ameliorated – at first by urea – and now much better by an impurity in urea, namely cyanate. Tablets or capsules of cyanate may be ingested to overcome the anemic hemolytic crisis.

"Cyanate can also be produced by hydrolysis of Laetrile, and conceivably it might be more sensible to obtain cyanate from ingested Laetrile – a working hypothesis yet to be demonstrated as efficacious, be it clearly noted, but which, if demonstrable, could be demonstrated with far less scientific effort than has been involved with Laetrile and cancer.

"This approach has been suggested to me by one of the most brilliant biochemists I know of in this country, who writes me further regarding his hypothesis: 'A relatively few simple clinical applications of Amygdalin in pure form or Laetrile in food rations should give us the answer.

" 'If the answer is confirmatory, I wonder if the FDA will attempt to perpetrate a discriminative genocide against the black population of this country who have sickle cell anemia?'

"He adds that 'Populations in Africa who have diets rich in vitamin B-17 (nitriloside) do not have sickle cell anemia no matter how loaded they are with sickle cells.' He further points out that there appears to be a remarkable difference in cancer incidence among Nigerian natives who do and do not have large amounts of vitamin B-17 in their diets, greatly in favor of those who do, with respect to absence of cancer –

according to reports by Dr. O. L. Oke, University of Ife, Ibadan, Nigeria.

"Sincerely yours,

"Dean Burke, Head,
"Cytochemistry Section, NCI

"**Disclaimer**: The above views of the oversigned research scientist may differ materially from those of administrators within HEW, and no such latter official support or endorsement is intended or should be inferred."

APPENDIX 12

HOW NUTRITION MAY AFFECT CELL DIFFERENTIATION

From: GENETIC CONTINUITY AND METABOLIC REGULATION AS SEEN BY THE EFFECTS OF VARIOUS MICROWAVE AND BLACK LIGHT FREQUENCIES ON THESE PHENOMENA

Sydney J. Webb*
Department of Bacteriology, University of Saskatchewan
Saskatoon, Saskatchewan, Canada

"Apart from these theoretic considerations, however, the data obtained do suggest that microwave spectroscopy, and perhaps Raman spectroscopy, could prove useful for identifying microbial cells and for rapidly differentiating tumor cells from normal ones. Whether microwave therapy can be used to control the growth of tumors in vivo must await much more experimentation.

"The concept outlined also seems to supply a possible mechanism by which cell differentiation may occur in higher organisms. In any organ, the nutrition received by an individual layer of cells is dependent on the metabolism of cells with which it is in contact. In a multicellular system, therefore, each layer of cells may have to adjust to a nutritional environment different from that of adjacent cell layers; thus, like bacteria, when each of these cells divides, it will produce a replica of itself and a daughter cell that contains a new dynamic system in harmony with the nutrition it receives. The daughter cell will be able to proliferate in accordance with its nutrition by normal fission, whereas each 'mother

**Present address: Department of Physics, University of South Florida, Tampa, Florida 33620. [Material offered by author.]*

cell' on division will continue to give rise to a replica of itself and a daughter cell that possesses the new differentiated system. This is in accordance with the known behavior of tissues in multicellular biologic systems. Such a proposal, however, suggests also that, during embryonic development, nutrition will be a very important factor in how various cells are differentiated and organs produced. Moreover, the spiraling motion induced by metabolic events will produce a similar motion of the entire daughter cell layer as it is produced, and this could play a part in the flowing motion of cells, which is known to occur during embryonic development as various stages are traversed."

APPENDIX 13

EARLY DETECTION – DIFFERING METHODS

The following is set forth, with permission, as it appeared in the International Health Council Booklet No. 70, November 1, 1974, entitled *A Program For Prevention, Detection and Reversal of Pre-Cancerous Conditions.*

"**Early Detection** is definitely the most important factor in the fight against cancer. Detection of a nutrition-related systems imbalance or precancer, long before cancer is discernible by the usual methods of observation, feel, Pap, x-ray or biopsy, can be the difference between life and death. Likewise, after an operation it is essential to know if the 'seeds' of the malignancy still remain in the system, and we have found very few that are clear.

"A quantitative urinalysis is available in the Philippines and other countries to determine the amount of Human Chorionic Gonadotrophin Hormone in the urine, in excess of natural amounts. This hormone is present with all types of cancer, including leukemia, and while it is generally considered a measure of tumor invasion, it is this writer's opinion that it can be a measure of 'malignancy pressure' against the 'body resistance,' or indicate tiny undetectable nodules. The test was developed in the U.S. and banned; it was further developed by Dr. Manuel Navarro, M.D., of the Santo Tomas University Medical School in Manila. Dr. Navarro found accuracy in extended tests from 97% to 100%. He found the test had forecast cancer up to two years before it could be detected by present medical techniques. The directions for taking the sample, partial processing and mailing are not too difficult for the average person. Dr. Navarro's diagnosis is easily understood by the layman and we have tied his diagnosis into our Program of revised living habits. Dr. Navarro's method was exhibited at the International Cancer Congress in

Tokyo, but our Government, the American Cancer Society and our medical profession showed little interest. Our observations indicate its value and accuracy.

"The mass testing of every person in the U.S. once or twice per year would be a desirable step in the eventual conquering of this disease. Samples from those with suspicious symptoms, follow-up, or direct involvement should definitely be sent in promptly.

"The suspicious symptoms we speak of above are the seven promoted by the American Cancer Society plus four of our own:

"1. Change in bowel or bladder habits.

"2. A sore that does not heal.

"3. Unusual bleeding or discharge.

"4. Thickening or lump in breast or elsewhere.

"5. Indigestion or difficulty in swallowing.

"6. Obvious change in wart or mole.

"7. Nagging cough or hoarseness.

"8. Any condition that doesn't respond to treatment.

"9. Following all cancer surgery or radiation therapy.

"10. Thrombophlebitis, inflammation from blood clotting in circulatory system.

"11. Putrid intestinal gas.

"**Cancer Immunologicial Test** (Philippine Urinalyses). Do not send a sample from a patient who is: pregnant, using birth control pills, estrogen, or other hormones, showing more than 100 mg of albumin, or a moderate amount of blood, is bedridden or severely deteriorated physically, has less than 50% normal liver function, or following chemotherapy. It takes one month to clear ingested hormones from the system so an accurate reading can be made.

"**Urine Sample Processing.**

"(1. Gather the following materials: glass household or lab measuring cups, one to measure 3.3 fluid ounces (100 cc) and one 13.2 fluid ounces (400 cc); glass funnel or wide-mouth jar; glass or stainless steel stirring rod or spoon; one gallon glass bottle — must be clean but do not use soap or detergents, get a domestic money order from the Post Office for $10.00 (subject to change); one pint or less of Glacial Acetic Acid from a drug store, chemical supply house or photo store handling dark room supplies; get one pint or more of Acetone from a chemical supply house, drug store, medical and surgical equipment supply house; a few sheets of filter paper (usually packaged in lots of 100) Whatman No. 41, 5 inch diameter, 12.5 cm., or the equivalent, from a chemical laboratory supply house, medical or surgical supply house, some drug stores, some hobby shops selling chemistry sets.

"(2. Collect all urine voided in a 24-hour period in the clean one-gallon glass bottle. Keep in a cool place. Shake well.

"(3. Take 3.3 fluid ounces (100 cc) of urine from the gallon bottle.

"(4. Add one tablespoon of Glacial Acetic Acid to the urine sample and stir well. Be careful, this is a powerful acid. Do not inhale and if splashed, use plenty of water for 15 minutes to flush.

"(5. Add this mixture to 13.2 fluid ounces (400 cc) of Acetone. Acetone is highly volatile and inflammable, so use it outside away from sparks and flame. Acetone will dissolve some plastics, so use only glass in handling.

"(6. Stir well and let stand outside for two or more hours.

"(7. Pour off most of the clear fluid, being careful not to lose any sediment.

"(8. Fold a circle of filter paper in half, then one quarter circle, then one eighth circle. Open partially and line the inner surface of a glass funnel loosely. If a funnel is not available, hold filter paper cone over a wide-mouth bottle. Pour the balance of the fluid with sediment through the filter paper, catching the sediment in the center of the paper.

Be sure to get all the sediment. In the event there is very little sediment, collect a new sample and rerun.

"(9. Cut off the surplus paper, leaving the sediment in the center.

"(10. Fold over the paper and place between two sheets of plastic while it is still damp. Trim off the surplus plastic, seal the edges with Scotch Tape to make it airtight and preventing it from drying out.

"(11. Insert the sample in an envelope with: the patient's name, address, sex, to whom report is to be sent, a brief case history, date sample was taken, $10.00 money order.

"(12. Air mail to: Dr. Manuel Navarro, M.D., 3553 Sining Street, Morningside Terrace, Santa Mesa, Manila D-403, Philippines. To avoid delay, have the post office weigh for proper postage. Do not send special delivery or registered.

"Interpretation of Report from Dr. Navarro

"Index Number	International Units	Interpretation
0	—	negative
1-3	—	doubtful
4	200-400	faintly positive
5	500-900	faintly positive
6	1,000-3,000	faintly positive
7	4,000	moderately positive
8	5,000	moderately positive
9	6,000	moderately positive
10-12	8,000-15,000	definitely positive
13-15	20,000-40,000	heavy positive
16-18	60,000-100,000	very heavy positive
19 and over	over 200,000	excessively positive

"Coordination with IHC Program

"Negative. Use Prevention Section of Program.

"Index 1-3 is doubtful because the quantity of HCG hormone being measured is so small there can be technical errors. It could be negative or show a precancerous condition, but it is generally considered negative unless other factors are evident.

"Index 4, 5, 6 are generally considered early or pre-cancer, a nutrition related systems imbalance. The Precancer Section of the IHC Program is used, unless other factors are evident.

"Index of 7 and above, and/or medical diagnosis, are considered advanced cancer and the Advanced Section of the IHC Program is used with professional therapy. Most Americans in the advanced stage who are knowledgeable leave the country for treatment by licensed physicians in Europe and elsewhere.

"Under some conditions a temporary 'flare up,' indicated by a rise in the index, will occur from a destruction or rupture of a tumor and will usually recede in a short time. A falling index generally indicates improvement if accompanied with a feeling of well being. A falling index concurrent with severe physical deterioration is sometimes experienced when a person is weak or bedridden because there is insufficient raw material present for the cancer cells to manufacture the HCG hormone being measured. Care must be taken to properly evaluate the report.

"Frequencies of tests used successfully by many people are as follows: for Prevention where they have never shown positive, once per year; for those showing positive, once every two months until three negatives are received and then every six months for the rest of their lives. Due to technical difficulties the lab may request another sample at an early date in index 3.

"From examination of hundreds of these test reports, it is this writer's opinion that this is a valuable asset to the individual and professional in the detection and control of cancer and the systems imbalance leading to cancer. Also, we believe this to be a measure of the malignancy pressure working against the body's resistance in the earlier stages. In other words, the malignancy pressure could break through at index 4 if the body's resistance is low and form a tumor. Yet at index 6, a detectable tumor might not form if the body's resistance is high. The IHC Program is designed to concurrently reduce the malignancy pressure and at the same time increase the body's resistance to disease.

"**Blood Test**. Many physicians outside the USA use this Blood Test in their day-to-day management of cancer. It is also useful in situations where the victim cannot use a urinalysis, as indicated previously, or as a double-check with the urinalysis. It is suggested that the advanced use both the urinalysis and blood test every one or two months until both are negative.

"**Materials required**: A few ounces of pure Methyl Alcohol – *no substitutes,* two or more new cleaned microscope slides from a hobby shop, a sterile lancet or pin, a $15.00 money order.

"**Instructions:**

"(1. If slides are not clean, clean with alcohol to remove dirt and grease film.

"(2. Clean finger tip or ear lobe with alcohol and let dry completely.

"(3. Puncture finger tip or ear lobe with *sterile* lancet or pin.

"(4. Wipe off first blood with Kleenex.

"(5. Deposit small drops of blood on the surface of one slide and quickly spread *very thin* with the sharp edge of a second slide. Thick or irregular smears *cannot* be used.

"(6. Allow blood smear to dry thoroughly.

"(7. Fix the smear by immersing in pure Methyl Alcohol for 20 minutes, let dry thoroughly.

"(8. Sandwich slide carefully between two thick pieces

of cardboard, Scotch Tape the edges, write name and address on the cardboard cover, enclose with money order in an envelope marked 'Hand Stamp,' send air mail (not registered or special)to: Laboratorio Del Mar, P.O. Box 2853, San Ysidro, California 92073.

"**Interpretation of report:**

"M Monocytes (damaged)	0-49% normal, over 50% Positive malignancy
"N Neutrophyls (damaged)	0-19% normal, over 20% Positive malignancy
"L Lymphocytes (small competant)	
"Body resistance:	Poor — 1-10% Fair — 11-25% Good — Above 25%

"Spiritual ignorance is a degenerating factor. A lack of understanding of where we came from, why we are here, where we are going, a fear of death, a feeling of being forsaken, insecurity from the atheistic rubbish thrown at us, ignorance of God's natural laws, are all degenerating. The ecology movement is helping us to understand the importance of getting right with nature, God's natural law. Many of the dying are just terrified and require a great deal of understanding and counseling, as this is an area generally avoided by their physician. Likewise, many clergymen are lax in this area. After all, death is a part of life and it is a privilege to get out of this crazy world and make the transition to a better life! Whether you follow one of the orthodox religions or not, get yourself right with God. (Orientation Course in the Paranormal, Walter Ermer.)

"Mental attitude is closely associated with the spiritual. A lack of positive thinking, inner tensions, outer tensions, are degenerating. Think sick and you will be sick. Think well and you will be well. Of course positive thinking can be carried to illogical extremes and become an escape from reality to the detriment of the person. Worry is actually a negative prayer, bringing about the very thing you are worrying about. In our interviews with many cancer patients, we find emotional trauma from childhood experiences or an ill-adjusted home life may have triggered the malignancy. Dr. Serov and Dr. Troskin of the Soviet Union demonstrated that negative emotions reduce the white blood count in an alarming manner, hindering a major body defense against disease. In the Bible, Paul said to transform your body by transforming your mind. It is very important that everyone review their own emotional condition in an objective manner, regardless if diseased or healthy. (*How to Live 365 Days a Year,* J. A. Schindler, M.D.)

"Drugs by prescription or purchased over the counter, including antibiotics, are foreign to the body and are important degenerating factors. Of course drugs and antibiotics are needed at times by all of us and, generally, temporary use is not too harmful. Degeneration usually does take place with extended use. The physicians' use of drugs is for the purpose of shocking the body into healing itself. No drug ever healed anything — nature heals. Where extreme pain is involved, the pain-killing drugs are the lesser of two evils. Sometimes the ill effects from drugs can be offset by the use of vitamins, particularly the 'B' series. One of the most vicious prescription items murdering our women today are birth control pills, estrogen and other female hormones. A medical doctor admitted that one person in ten will get cancer from female hormones, but he still prescribes them.*

"Recent studies indicate the use of female hormones by pregnant women is causing vaginal cancer in their teenage daughters. The leukemia rate is reported highest in the more affluent areas where they get the best medical care, and lowest in the poor areas where medical care is lacking —

**Author's note: This is not scientific evidence.*

suggesting depletion by drugs. (*Cleveland Plain Dealer,* 5/22/72.) Antibiotics destroy the beneficial bacteria in the digestive system, hampering the assimilation of vitamins and minerals with long term degeneration. (The Truth Crusader No. 44; Women's Medical College of Pennsylvania; *The Dictocrats,* Omar Garrison; *The Case for Unorthodox Medicine,* Brian Inglis.)

"Food additives like MSG, BHT, BHA, DES, and others are foreign to our bodies, so read the labels and avoid. Many of these chemicals do not appear on the labels because the FDA considers them as 'Generally Regards as Safe.' (FDA GRAS List.)

"Modern processing, canned foods and the cooking habits we are addicted to, destroy enzymes as low as 106° and many at 120°. Keep foods that have been subjected to heat to a minimum because they are apt to throw an overload on the pancreas, robbing the body of pancreative enzymes needed to digest wandering cancer cells. Eat as much raw fruit and vegetables as possible with a large proportion being juiced. Juicing improves assimilation by the body; because when the juices are in colloidal form they are easily digested and pass through the walls of the stomach and intestines. One tall glass of raw carrot juice, with a teaspoon of safflower oil to improve assimilation, contains carotene, the precursor of vitamin A. One tall glass of cider or apple juice will add potassium and help keep the sodium-potassium balance correct. One small glass of unsweetened grape juice will add needed trace elements including chromium. Drs. Gurvtch and Kirlian of the Soviet Union found an unexplainable energy field emanating from raw fruits and vegetables that may some day further explain the value of living foods. Be sure to drink the cooking water from vegetables that you do cook and do not throw the nutrients down the drain. Cancer cures have been traced to this source. (*A Biologist's Handbook of Health,* John Kimball; *Psychic Discoveries Behind the Iron Curtain,*

Ostrander and Schroeder.)

"**Nitriloside Foods**

Kernels of all fruits (except citrus)	Millet
Buckwheat	Raspberries
Lima Beans	Elder Flower Tea
Cherry Brandy	Rabbit (clover fed)
Apricot Brandy	Chick Peas
Plum Brandy	Flax Seed
Peach Brandy	Stewed Apricots
Elderberry Wine	Bamboo Sprouts

"The brandy and wine are not recommended except for those who refuse to stop drinking alcohol.

"**Radiation Cocktail.** There is no safe level of radiation from x-ray or isotope diagnosis, radiation therapy or environmental sources. Radiation is accumulative. All advanced cancer victims have been damaged by radiation, antibiotics or toxic chemotherapy. Damage is to the intestinal villi and beneficial intestinal bacteria, resulting in reduced assimilation of vital nutrients. The result is tiredness, extreme weight loss, and possibly pain. The following nutritional program is an attempt to compensate for this damage with materials available in most health food stores. The recipe makes two servings, one at lunch and one at dinner, or it can be used advantageously one-half hour before radiation therapy and one-half hour after.

"Recipe for 'A Radiation Cocktail'

1 tbsp. Acidophilus

1/2 tsp. or 2 tablets Acidophilus Food

1½ tsp. Alginate

1 tsp. Granulated Kelp or crushed tablets

3 RNA tablets based in Brewer's Yeast

1 Tbsp. Brewer's Yeast

"Mix the above in two tall glasses of vegetable juice, such as tomato, V-8, fresh, or other, preferably salt-free. Thin with more juice if too thick. Also mixing the ingredients with cold, salt-free boullion makes an excellent drink. (*The Hidden Truth of Cancer,* Dr. K. Morishia, M.D.; *Prevention Magazine.)*

"Antibiotics hamper assimilation of nutrients by destroying the useful bacteria in the intestine. Acidolphus materials can be used on a temporary basis to offset this damage.

"Hormones of the opposite sex are still used by some doctors but we have never seen a surviver living more than a couple of years. Dr. Gerson stated that he lost twenty-five of his best patients on this therapy.

"Hydrazine Sulphate is an experimental drug that is claimed to show great promise, particularly on terminal patients, but it is too soon to draw definite conclusions. (Syracuse Cancer Research Institute, 600 E. Genessee St., Syracuse, N.Y.) We have seen no one who benefitted.

"Therapy outside the U.S. is much greater in scope. It is claimed that some physicians are years ahead of those in this country, having given up American methods in 1960. However, we do find some using radiation and toxic chemotherapy, so victims should be fully aware of the possible consequences if they permit its use. Because of frequent changes, the names of these licensed physicians in other countries are not given here, but this writer will gladly give up-to-date information to anyone in need upon receipt of a self-addressed and stamped envelope. The total number of therapies available outside the U.S. possibly exceeds 70, but we will list only the most popular here.

"Proteolytic Enzymes are natural to the body and essentially non-toxic. They were in use prior to the turn of the century, and have been updated by many researchers and clinical physicians all over the world. The late Dr. F. L. Shively, of Dayton, Ohio, did some excellent work on these enzymes, but was shut off by the FDA in 1964. He was able to start dissolving the tumor on the third day of treatment without harm to the body. Elsewhere, they have been used with remarkable results on tens of thousands of people, and are available to the physician in many countries, but not in the U.S. Trypsin and Chymotrypsin are most important, but they are more effective if other enzymes are present, also the most effective administration is by enema. (*Multiple Proteolytic Therapy of Cancer,* F. L. Shively; *Enzyme Therapy,* Drs. Wolf and Ransberger.)

"The biggest problem facing physicians in other countries is to repair the damage done by orthodox therapy received in the U.S. The problem is to survive the treatment, not the disease. It is preposterous to expect these physicians to perform miracles with a cancerous body badly depleted by cutting, burning and poisoning in the U.S. There are several approaches used to repair this damage, however, and results are sometimes fantastic. We frequently hear of stretcher cases who walk out under their own power after treatment.

"Amygdalin, known as B-17 and Laetrile, has been used in the Western world for 150 years and in China for 3,500 years. It is a nitriloside food product and very popular outside the U.S. It is now manufactured in six countries and used in twenty-two, with production measured in tons. Frequently, doctors inject IV or IM, 9 grams per day for the first week, 3 grams a day for the next two weeks, 1 to 3 grams oral thereafter. Thousands of patients have used the material and testify to its worth. Generally, injections are considered quite effective on lung tumors; injections and oral material are used on all slow growing tumors, and not recommended at all on brain tumors. In many instances, injections will relieve severe pain. Thiamin Hydrochloride (B-1), 50 mg, is claimed to act as a synergist and increase the effective potency of Amygdalin. While on this material, it is advisable to use Dr. Gerson's coffee enema described previously. Amygdalin is essentially non-toxic, but the scientific testing was blocked by FDA in 1970. (*Physician's Handbook of Vitamin B-17 Therapy,* McNaughton; *A New Approach to Etiology, Diagnosis, Treatment and Prevention of Some Degenerative Diseases,* Dr. Howard Beard; *Laetriles – Nitrilosides in Prevention and Control of Cancer,* McNaughton.)

"Glyoxilide is a homeopathic oxidation catalyst and has been used since 1919. It is interesting that the oxidation characteristics of this material used so long ago, has a similarity to the relatively new work of Dr. Otto Warburg – that cancer cells can be replaced by normal cells when they expire if the oxygen respiration can be reinstated. This therapy is available in Europe and Latin America, but it is banned in the U.S. Many survivors attest to its value. Glyoxilide is considered safe and useful on all tumor types, particularly the fast moving lymphomas and tumors of the brain. (*Cancer Cures Crucified,* Craum; *The Survival Factor in Neoplastic and Viral Disease,* Dr. Koch; *The Prime Cause and Prevention of Cancer,* Dr. Otto Warburg.)

"The Hoxsey material is used in other countries but is banned here by FDA, even though an AMA representative testified in a Dallas court in 1953 that it was effective on skin cancer.

"Skin cancer is being treated with cotton soaked in 190 proof alcohol, left on overnight, and castor oil is applied in the morning. Pancreatic enzymes dissolved in water are applied as a compress overnight. Amygdalin is also dissolved and used as a compress. Of course body-building techniques and internal therapies are used at the same time.

"Vitamin C Complex, including rutin, bioflavinoids and hesperidin, is used to control bleeding, particularly from the bladder or lungs.

"Calcium Dioratate (oratate) was developed in Germany to recalcify bone damaged by a malignancy and is used as a preventive to prevent bone metastasis that often follows breast prostate and thyroid cancer.

"BCG and the AC Factor are used to activate or build up the immunization system in the body, particularly where body resistance has been damaged by the disease, radiation or chemotherapy.

"Bromelaine is becoming popular abroad and is covered elsewhere in this book. It is considered essential by some physicians. They are reporting success, but we have not found anyone who benefitted.

"Both the urinalysis and the blood test are being used abroad by physicians in their daily management of the disease.

"The eventual answer to the cancer problem lies in: (1) prevention; (2) a mass testing of the general public; (3) a reversal of the nutrition-related systems imbalance that precedes the disease itself, by a correction of faulty living habits. For those careless enough to allow the disease to develop into the advanced stage, they should leave the U.S. for professional therapy in some other country. This exodus should continue until American techniques catch up with therapy abroad."

The address of Dr. Ernesto Contreras is No. 20 Pasco de Tijuana, Playas de Tijuana, Mexico, telephone 903-387-1850.

STRICT LAETRILE DIET

Strict Laetrile Diet	Forbidden Food
Beverages: Chamomile tea, clear tea, mint tea, papaya tea.	Alcohol, cocoa, coffee, milk, soft drinks.
Bread: Rye bread, soya bread, whole wheat or bran muffins, whole wheat bread.	Others, white bread.
Cereals: Buckwheat, cornmeal, cracked wheat, millet, oatmeal, sesame, fine ground grits.	All other. Refined and bleached flour.
Cheese: None.	All forbidden.
Dessert: Fresh fruits, stewed fruits, Jello.	All pastries, puddings, custards, junket, sauces, ice cream.
Eggs:	In any form.
Fat: Cold pressed oils, preferably safflower or soya oil soya lecithin spread.	Butter, shortening, margarine, saturated oils and fats.
Fish: White flesh fish only (very fresh).	All other fish and sea foods.
Fruits: Fresh fruits only: apples, pears, apricots, bananas, cherries, currants, grapes, guava, mangos,	Canned fruits.

Strict Laetrile Diet	Forbidden Food
melon, nectarines, papaya, peaches, plums, ripe oranges, quince, tangerines, avocados, ripe pineapple. Following dried fruits (unsulfured) can be stewed: apples, apricots, dates, figs, prunes, peaches, pears, plums, raisins.	
Juices: Only fresh juices. May be selected from lists of fruits and vegetables permitted, including the following green leaves: chicory, endives, escarole, lettuce, swiss-chard, and watercress.	All canned juices, and juices with artificial coloring and sweetening.
Meat: Lean, grilled, broiled, roasted, or baked beef, chicken, lamb, turkey, and veal. Internal organs; only heart and extra fresh calf liver permitted.	No pork, fat, fried and smoked meat sausages.
Milk:	Dairy products.
Nuts: All types of fresh, raw nuts (except peanuts), almonds, 6 to 10 a day.	Roasted and salted nuts and peanuts.

Strict Laetrile Diet	Forbidden Food
Potatoes: Baked, boiled and mashed. Potato salad seasoned with salad dressing substitute, brown rice or corn.	French fried, chips, white rice.
Salads: The following raw vegetables, shredded or finely chopped, separated or mixed: carrots, cauliflower, celery, chicory, green pepper, lettuce, radishes, swiss-chard, watercress, onions, ripe tomatoes, turnips, brussel sprouts, broccoli.	Any other.
Seasoning: Chives, garlic, onion, parsley, herbs, laurel, marjoram, sage, thyme, savory cumin, oregano, salt substitutes such as Co-salt or other potassium salt.	Spices, pepper, paprika, sodium salt.
Soups: Vegetable soup, barley, brown rice and millet can be added.	Canned and creamed soup, fat stock, consomme.
Sweets: Unpasteurized honey, unsulphured molasses, raw sugar or dark brown sugar, Carob.	Candy, chocolate, white sugar.

Strict Leatrile Diet	Forbidden Food
Vegetables: Raw of freshly cooked: Artichokes, asparagus, carrots, cauliflower, celery, chives, corn, endives, green leeks, spinach, green peas, green pepper, leeks, lentils, lima beans, potatoes, radishes, tomatoes wax beans, yama, egg plant, squash. Any vegetables listed under salads.	All canned ones.

MODIFIED LEATRILE DIET

Modified Leatrile Diet	Forbidden Food
Beverages: Chamomile tea, clear tea, mint tea, papaya tea, Sanka.	Alcohol, cocoa, coffee, milk, soft drinks.
Bread: Rye bread, soya bread, whole wheat or bran muffins, whole wheat bread	Others, white bread.
Cereals: Buckwheat, cornmeal, cracked wheat, millet, oatmeal, sesame, fine ground grits.	All other. Refined and bleached flour.
Cheese: Cottage cheese only in limited quantities.	All others forbidden.
Dessert: Fresh fruits, stewed fruits, Jello.	All pastries, puddings, custards, junket, sauces, ice cream.

Modified Laetrile Diet	Forbidden Food
Eggs: Poached or boiled, not fried, one a day.	Any other form.
Fat: Cold pressed oils, preferably safflower or soya oil soya lecithin spread.	Butter, shortening, margarine, saturated oils and fats.
Fish: White flesh fish only (very fresh).	All other fish and sea foods.
Fruits: Fresh fruits only: apples, pears, apricots, bananas, cherries, currants, grapes, guava, mangos, melon, nectarines, papaya, peaches, plums, ripe oranges, quince, tangerines, avocados, ripe pineapple. Following dried fruits (unsulfured) can be stewed: apples, apricots, dates, figs, prunes, peaches, pears, plums, raisins.	Canned fruits.
Juices: Only fresh juices. May be selected from lists of fruits and vegetables permitted, including the following green leaves: chicory, endives, escarole, lettuce, swiss-chard, and watercress.	All canned juices, and juices with artificial coloring and sweetening.

Modified Laetrile Diet	Forbidden Food
Meat: Lean, grilled, broiled, roasted or baked beef, chicken, lamb, turkey, and veal. Internal organs: only heart and extra fresh calf liver permitted.	No pork, fat, fried and smoked meat sausages.
Milk: Yogurt, buttermilk and non-fat milk allowed in limited quantities.	Other dairy products.
Nuts: All types of fresh, raw nuts (except peanuts), almonds, 6 to 10 a day.	Roasted and salted nuts and peanuts.
Potatoes: Baked, boiled and mashed. Potato salad seasoned with salad dressing substitute, brown rice or corn.	French fried chips, white rice.
Salads: The following raw vegetables, shredded or finely chopped, separated or mixed: carrots, cauliflower, celery, chicory, green pepper, lettuce, radishes, swiss-chard, watercress, onions, ripe tomatoes, turnips, brussel sprouts, broccoli.	Any other.

Modified Leatrile Diet	Forbidden Food
Seasoning: Chives, garlic, onion, parsley, herbs, laurel, marjoram, sage, thyme, savory, cumin, oregano, salt substitutes such as Co-salt or other potassium salt, and sea salt in small amounts.	Spices, pepper, paprika, salt.
Soups: Vegetable soup, barley, brown rice and millet can be added.	Canned and creamed soup, fat stock, consomme.
Sweets: Unpasteurized honey, unsulphured molasses, raw sugar or dark brown sugar. Carob.	Candy, chocolate, white sugar.
Vegetables: Raw or freshly cooked: artichokes, asparagus, carrots, cauliflower, celery, chives, corn, endives, green leeks, spinach, green peas, green pepper, leeks, lentils, lima beans, potatoes, radishes, tomatoes, wax beans, yama, egg plant, squash. Any vegetables listed under salads.	All canned ones.

The foregoing diets appeared in the *Natural Food News,* "The Newspaper For Your Health," published monthly by Natural Food Associates, and distributed through the nation's health food stores. They appeared in Vol. 14, No. 6, in April, 1976.

APPENDIX 14

DR. MAX GERSON REPORTS ON CANCER

The following article appeared in the *Cancer Control Journal*, Vol. 3, Nos. 1 and 2, 1975:

"Dr. Max Gerson Reports on Cancer

"The method outlined by Max Gerson, M.D., of New York City, for treatment of cancer sounds relatively simple. And the physician states the most gratifying results have been obtained in 50 percent of the cancer patients who have been treated at his clinic. Many of these persons were reported to have been in advanced stages of the disease.

"Regimen

"Dr. Gerson's treatment is based on complete detoxification, or cleansing of the body, and the use of proper foods which are procured from the best sources possible. Tools for this process include a soup known as Hippocrates' soup, coffee enemas, a total absence of sale and fats from the diet, and the use of enzymes, vitamins and minerals in the food.

"Two components

" 'Two components are to be considered when dealing with cancer,' the physician said. 'One is the general, or whole body; the other is a local one or symptoms. What must be treated is the general which includes the digestive tract and the liver. The trouble begins in the liver. When we are able to bring the digestive tract and the liver into order the local symptoms disappear.'

"Specifically, Dr. Gerson blames changes that take place in the balance of the sodium ratio in the liver for the inception of cancer. These changes affect the metabolism of fats and proteins, poisonous substances develop and trouble begins. . ." (from *Let's Live,* 1956*.)

For more complete information, write Cancer Control Society, 2043 N. Bevendo, Los Angeles, CA 90027, Tel. 213-663-7801.

***Coffee Enemas**

"The digestive tract takes a great deal of punishment in cancer, Dr. Gerson said. The stomach juices are not functioning, and so one of his first steps in healing is to eliminate all waste and poisonous matter from the system. He finds coffee enemas extremely beneficial . . . The coffee enema is made by boiling three heaping tablespoonfuls of ground (not powdered) coffee in one quart of water for three minutes, then simmering 10 to 20 minutes. The enema is given at bodily temperature. In addition to its cleansing properties he discovered that it also acts as a sedative.

"At the beginning of their treatment, Dr. Gerson immediately takes from his patients all drug sedation. He said that some of his patients take the coffee enemas every two hours day and night instead of every four, as he prescribed, and that after a few days they have almost no pain at all."

APPENDIX 15

COLON CANCER AND CHOLESTEROL

Worth Noting

Colon Cancer and Cholesterol

"*Colon Cancer and Blood-Cholesterol.* Rose, G., H. Blackburn, A. Keys, H. L. Taylor, W. B. Kannel, O. Paul, D. D. Reid, and J. Stamler, *Lancet* 1:181-183, 1974. A strong positive correlation between mortality rates for colon cancer and coronary heart disease (CHD) among some populations of the world is well recognized. Because blood cholesterol level has been regarded as a powerful indicator of CHD risk, this study sought to confirm the hypothesis that it could also be a predictor of colon cancer.

"Six surveys of CHD provided blood cholesterol levels of 90 males who died of colon cancer. Pooled data from these studies revealed a negative correlation within populations between blood cholesterol and colon cancer. This observation was rationalized in two ways. First, individuals with lower blood cholesterol levels may form more bile salts, possibly as a result of a higher intake of polyunsaturated fatty acids; the risk of colon cancer increases since more bile salts are made available for carcinogenic-forming bacteria. Second, this negative correlation between cholesterol and colon cancer risk may be due to the presence of bile-degrading bacteria, perhaps as a result of high polyunsaturated fatty acid intake or lower intake of fiber. Extensive degradation of bile can result in a decrease in blood cholesterol level since the bile pool requires replenishing from blood cholesterol.

"The authors pointed to the need to study the relationship between carcinogen-producing bacteria and the dietary intake of polyunsaturated fatty acids and fiber."

Fermented or Sour Milk and Cholesteremia

"*Studies of a Surfactant and Cholesteremia in the Maasai.* Mann, G. V., and A. Spoerry, Am. J. Clin. Nutr. 27: 464-469, 1974. The present study tested the hypothesis that surfactant food additives, in amounts found in human foods, cause hypercholesteremia in people not previously receiving them. The Maasai people were chosen as appropriate subjects since they have low levels of serum cholesterol despite their diet of milk and meat. Furthermore, they do not receive surfactants in their foods despite the large amount of cholesterol in their diet.

"Two groups of 12 men each were fed fermented milk for 21 days. The control group received fermented milk with an olive oil placebo additive while the treatment group received milk with the surfactant Tween 20. Because of the enormous consumption of milk, the subjects gained weight and body fat. Despite this weight gain and contrary to the surfactant hypothesis, the level of serum cholesterol in both groups decreased significantly. The more fermented milk consumed, the larger the decrease in serum cholesterol. The most reasonable explanation seems to be that large fermented milk intakes furnish a factor that impairs endogenous synthesis of cholesterol, thus lowering the serum level. The effect of this factor must overshadow the expected elevating effect of the surfactant.

"The authors stressed the need to re-examine the effects of surfactants and to identify the factor in fermented milk, since these two hypothetical agents may have competing effects on cholesteremia."

Fiber in Cholesterol Metabolism

"*Isocaloric, Isogravic Diets in Rats. Effect of Non-nutritive Fiber (Alfalfa or Cellulose) on Cholesterol Metabolism.* Kritchevsky, D., S. A. Tepper, and J. A. Story, Nutr. Rep. Int. 9:301-308, 1974. Observations that various non-nutritive fibers (NNF) have different degrees of cholesteremic and atherogenic effects have been reported. The present study compared the effects of two NNF (alfalfa and cellulose) on the weight gain and cholesterol levels in rats maintained on isocaloric, isogravic diets.

"The animals gained less weight and had lower serum and liver cholesterol levels when alfalfa, rather than cellulose, was the NNF in the diet. Based on the fecal steroid excretion patterns, two possible explanations for the observed changes in serum cholesterol levels are given. First, alfalfa contains saponins which have the ability to bind cholesterol, thus preventing its absorption. Second, alfalfa binds bile acids and bile salts resulting in a loss of sterol which depletes the body pool.

"The importance of the role of NNF as well as the complexity of interactions between dietary components in cholesterol metabolism was stressed in this investigation."

Protein-Sparing Effect in Obesity

"Protein-Sparing Effect in Obese Women Fed Low Calorie Diets. Jourdan, M., S. Margen, and R. B. Bradfield, Am. J. Clin. Nutr. 27:3-12, 1974. The well-documented interrelationship between protein and total calorie consumption can be briefly stated: the optimum utilization of a given amount of dietary protein depends upon an adequate intake of calories; that is, the efficiency of protein utilization drops as the intake of calories falls below a certain level. Conversely, when dietary protein intake is zero, breakdown of body protein is minimized when an optimum caloric intake is provided. Because obese subjects have a large endogenous reserve of calories in the form of fat, they should, theoretically, be able to minimize body protein breakdown even when they are fed low-protein, low-calorie diets.

"Six obese women were fed liquid diets which varied in nitrogen and caloric content. During the stabilization period of 15 days, the subjects were fed 12 g protein nitrogen per day and enough calories to permit maintenance of constant weight (100% calories). In the second metabolic period of 12 days, no protein nitrogen was fed but the caloric content was maintained at 100%. During the next three metabolic periods of 12 days each, the liquid diets contained: 50% kcal and 12 g N; 25% kcal and 0 g N; and 25% kcal and 3 g N.

"At the end of the 63-day period, there was an increase in serum uric acid; a decrease in urinary excretion of urea nitrogen, creatinine, and uric acid; and no significant change in serum creatinine.

"On the basis of these findings, it was concluded that obese women can minimize breakdown of body protein on diets providing as little as 3 g nitrogen and 25% of the energy needed for weight maintenance.

Calcium Interrelationships

"A Recognition of the Interrelationships of Calcium With Various Dietary Components. McBean, L. D., and E. W. Speckmann, Am. J. Clin. Nutr. 27:603-609, 1974. The purpose of this review was to recognize the scope and significance of calcium interrelationships with other dietary factors. This review emphasized the varied calcium allowances adopted throughout the world as well as the role of calcium in the etiology of osteoporosis. Various means of establishing an optimal calcium allowance, including metabolic balance studies, radioisotopic studies, and surveys of dietary intakes, are discussed. The dietary components discussed in this review include vitamin D, phosphorus, calcium-to-phosphorus (Ca:P) ratio, protein, lactose, magnesium, fat, oxalic acid, and phytic acid.

"A direct correlation between urinary calcium excretion and dietary protein intake has been reported. However, the effect on calcium absorption and retention is not well demonstrated, and thus there is a need for long-term studies in human adults.

"Lactose has been reported to improve calcium absorption in subjects with normal intestinal lactase. The acidic environment resulting from the formation of lactic acid from lactose by the intestinal microflora could possibly favor calcium absorption.

"Human subjects consuming a constant fat intake showed increased calcium and fat excretion as dietary calcium increased. Decreased fat, bile, and bile salts may decrease calcium absorption directly by the formation of insoluble calcium soaps, and indirectly by retarding exogenous cholecalciferol absorption. This interrelationship is complex and not fully understood.

"The authors conclude that while these nutrient interactions make it difficult to formulate valid recommended allowances, the available information lends support to a calcium RDA for adults of at least 800 mg."

From the Press –

The author of this book takes no editorial responsibility for these statements.

"Cancer-Prevention Center Opened in Westchester

By James Feron

"Valhalla, N.Y., June 20 – A research institute described by Dr. Frank J. Rauscher, director of the National Cancer Institute, as the nation's primary institution concerned solely with the prevention of the disease, was dedicated here today.

"Situated on the Grasslands reservation, which houses the Westchester County Medical Center, the new Naylor Dana Institute for Disease Prevention will operate as the technical research arm of the American Health Foundation.

"The single-story structure, built at a cost of $6 million, will also be linked through teaching and research arrangements with the medical center, which is to be the focal point of a seven-county health-planning region, one of eight in the state.

"Dr. Rauscher said, 'It would be nice if we could do this well around the country.' He spoke of the institute as the 'possible quarterback, or organizing center of other such facilities nationwide.'

"The move of the research institute to Westchester was encouraged by the former County Executive, Edwin G. Michaelian, who aided in the move by the New York Medical Center to this suburban community.

"Alfred B. DelBello, Mr. Michaelian's successor, said the cancer research unit would contribute to the 'total effort' of the medical center.

"Dr. Ernst L. Wynder, the president of the American Health Foundation said they would be concentrating on smoking and health, occupational-related cancers and endocrine-related and gastrointestinal cancers. Dr. Wynder left the Sloan Kettering Institute for Cancer Research to form the health foundation in Manhattan seven years ago.

"'Cancer and cardiovascular diseases, we know, are related to manmade factors.' Dr. Wynder said. 'We also know that man has never eradicated a disease by therapy alone, but through prevention. Our main task here, as a Greek proverb says, will be to help people die young as late as possible.'"

The following article appeared in the *American Laboratory,* August, 1976, page 71, by S. Harguindey and R. C. Kolbeck. Dr. Harguindey is Fellow, Division of Metabolic and Endocrine Disease, and Dr. Kolbeck is Instructor, Division of Cardiology, Department of Medicine, Eugene Talmadge Memorial Hospital, Medical College of Georgia.

From: "Cancer – A Generalization

"Both Warburg (1), from a biochemical and metabolic point of view, and Gerson (2) understood cancer as a systemic disease affecting the entire metabolism of the body. To quote Warburg's basic premise, this thought Is summarized at the end of the preface of his book, *The Metabolism of Tumors.* (1).

"'Interference with the respiration in growing cells is, from the standpoint of the physiology of metabolism, the cause of tumors. If the respiration of a growing cell is disturbed, as a rule the cell dies. If it does not die, a tumor cell results. This is not theory, but a comprehensive summary of all the measurements at present available.'

"Warburg compared cancer to lower forms of life, primarily yeast (3) (1). If his opinion is valid, it seems to interpret cancer as being an infestation of *vegetable life* into *animal life.*"

References:

1. Warburg, O., *The Metabolism of Tumors* (Constable & Co., Ltd., London, 1930)
2. Gerson, M., *A Cancer Therapy* (Totality Books, Del Mar, Calif., 1975).
3. Warburg, O. *Science* 123, 309 (1956).

APPENDIX 16

SPACE, NOT TIME, MAY BE RELATIVE

An Approach to Cancer Based Upon Time as a Wave

The development of life upon this planet introduced *time* as a new dimension, as compared with inanimate matter.

Much of the observable universe which may be measured may be reduced to waves of some form. The hypothesis adduced here assumes also that time is a wave, of a velocity different from that of light or sound, or any other thing.

The approach to cancer involved here is based upon this assumption.

What is the velocity of time?

Light may, in effect, be reduced to matter through photosynthesis. According to the theory presented here, matter must become light upon achieving the velocity of light.

Velocity of vibration determines the nature of anything within the universe we may observe.

Sound, like the waves of the sea, represents a specialized form of matter.

Basically, we have matter, light, time, and thought wavelengths of different velocities.

How to measure these? Through structural logic.

Structural logic assumes that changes involving infinity must follow an identical mathematical pattern. It also assumes that like orders of complexity may be compared; unlike may not. A less complex order of complexity contained within a more complex order may be compared with that aspect of the more complex order with which it is identical, and no other.

"Changes involving infinity" may be explained in this way. Start with a point of zero dimension. Move the point and it becomes a line, an infinity of points.

Zero represents the infinitely small. Yet the line represents finite dimension, composed of infinitely small dimension. Certainly the change involves infinity, movement through it, in fact.

Move the line about a point or center, and the line must become a circle. Describing the line, mathematically, in terms of circle must involve pi (π).

Pi is an infinite number. Again change involves infinity, something beyond human ability to measure.

The area of the circle also represents the radius of the circle to the second power. The second power describes the order of complexity of the circle, in terms of area.

The area represents an infinity of points and an infinity of lines, two infinities.

Move the circle about a fulcrum, and a sphere develops, through an infinite number of circles, an infinite number of lines, and an infinite number of points. Yet a sphere is not a circle, a line, or a point.

In terms of structure, a sphere may not be compared with a circle, save regarding the plane attributes to its inner structure. A circle may not be compared to a line, save in terms of a line. And a line may not be compared to a point save in terms of a point.

Different complexities may be compared only in terms of like complexity.

The order of complexity of the sphere, in terms of cubic measurement, must represent the radius to the third power.

Only space may be relative; not the velocity of light, time, or thought.

According to the hypothesis presented here, the more complex must encompass the less complex (or *vice versa*), as matter is encompassed by light.

The higher velocity must contain the lesser.

In the perceptible universe, unity moves toward infinity,

and infinity moves toward unity.

Should this theory prove correct, or be correct, life must reach beyond the inanimate in complexity. The inanimate must be contained within the animate, by this hypothesis.

(Life must contain the universe. The universe contains life.)

If physical energy may relate to the speed of light to the second power, then the speed of time may represent the speed of light at least to the third power, many billion times the speed of light.

(The speed of thought may represent the velocity of light at least to the fourth power, thousands of trillion times the speed of light.)

As a masterpiece of understatement, the speed of time in terms of waves might be difficult to demonstrate in a physical experiment, even though many things have been done previously considered far beyond human achievement. (Astronomy might help.)

On the other hand, time-waves, themselves, may not be so difficult to demonstrate. Perhaps only the proper frame of reference may be lacking now.

For instance, the truth of falsity of structural logic might be demonstrated through various experiments, to make a scientific method of extrapolation.

I began with cancer as a subject for empirical examination. My reasons I shall not endeavor to explain here.

Let us begin with the examination of time as a wave without regard to its absolute dimensions.

All of life, even heredity, itself, must depend upon rhythms of one kind or another. I will illustrate this through an interpolation from the *Scientific American*, April, 1971, in the form of an article by Eric T. Pengelley and Sally J. Asmundson, entitled: *Annual Biological Clocks.*

"Annual Biological Clocks

"Many organisms have a built-in circadian, or daily, clock. It has now been demonstrated that some also have a circannual, or yearly, clock that operates even when environmental signals are eliminated."

The article, as I understand it, appears to knock out light as a controlling factor in the hibernation of some animals, and perhaps even heat. If not light or heat, what does control, if not time, with some vibration of its own?

Should the foregoing theory prove correct, cancer may be spotted or plotted as to its complexity in relation to evolutionary development, or time. The evolutionary level of the cancer may be studied without regard to the cancer, itself.

This I have endeavored to do, in a limited way.

Should time prove to be a wave much faster than light, the action of protons in relation to electrons might be better explained.

Should time prove to be a wave capable of more than one direction, progression and regression might be better explained, including Dr. Garb's remarkable description of a circulatory system developing to meet the requirements of regressive cells.

APPENDIX 17

NEW DANGERS DEVELOPING

The following article appeared in the September, 1976, edition of the *Bulletin of the Atomic Scientists,* by John T. Edsall, M.D., who is professor of biochemistry, emeritus, at the Biological Laboratories of Harvard University.

"Cancer in workers exposed to plutonium

"It has often been stated that there is no clear evidence of cancer induced by exposure to plutonium in human subjects (1). This view has recently been challenged by Dr. Sidney M. Wolfe, of the Public Citizen's Health Research Group in Washington, D.C., in a letter submitted to *Lancet.* Dr. Wolfe makes use of data from the U.S. Transuranium Registry in Richland, Washington, established by the U.S. Atomic Energy Commission in 1968. The Registry is accumulating data on the uptake, distribution, and retention of plutonium and other transuranium elements among AEC employees whose work has exposed them to these substances.

"Of some 5,800 workers identified under this program, 819 have agreed to be autopsied. The results of the first 30 autopsies have been reported (2), and the authors of this report inferred nothing unusual in the resulting pattern of deaths. Dr. Wolfe, however, making use of the same data, noted that 11 of the 30 subjects had cancer or leukemia, whereas the predicted number of such cases, in a sample of individuals with the same age distribution, drawn from the general public, would have been just over 6.

"The difference appears highly significant, in spite of the smallness of the sample. Moreover, only one of the 11 subjects was found to carry a body burden of plutonium greater than the officially permitted maximum of 40 nanocuries. One of the others was just above 1 nanocurie, and the values for the rest were far below this. Wolfe concluded that these data offered a powerful argument for reducing the permitted body burden for plutonium, perhaps by a factor of 1,000.

"Although the editorial review of this paper has not yet to my knowledge been completed, I believe that this matter should be noted here."

References:

(1) Medical Research Council, *The Toxicity of Plutonium,* (London; Her Majesty's Stationery Office, 1975; and National Council on Radiation Protection and Measurements, *Alpha Emitting Particles in Lungs,* NCRP Report No. 46 (Washington, D.C.; NCRP, Aug. 15, 1975).

(2) W. E. Norwood and C. E. Newton, Jr., *U.S. Transuranium Registry; Study of Thirty Autopsies,* Health Physics; 28 (1976), 609-675.

APPENDIX 18

NEW ANSWERS FORTHCOMING

The following article appeared in the *American Laboratory,* July, 1976, Vol. 8, No. 7, pages 56-60, by John E. Illingworth, who is an Independent Researcher.

"Ultraviolet – Initiator of Cancer

"Research into the literature of the various scientific disciplines over the past several years has indicated that there exists a relatively unexplored basic cause of cancer; electromagnetic radiation in the ultraviolet range of the spectrum. It is suggested that this ubiquitous radiation, occurring in situ, may be a basic cause of cancer.

"Conclusion.

"For many years, certain foods and chemicals have been designated as radiomimetic because of their ability to produce radiationlike carcinogenic effects in living tissue. It has been determined that radiomimetic chemicals actually do emit radiation in specific wavelengths which do cause cancer. It is only logical to believe that radiomimetic foods also emit radiation in this specific wavelength.

"Add to this such phenomena as bioluminescence, chemiluminescence, sensitization, photoallergy, phototoxicity, and synergism, and it may well be proved that this ubiquitous ultraviolet radiation is a basic cause of cancer."

APPENDIX 19

THE BABY IS BLESSED WHEN FED FROM THE BREAST

The following article appeared in *Modern Problems in Pediatrics,* Vol. II, by P. Gyorgy, Professor of Pediatrics, School of Medicine, University of Pennsylvania, Philadelphia, Pennsylvania.

"Development of Intestinal Flora
in the Breast-Fed Infant

"Infants fed human milk distinguish themselves, at least in two respects from those fed cow's milk. First, breast feeding reduces both the morbidity and especially the mortality rates. In general, this increased resistance of infants fed human milk to a variety of infections was ascribed not so much to the presence of specific antibodies, but more to the action of unspecific factors of unknown origin. Transfer of immunbodies from ingested human milk through the intestine into the blood is a negligible factor in resistance to disease, if it occurs at all.

"The second distinctive feature regarding infants fed human milk as compared to cow's milk refers to the intestinal flora and the reaction of the feces. In contrast to the acid reaction of the feces of normal breast-fed infants, the pH of the feces of those infants given the usual cow's milk formulae fell in the neutral or alkaline range. Unlike the mixed intestinal flora of infants on cow's milk formulae, the intestinal flora of healthy breast-fed infants is characterized by the prevalence of a particular sub-species of Lactobacillus, i.e., bifidus. A gram-stained fecal smear obtained from healthy breast-fed infants appears to be almost uniform, as if it would represent a pure culture of gram-positive rods, characteristic of L. bifidus. On the average, the proportion of gram-positive rods is around 98 percent, with only slight variation, in normal breast-fed infants."

The following article appeared in the *Los Angeles Times* "Home Magazine," October 20, 1974:

"Just What the Doctor Ordered: Mother's Milk

For Natural Immunization

S	F	H
SCIENCE	FOOD	HEALTH

By Roslyn B. Alfin Slater, Ph.D. and
Derrick B. Jelliffe, M.D.

"Recent work has shown that the protective effect of breast milk against infection in the newborn is much more powerful and subtle than had been appreciated previously. In fact, human milk is literally a live fluid. Microscopic examination shows that living and active white cells, similar to those present in the blood, are also present in human milk and can dispose of bacteria which may enter the terminal lacteals of the breast or the baby's mouth and throat.

"The bifidus factor is 40 times higher in concentration in human milk than cow's milk. It is so called because it encourages the growth of 'friendly flora,' or *Lactobacillus bifidus,* in the baby's intestine. Once established, this prevents invasion and growth of harmful organisms. It is also responsible for the different color, consistency and chemical composition of the stools of breast-fed babies as compared with formula-fed or cow's milk-fed infants."

APPENDIX 20

EVEN IN EVENT OF ATOMIC WAR COWS MUST BE PROTECTED

The following is a news release, 11 a.m., Tuesday, January 14, 1964:

"The Fallout Shelter
(A Gesture Related to Social Cancer)

"Today, the Office of Civil Defense in Washington, D.C., said, 'thank you,' to a man who has been instrumental in developing fallout shelters for cattle in America. Mr. J. Gordon Roberts, president of the Roberts Diary Company, was awarded the OCD's Distinguished Service Citation during a brief ceremony held at the company's general office in Omaha, Nebraska. The citation, signed by the Hon. Steuart L. Pittman, assistant secretary of defense (civil defense), is for 'outstanding leadership and cooperation in the National Civil Defense Program.'

"As Mr. Roberts had been called out of town on business, Acting Regional Director David G. Harrison of OCD's Denver Region made the presentation to Oscar W. Zinsmaster, dairy general manager.

"Mr. Roberts first became concerned with the dangers of nuclear war as a result of witnessing the Atomic Energy Commission's atomic test at Yucca Flats, Nevada, in 1955. Since that time, he and his company have taken many steps to help educate people to the dangers of nuclear war, a program which culminated in the construction of a pioneer fallout shelter for dairy cattle in 1961 and 1962, at the Roberts Diary Farm near Omaha.

"During the summer of 1963, the company conducted a two-week occupation test of the cattle shelter – the first of its kind in this country — working with the Office of Civil Defense and U.S. Department of Agriculture. During this 'live' test, varied data were collected, from the amount of air needed by animals and their attendants, to the best way to reduce humidity in the shelter, to the question of 'would cattle accept underground living peacefully?'

"One-third of the 108 feet x 45 feet concrete shelter was blocked off and occupied by one-third of the cattle the shelter could hold . . . thirty-five Guernsey cows, one bull named 'Aristocrat' and two attendants from the University of Nebraska. During the two-week period (August 6 - 20, 1963), the animals were fed and watered from supplies stored underground, and were exercised outside their underground home each day, after the first forty-eight hours, for gradually lengthening periods of time.

"One of the many interesting features of the occupation test was use of 'artificial weather,' manufactured mechanically above ground, during the second week. When temperatures dipped below normal, Civil Defense engineers from the University of Florida introduced hot weather into the shelter through an air intake, with heat and humidity paralleling the Weather Bureau's 'normal' range of 69° low and 90° high. As the test's second week progressed, hotter air was blown into the shelter until it peaked at a sizzling high of 100°.

"The two college students who cared for the cattle fared well during their underground stay since they were busy most of the time. Their many duties included changing hundreds of pounds of straw daily, feeding the animals, keeping detailed reports, cooking and the other incidentals of life above or underground.

"Results of the test were disseminated to personnel of the Department of Agriculture and Office of Civil Defense shortly after the test was concluded.

"At its conclusion, Mr. Roberts observed, 'In a Democracy, the citizens ultimately determine what foreign policy should be. If we have our people prepared for the worst, and tests like this one can contribute a great deal to that preparedness, then both Russia and China must think twice about using atomic weapons on our country.'

"As part of the company's program of public education, more than three hundred Cub Scouts and their leaders will tour the cattle fallout shelter during Scout 'Home Alert Month,' on January 18, 1964."

APPENDIX 21

THE RIGHT OF FREE SPEECH IS FOREVER BEING CHALLENGED

Written in 1966 and run in the *Washington Post,* District of Columbia.

"How a Proposal by the Federal Food and Drug Administration May Affect YOU

"Roberts Dairy is an old company (1). In a way, it may represent an era, an era you may not wish to end.

"Roberts Dairy Company introduced pasteurized milk into Nebraska shortly after the turn of the century.

"At that time some conscientious people recommended that our company be prevented from selling pasteurized milk. Had these people had the power to do so, they would have stopped its sale.

"Had the same conditions been present at the turn of the century which are being contemplated now, the sale of pasteurized milk might very well have been blocked.

"What Is Proposed?

"A proposal has been offered by the Federal Food and Drug Administration to be effective 180 days from June 18, 1966, whereby neither truth in advertising nor wholesomeness of product may protect against obstruction by this branch of government. Authoritative opinion is to serve as a substitute for determination of truth.

"Specifically prohibited are statements about any food, fortified in any way to the effect.

"That a diet of ordinary foods will not supply adequate amounts of vitamins and minerals (2).

" 'That significant segments of the population of the

United States are suffering or in danger of suffering from a dietary deficiency of vitamins or minerals.

"'That a dietary deficiency or threatened dietary deficiency of vitamins and/or minerals is or may be due to loss of nutritive value of food by reason of the soil on which the food is grown, or the storage, transportation, processing and cooking of food.'

"How such *prohibition* against the foregoing statements may be compatible with the facts established about vitamin C, for example, might be difficult to conceive, in our opinion.

"The foregoing prohibition is to be accepted, nevertheless as based upon indisputable, scientific fact established predictably by scientific method to be true, beyond question, under any and all conditions which might arise, for whatever indefinite period the ruling may be in effect.

"How this Issue May Affect your Citizenship

"Because freedom of inquiry as well as political liberty may depend upon freedom to tell the truth, rather than administrative expediency, the issue here may be the most significant facing this nation since the writing of the Constitution. For the right to vote may be no more protective than access to information without distortion may permit.

"Those who wrote the Constitution apparently believed that the benefits of liberty may be protected only by freedom, itself. Because human knowledge must always be limited, however authoritative, unlimited power to regulate in the hands of the administrators, however conscientious, may not allow for limitations upon human judgment and foresight.

"This advertisement shall represent an effort to develop this principle more fully. For the issue here is one of human nature, rather than party politics or personalities, and as old as humankind.

"Vitamin D Milk Represents Freedom in Action

"Our company was the first in the nation successfully to introduce vitamin D into fresh milk. A few had tried, half-heartedly.

"Not too many will undertake a project of this kind, and take the inevitable back-lash of resistance to change. My own father told me that the American diet had been 'perfected' with the advent of pasteurization, and cited authorities to prove it.

"Prior to embarking upon this enterprise, however, we investigated the need for vitamin D. We found that an alarming percentage of children in low-income families were suffering from crippling rickets.

"This was particularly true in the non-white elements of our society, most of whom at that time could not afford vitamin D by prescription. Nevertheless, we were accused of trying to be medicine men rather than milk men. The majority of doctors, themselves, however, supported us. Otherwise the product just would not have sold, irrespective of any governmental action.

"At that time, though I became convinced that the only protection against pressure groups in government within a Democratic society is the right to tell the truth.

"For pressure groups have always been active since the founding of the Republic, and apparently always will be. What such people might have done to vitamin D milk under the proposed regulation must be a moot question. But more about pressure groups later.

"Today, rickets has disappeared almost completely from the American scene. But some of our finest athletes today might otherwise have been afflicted with twisted limbs. For our company successfully introduced vitamin D milk back in the early 30's, in the depth of the depression. Other companies of course later followed our lead.

"Homogenized Milk Another Nutritional Improvement

"Prior to the introduction of homogenized milk by Roberts Dairy, dairymen said that milk had always been and always would be sold on the basis of cream-line. And again we were accused of resorting to a gimmick, the nastiest of all words in nutritional jargon.

"Actually, we were trying to make cow's milk as nearly like human milk as we could. We did not then, and do not now subscribe to the theory that cows' milk as it comes to the calf is an ideal food for human beings.

"For example, the curd of unhomogenized cows' milk is the size of a walnut, suited to the four stomachs of a calf. The curd of homogenized milk is the size of a pea, and the curd of human milk is even much smaller.

"Some people need milk with the milk-sugar removed, which is not being done very satisfactorily now. Many things need doing.

"Although this may not be proved, it is our theory that as cows' milk may be made to approach human milk, human health may also improve. Such a goal may hardly be described to meet 'special dietary need' according to the terms of proposed regulation.

"So far as vitamin C is concerned, the amount of vitamin C in either cows' milk or human milk must depend upon the kind of food fed to the mother. At least one textbook comparison of maximum quantities of vitamin C, however, in human as compared to cows' milk, shows that human milk may be nearly eight times richer than cows' milk in this vitamin (3). The well-documented fact that breast-fed babies have an advantage, on the average, over babies fed any kind of cows' milk indicates beyond question that cows' milk may hardly be described as ideal. But spelling out the difference in terms of 'special dietary need' might be difficult (4). For who knows the sum total of such needs as a basis for comparison?

"Should Vitamin C Be Added to Milk?

"At about the time we started investigating the addition of vitamin C and other micronutrients to milk, highly fortified 'reducing' foods were coming into vogue.

"I asked myself, 'Why should the benefits of vitamin fortification be limited to the rich?'

"My experience with vitamin D milk made me feel that I might accomplish some good.

"In a later conversation, a representative of the Boys' Clubs in Omaha described the deplorable teeth of many of his young charges from areas of economic disadvantage. I could not give away enough product to affect this problem materially, but I could help with the diet . . . and education as to need.

"Our research indicated that many low-income family groups eat very few fresh fruits.

"And many members of low-income groups suffer from very bad teeth. Yet, at the very least, vitamin C affects the problem of healthy teeth and gums through affecting general health. For vitamin C is 'cement' in the body.

"The need of elderly people, particularly those with fixed income, for a low-cost source of vitamin C in milk should be too obvious for comment (5). Many such people practically live on milk because of bad dentures, for economic and other reasons.

"To our knowledge, there is no evidence that vitamin C, even in very large quantities, may be harmful to health in any way. And hazard of vitamin C shortage for the very young and very old may be found described in a medical textbook (6).

"Research (7) demonstrates that vitamin C is extremely important in overcoming infections, through attacking some bacterial toxins, as well as bacteria themselves, and conceivably some virus."

—by J. Gordon Roberts

References:

(1) Roberts Dairy supervises quality control for Stearns Dairy in Denver, Colorado.

(2) This would probably preclude research into adequacy of diet with federal funds and discourage it at any level.

(3) Waldo E. Nelson, M.D., D.Sc., ed., *Textbook of Pediatrics,* 8th ed. (Phil., 1964), p. 135.

(4) By one interpretation, technically, human milk might be considered illegal because of natural fortification with vitamin C. The inclusion of vitamin C in milk, as found in human milk, is not the same as inclusion elsewhere in the diet.

(5) Eva D. Wilson, Katherine H. Fisher, Mary E. Fuqua, *Principles of Nutrition,* (N.Y., 1965), p. 245.

(6) *Ibid.*

(7) For example see: C. W. Jungeblut, *J. of Immunol.*, vol. 33, p. 203 (1937); and E. Cottingham, *J. of Immunol.*, vol. 47, p. 493 (1943).

APPENDIX 22

THE ROSETTA STONE* OF CANCER

By and large, monkeys don't have cancer, within their own environment, according to my reading. Humans do.

Presumably, physiological requirements of both are much the same. Should the dietary theory of cancer prove correct, monkeys may be smarter than people. For instance, monkeys are reputed to prefer the pits of fruit seeds to the outside covering. Humans of course crave the "meat" of the fruit, without regard to pits.

The foregoing example of dietary difference is not intended to prescribe fruit pits as a "medication" to prevent or cure cancer. In my admittedly fallible opinion, the limited-nutritional medication approach is a "pitfall" so to speak, absurd as a one-note symphony, or the outlawing of any one note.

Leaving out the "medication" approach, should we look at the entire monkey diet as compared to the average human diet to see what may be observed?

If this book may serve any purpose at all, it must convince the reader that a much broader area should be examined relevant to cancer, in order to avoid ignoring possible ways to wipe out cancer. For example: an Associated Press release, printed in the Lincoln, Nebraska, *Journal*, on January 1, 1977, cites *Atlas World Press Review* as stating that "diet apparently plays a key role in the comparatively lower death rate of Seventh Day Adventists from cancer (only 1/3 to 1/2 as many as their fellow Americans)," noting that "Adventists do not smoke or drink alcohol or coffee." This could be one of these broader areas.

Should the monkey diet prove a "norm" whereby to measure goals of human nutrition, it would, indeed, be a

Rosetta stone, translated into better health, conceivably even precluding cancer, as the ideal benefit.

However strong the evidence contained in this book favoring any approach, the goal is to point to totality of nutritional need, to be blueprinted first, then turned into reality.

*For many hundreds of years after the fall of the last ancient Egyptian empire about 500 B.C., the strange hieroglyphic picture-writings of the Egyptians could not be read. Then, in 1779 A.D., a carved stone was found near Rosetta on the Nile, giving the same message in hieroglyphics; in a simpler form of hieroglyphics, called demotic; and in Greek, which was well understood by scholars. Using the Greek message, men were able to learn to read the hieroglyphics and demotic and thus to translate many carvings telling the fascinating history of Egypt. Thus, something that unexpectedly leads to the understanding of a formerly-puzzling situation is sometimes referred to as a "Rosetta stone."

Footnote to entire book:

The works of Alfred Szent-Gyorgy of the National Foundation for Cancer Research, 4706 Bethesda, Md. 20014; telephone 301-654-1250 – should not be overlooked by the serious student of cellular mechanics, assuming availability.